Challenging and Emerging Conditions in Emergency Medicine

Challenging and Emerging Conditions in Emergency Medicine

Edited by

Arvind Venkat, **MD, FACEP**

Director of Research
Department of Emergency Medicine
Ethics Consultant
Allegheny General Hospital
Pittsburgh, PA;
Associate Professor of Emergency Medicine
Drexel University College of Medicine
Philadelphia, PA
USA

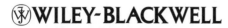

WILEY-BLACKWELL

A John Wiley & Sons, Ltd., Publication

Contents

List of contributors

Jonathan S. Anderson, MD
Attending Physician
Department of Emergency Medicine
Beth Israel Deaconess Medical Center and Milton Hospital;
Instructor in Medicine (Emergency Medicine)
Division of Emergency Medicine
Harvard Medical School
Boston, MA
USA

Melissa B. Bagloo, MD
Fellow
Section of Laparoscopic and Bariatric Surgery
Department of Surgery
Weill Medical College of Cornell University
New York Presbyterian Hospital
New York, NY
USA

Andra L. Blomkalns, MD, FACEP
Vice Chair, Academic Affairs
Associate Professor of Emergency Medicine
Department of Emergency Medicine
University of Cincinnati College of Medicine
Cincinnati, OH
USA

Clifton W. Callaway, MD, PhD, FACEP
Associate Professor and Executive Vice Chair of Emergency Medicine
Ronald D. Stewart Endowed Chair in Emergency Medicine
Department of Emergency Medicine
University of Pittsburgh School of Medicine
Pittsburgh, PA
USA

Esther K. Choo, MD, MPH, FACEP
Attending Physician
Department of Emergency Medicine
Rhode Island Hospital and The Miriam Hospital;
Assistant Professor of Emergency Medicine
Department of Emergency Medicine
Warren Alpert Medical School of Brown University
Providence, RI
USA

Craig R. Cohen, MD, FACC
Medical Director
Arizona Pediatric Cardiology Consultants
Phoenix, AZ
USA

Moira Davenport, MD
Director of Simulation
Associate Residency Program Director
Department of Emergency Medicine
Attending Physician
Division of Sports Medicine
Department of Orthopedic Surgery
Allegheny General Hospital
Pittsburgh, PA;
Assistant Professor of Emergency Medicine and Clinical
Instructor of Orthopedics
Drexel University College of Medicine
Philadelphia, PA
USA

Ankur A. Doshi, MD, FACEP
Attending Physician
Department of Emergency Medicine
UPMC Presbyterian and Mercy Hospitals;
Assistant Professor of Emergency Medicine
Department of Emergency Medicine
University of Pittsburgh School of Medicine
Pittsburgh, PA
USA

Shamai A. Grossman, MD, MS
Attending Physician
Department of Emergency Medicine
Beth Israel Deaconess Medical Center;
Assistant Professor of Medicine (Emergency Medicine)
Division of Emergency Medicine
Harvard Medical School
Boston, MA
USA

Ward Hagar, MD
Director, Adult Sickle Cell Center
Children's Hospital and Research Center
Oakland, CA
USA

Mary Ann Howland, PharmD, DABAT, FAACT
Clinical Professor of Pharmacy
College of Pharmacy
St. John's University;
Adjunct Professor of Emergency Medicine
New York University School of Medicine
Bellevue Hospital Center and
New York University Langone Medical Center;
Senior Consultant in Residence
New York City Poison Center
New York, NY
USA

Kara M. Iskyan, MD, MPH
Clinical Faculty
Department of Emergency Medicine
Maricopa Medical Center
Phoenix, AZ
USA

Elan Jeremitsky, MD, FACS
Attending Physician
Division of Trauma Surgery
Department of Surgery
Allegheny General Hospital
Pittsburgh, PA
USA

Daniel M. Lindberg, MD, FACEP
Attending Physician
Department of Emergency Medicine
Brigham and Women's Hospital;
Instructor in Medicine (Emergency Medicine)
Division of Emergency Medicine
Harvard Medical School
Boston, MA
USA

Joseph B. Miller, MD
Senior Staff Physician
Department of Emergency Medicine
Henry Ford Hospital;
Clinical Assistant Professor of Emergency Medicine
Wayne State University School of Medicine
Detroit, MI
USA

Claudia R. Morris, MD, FAAP
Attending Physician
Director of Fellowship Research
Department of Emergency Medicine
Children's Hospital and Research Center
Oakland, CA
USA

John M. O'Neill, MD
Assistant Director, Combined Emergency Medicine/Internal
Medicine Residency Program
Trauma Liaison
Department of Emergency Medicine
Attending Physician
Department of Medicine
Allegheny General Hospital
Pittsburgh, PA;
Clinical Instructor of Emergency Medicine
Drexel University College of Medicine
Philadelphia, PA
USA

Joseph M. Pilewski, MD
Co-Director, Adult Cystic Fibrosis Program
Antonio J and Janet Palumbo Cystic Fibrosis Center
Children's Hospital of Pittsburgh of UPMC;
Associate Professor of Medicine, Cell Biology,
Physiology and Pediatrics
University of Pittsburgh School of Medicine
Pittsburgh, PA
USA

Alfons Pomp, MD, FACS, FRCSC
Leon C. Hirsch Professor of Surgery
Vice Chair for Quality and Patient Safety
Department of Surgery
Chief
Section of Laparoscopic and Bariatric Surgery
Weill Medical College of Cornell University
New York Presbyterian Hospital
New York, NY
USA

Jeffrey A. Rudolph, MD
Attending Physician
Children's Hospital of Pittsburgh of UPMC;
Assistant Professor of Pediatrics
Division of Pediatric Gastroenterology
Department of Pediatrics
University of Pittsburgh School of Medicine
Pittsburgh, PA
USA

Richard A. Saladino, MD
Medical Director
Emergency Department
Children's Hospital of Pittsburgh of UPMC;
Associate Professor of Pediatrics
Chief
Division of Pediatric Emergency Medicine
Department of Pediatrics
University of Pittsburgh School of Medicine
Pittsburgh, PA
USA

David W. Silver
Resident
Department of Emergency Medicine
University of Cincinnati College of Medicine
Cincinnati, OH
USA

Lauren T. Southerland, MD
Resident
Division of Emergency Medicine
Department of Surgery
Duke University School of Medicine
Durham, NC
USA

Sukhjit S. Takhar, MD
Attending Physician
Department of Emergency Medicine
Brigham and Women's Hospital;
Instructor in Medicine (Emergency Medicine)
Division of Emergency Medicine
Harvard Medical School
Boston, MA
USA

Victoria L. Thornton, MD, MBA, FACEP
Director, Pain Management and Palliative Care
in Emergency Medicine
Attending Physician
Department of Emergency Medicine
Duke University Medical Center;
Assistant Professor of Surgery (Emergency Medicine)
Division of Emergency Medicine
Department of Surgery
Duke University School of Medicine
Durham, NC
USA

Arvind Venkat, MD, FACEP
Director of Research
Department of Emergency Medicine
Ethics Consultant
Allegheny General Hospital
Pittsburgh, PA;
Associate Professor of Emergency Medicine
Drexel University College of Medicine
Philadelphia, PA
USA

K.K. Venkat, MD
Senior Staff Physician
Division of Nephrology and Hypertension
Department of Medicine
Henry Ford Hospital;
Clinical Associate Professor of Medicine (Nephrology)
Wayne State University School of Medicine
Detroit, MI
USA

Melissa A. Vitale, MD
Attending Physician
Children's Hospital of Pittsburgh of UPMC;
Assistant Professor of Pediatrics
Division of Pediatric Emergency Medicine
Department of Pediatrics
University of Pittsburgh School of Medicine
Pittsburgh, PA
USA

Acknowledgments

The preparation of this book has been one of the most rewarding experiences of my professional life. For that, I have many people to thank. First and foremost, I wish to acknowledge the work of the contributing authors of the various chapters in this book. All of them are experts in their fields of medicine, surgery and pediatrics who have taken the time to write chapters that I truly believe bring together their knowledge with the practical needs of emergency physicians. They also have worked extremely hard to meet tight deadlines, allowing this book to be published in a timely manner without sacrificing scope or content.

In developing the central premise behind this book of educating emergency physicians on the acute care issues of challenging and emerging patient populations, I have been fortunate to have had the mentorship and support of Dr. W. Brian Gibler of the University of Cincinnati College of Medicine. Dr. Allan B. Wolfson of the University Pittsburgh School of Medicine also provided critical suggestions on chapter selection and authors during the book's development. Finally, Dr. Fred Harchelroad, Chair of the Department of Emergency Medicine, and my colleagues at Allegheny General Hospital – both within my department and throughout the institution – have been generous in their time to support this project from its inception to its completion.

Wiley-Blackwell Publishing has been a great professional partner in the preparation of this textbook. From the time of my initial proposal, Mary Banks, Senior Publisher, along with Simone Dudziak and Jon Peacock, Development Editors; Cathryn Gates, Production Editor; Don Kehoe and Neil Burling, Marketing; and Shalini Sharma, Aptara Corporation, have been critical in taking this idea from mere conception to actual published book. They have worked very hard to ensure that the finished product represents our joint vision of what this textbook would be.

Finally, and most sincerely and affectionately, I want to thank my family for their constant encouragement and support of this endeavor. To my parents, K.K. and Hema Venkat, and my brother Deepak and sister-in-law Divya, thank you for always supporting me in both times of triumph and sorrow. To my wife Veena and my children, Avani, Jahnavi and Ashok, thank you for your understanding and love while I worked on this project and at all other times in my personal and professional life. This book is dedicated to all of you.

CHAPTER 1

Introduction

Arvind Venkat
Allegheny General Hospital, Pittsburgh, PA, USA; Drexel University College of
Medicine, Philadelphia, PA, USA

The emergency department (ED) serves as the gateway for medical care for
the preponderance of acutely ill patients. Whether due to medical, surgical,
pediatric, obstetric, neurologic, or psychiatric conditions, patients presenting with acute ailments expect that the ED and emergency physicians in
particular will be able to diagnose and initiate management of critical conditions. In the United States, as of 2007, there were 117 million annual
visits to the ED with 39.4 visits/100 persons [1]. Worldwide, there has
been increasing recognition of the need for quality emergency care and the
resultant recognition of emergency medicine as a medical specialty in nations as diverse as India, Turkey, and Malaysia. With this explosive growth
in emergency care, it is increasingly common for patients to view the ED
as the location for entrance into the health care system when confronted
with unexpected and severe medical complaints.

This recognition of the ED is well warranted, but it does create a dilemma
for emergency physicians who in their practice must be aware of the vast
complexities of ailments that can cause patients to present for emergency
care. While emergency physicians are clearly well trained to deal with the
most common diseases that require emergency interventions, such as cardiovascular disease and trauma, providers in the ED must now become
facile with managing patients whose disease entities are either only now
being recognized and treated or whose therapies have only recently been
developed. During a typical clinical shift, an emergency physician may
have to manage acute issues in patients whose co-morbid illnesses may
include transplantation, congenital heart disease, end-stage renal disease
or cancer. Without awareness of the new treatments and procedures in
these areas as well as the implications of increased longevity in patients
who previously may have never required emergency care in the past, it is

Challenging and Emerging Conditions in Emergency Medicine, First Edition. Edited by Arvind Venkat.
© 2011 by John Wiley & Sons, Ltd. Published 2011 by Blackwell Publishing Ltd.

easily foreseeable that emergency physicians may not correctly diagnose and initiate treatment in conditions that require acute intervention with resultant detriment to the patient.

At the same time, the literature and educational process in emergency medicine has understandably largely focused upon patients who present most commonly for ED care. Research in emergency medicine largely, though not exclusively, focuses on the most prevalent conditions, such as acute coronary syndromes, pulmonary embolism, stroke, trauma, and sepsis, while textbooks in emergency medicine are largely comprehensive surveys of the entire gamut of diseases that can cause presentation to the ED. Similarly, the core curriculum in emergency medicine for residency training in the United States attempts to cover the entire range of conditions to the ED, but in the process does not allow for more in-depth consideration by trainees of patient populations that are either on the horizon or whose therapies are quickly evolving to result in increased longevity and changed pathophysiology.

This book attempts to address this educational need for emergency physicians to understand patient populations whose ailments either are being treated in new ways or to rectify a lack of common recognition both in diagnosis and the implications of increasing longevity. In selecting topics for inclusion, three themes emerge that underline the challenge facing emergency physicians.

Increased longevity

As seen in the chapters on adults with congenital heart disease, the geriatric trauma patient, adults with cystic fibrosis, the intellectually disabled patient, adults with sickle cell disease, and children with intestinal failure, evolving medical care and understanding of the pathophysiology of disease has resulted in a vast improvement in the life expectancy of patients who previously have not survived to adulthood or whose survival to late adulthood has resulted in their exposure to illnesses that will now require ED care. For emergency physicians, this increased longevity will result in the need to reconsider the pathologic processes that can result in illness as well as new complications of late-stage disease. For example, survival to adulthood of patients with congenital heart disease means that emergency physicians will have to recognize the late complications of surgical procedures that were used to correct these defects in infancy as well as the late cardiovascular and pulmonary issues that may not arise until adulthood. The aging of the general population means that emergency physicians will have to understand the more complex pathophysiology of trauma when interacting with other age-related illnesses. Children with intestinal failure may now survive for longer periods of time and present with complications that were only seen in the past in specialized centers shortly after birth. For all the patient populations discussed in these chapters, the underlying theme is that the emergency physicians have to conceive of these patients as surviving well beyond what was previously recognized in day-to-day medical practice and consider how that may cause these individuals to present with novel complications not seen in the past.

Novel treatment modalities

As seen in the chapters on the bariatric surgery patient, HIV-positive adults on highly active antiretroviral therapy, emergency complications of chemotherapeutic regimens, the post-cardiac arrest patient, renal dialysis patients and renal transplant patients, evolving medical and surgical care for patients who previously either had different or ineffective treatment modalities has resulted in emergency complications that require recognition by ED providers. Such treatments have often provided wonderful benefits to these patient populations in terms of quality of life and longevity, but have made the ED the venue in which acute diagnosis of treatment failures or complications will take place. For example, the astronomic growth of bariatric surgical procedures requires emergency physicians to recognize the resultant anatomic and physiological changes that take place post-operatively and the side effects and treatment issues that can arise. The increased longevity of HIV-positive adults on highly active antiretroviral therapy has resulted in completely new disease processes that more commonly affect this patient population. With the development of hypothermia treatment post-cardiac arrest, emergency physicians are being called upon to manage patients previously thought to be neurologically devastated in a novel and potentially life-changing way. For all these patient populations, the underlying theme is that new and evolving therapies have created a novel set of disease processes and treatments with which emergency physicians must become familiar.

Complications of social pathologies and lack of medical resources

As seen in the chapters on conditions causing chronic pain, family violence, and the obese patient, the ED also serves as the "canary in the mine" for pathologies that often extend beyond the medical realm [2]. To some extent, this may be seen as the dark side of the increased recognition of the ED as the gateway to the health care system. As such, emergency physicians now must contend with the consequences of failures in our medical system and complexities that result from the breakdown in family relationships or societal forces well beyond their control. For example, the growth in the number of patients with conditions that cause chronic pain coupled with a lack of medical training in pain management and a shortage of pain management physicians has left the ED as the venue of last resort for patients who require analgesia, perhaps best managed ideally in the outpatient setting. Increased recognition of child abuse and intimate partner violence has imposed a burden on emergency physicians to treat the medical and social dangers imposed by these conditions. The epidemic of obesity has profound implications for the diagnostic assessment and therapeutic management of patients in the ED. Together, these emerging patient populations represent a profound challenge for emergency care in the twenty-first century.

Chapters in this book are structured so that the reader will have an understanding of the epidemiology, procedural interventions, and disease presentation and management in these patient populations in the ED. Each chapter concludes with a section entitled "The next five years" which is meant to provide the reader with a prediction of where these fields will likely evolve in the near future and the implications of those changes for emergency practice. The contributing authors to this book and I hope that the reader will find that this serves as a starting point for consideration in training programs and clinical EDs as to how best to address the numerous challenging and emerging conditions that will cause patients to present for emergency care.

References

1. Niska R, Bhuiya F, Xu J. National Hospital Ambulatory Medical Survey: 2007 emergency department summary. *National Health Statistics Reports* 2010 Aug 6; 26: 1–32.
2. Venkat A. Health insurance: canary in the mine. *Cincinnati Enquirer* 2004 Jul 1: C10.

CHAPTER 2

The post-cardiac arrest patient

Ankur A. Doshi[1,2] and Clifton W. Callaway[2]
[1]UPMC Presbyterian and Mercy Hospitals, Pittsburgh, PA, USA
[2]University of Pittsburgh School of Medicine, Pittsburgh, PA, USA

Introduction

Heart disease is the leading cause of death in the industrialized world [1]. Consequently, the presentation of end-stage heart disease—cardiac arrest—is well known to emergency physicians. Similarly, emergency providers, both in the prehospital setting and in the emergency department (ED), are well versed in the treatment algorithms for patients during cardiac arrest. Over the past 35 years, organizations such as the American Heart Association (AHA) and International Liaison Committee on Resuscitation (ILCOR) have developed recommendations for care of patients in cardiac arrest [2, 3]. These references, including Advanced Cardiovascular Life Support (ACLS), provide standardized care of patients in cardiac arrest. Even though the baseline characteristics of patients in cardiac arrest are fairly uniform, the rates of survival for these patients still vary geographically [4]. Moreover, from the 1970s through the early 2000s, despite a variety of newly researched and implemented interventions, there was no change in long-term survival of cardiac arrest patients [5–10].

In the past 10 years, scientists have begun to better describe the pathophysiology of cardiac arrest leading to research that has demonstrated that physiologic derangements occur not only during but also after cardiac arrest [11]. Consequently, clinicians have begun to recognize the need to coordinate care of patients during and after cardiac arrest to maximize patients' survival [11]. In many cases, early, aggressive treatment directed at the specific pathology after cardiac arrest (post-cardiac arrest care) is essential to allow patients the maximum likelihood of beneficial neurological outcomes [11]. This strategy of beginning post-cardiac arrest care promptly is now advocated by guidelines published by the AHA and ILCOR such as

Challenging and Emerging Conditions in Emergency Medicine, First Edition. Edited by Arvind Venkat.
© 2011 by John Wiley & Sons, Ltd. Published 2011 by Blackwell Publishing Ltd.

ACLS [2, 3]. Yet, less than 20% of US emergency physicians have treated patients with post-cardiac arrest care [12]. This chapter outlines the evidence supporting aggressive post-cardiac arrest care in the ED, protocols for performing efficient post-cardiac arrest resuscitation in the acute setting, and future directions in the evolution of care of the post-cardiac arrest patient.

Epidemiology and pathophysiology

An estimated two-thirds of US citizens are at high lifetime predicted risk for atherosclerotic cardiovascular disease [13]. Consequently, cardiovascular disease was the cause of one in six deaths in the United States in 2006 [1]. The end point of cardiovascular disease is sudden cardiac arrest, which most often occurs in the out-of-hospital setting [14]. The incidence of out-of-hospital cardiac arrest is estimated to range from 55 to 120 events per 100,000 persons per year [14, 15]. A recent North American sample demonstrated the median incidence of out-of-hospital cardiac arrest to be 52.1 events per 100,000 persons per year. The mean survival in this cohort was 8.4% [4]. As expected, the demographics of cardiac arrest mirror those of other coronary heart disease. The mean age for patients with sudden cardiac arrest is between 65 and 70 years of age, and death from sudden cardiac arrest is more common in men than women [4, 14]. Patients with ventricular fibrillation arrests, those who received bystander CPR (cardiopulmonary resuscitation), and those with rapid return of spontaneous circulation, survive at a greater rate than those who do not meet these criteria [11]. However, there is great variability in survival, with some regions of North America reporting overall survival after out-of-hospital cardiac arrest to be greater than 15% and others reporting survival of less than 2% [4]. This variation persists even after controlling for patient and resuscitation variables, such as witnessed collapse, bystander CPR, ambulance response times, and initial rhythm [4]. Part of this variation may be explained by differing ED and in-hospital care [16].

The causes of death for patients after cardiac arrest can be broadly divided into two categories—"cardiac death" and "neurological death." Cardiac death is due to intrinsic cardiac failure, either the inability to restart spontaneous cardiac contraction or the inability to maintain systemic perfusion after significant myocardial damage. Neurological death is due to accumulated cellular damage to the central nervous system (CNS). Standard care of the cardiac arrest patient prior to 2002 focused only on the restoration of circulation and did not address the continued pathology of cardiac arrest after return of spontaneous circulation [17]. For the past 30 years, despite newer medications and devices to treat out-of-hospital cardiac arrest, only approximately one-third of patients have return of spontaneous circulation long enough to be admitted to the hospital [14]. Almost by definition, patients who do not survive to hospital admission are considered to have cardiac death [11].

Of the out-of-hospital cardiac arrest patients who survive to hospital admission, another two-thirds will die prior to hospital discharge. Although some patients develop secondary cardiac failure or other complications of severe illness, the primary etiology of in-hospital mortality is severe neurological injury [18, 19]. The CNS cellular damage in this group is not simply due to ischemic cell necrosis but also due to reperfusion injury. Reperfusion injury is a second wave of cellular damage that is characterized by dysregulation of CNS protective mechanisms and plays out for hours to days after return of spontaneous circulation. Consequently, the previous treatment of cardiac arrest, as limited to the achievement of return of spontaneous circulation, did not address this secondary neurological injury [11]. Although CNS reperfusion injury had been identified for a number of years, until recently, no therapy had been found to minimize its effect. Randomized trials tested treatment such as calcium-channel blockers, benzodiazapines, and even specific antibodies without demonstrating benefit in humans [20–22]. The first successful clinical trials demonstrating successful treatment of CNS reperfusion injury after out-of-hospital cardiac arrest were published in 2001 and 2002 [23–25]. These three trials evaluated the use of induced therapeutic hypothermia (ITH) in patients after return of spontaneous circulation from out-of-hospital cardiac arrest.

Over the past 20 years, ITH has been used to treat neurologic disorders, such as traumatic brain injury and stroke, and has been shown to be of benefit to prevent brain injury during cardiac bypass surgery [26–28]. ITH is theorized to minimize CNS reperfusion injury via a number of mechanisms. Possibilities include decreasing cerebral metabolism, reducing brain edema, and therefore, increasing perfusion, diminishing free radical production, suppressing neuroexcitatory toxins, controlling apoptosis, improving brain glucose metabolism, and reducing seizures. This multifactorial effect on the CNS is likely why ITH has shown benefit, when other specific therapies have not [11].

The three original cardiac arrest ITH trials demonstrated that the use of ITH after out-of-hospital cardiac arrest could significantly increase patient survival to hospital discharge. A meta-analysis of these studies showed an almost 30% relative risk reduction for death or poor neurological outcome in survivors of cardiac arrest treated with ITH [29]. Early use of ITH (within the first 8 hours of cardiac arrest) increased patients' absolute survival to discharge with good neurologic functioning by 16% [24, 25, 29]. Additionally, the early use of ITH resulted in the same magnitude of benefit at 6 months post-arrest [24]. A number of further studies have confirmed this benefit [30, 31]. On the basis of these data, the AHA and ILCOR recommend that patients after out-of-hospital cardiac arrest receive specific post-arrest management [2, 3].

Supportive treatment to minimize secondary CNS injury during reperfusion has also been associated with improved patient survival with good neurological status. These therapies have been modeled after successful treatments in the intensive care setting, such as minimizing hypoxia, hypotension, and hyperglycemia, in other critical illnesses [32–34]. Bundling these interventions with ITH into treatment pathways has been labeled as "post-cardiac arrest care." A truly integrated protocol to neuroresuscitation for the post-cardiac arrest patient should include these interventions. There have been several small studies that have demonstrated the efficacy of integrated post-cardiac arrest care in the intensive care setting to increase patient survival [35–37].

Despite the known benefits of post-cardiac arrest care, there remains large local variability of in-hospital care after out-of-hospital cardiac arrest. For example, when similar out-of-hospital cardiac arrest patients were taken by ambulance to different hospitals, their survival to hospital discharge differed simply based upon the hospital where treatment occurred [35, 38]. This difference was postulated to be due to the different in-hospital care patients received, including the use, or lack thereof, of ITH. It is postulated, then, that regional variability in out-of-hospital cardiac arrest survival is also partially due to in-hospital care differences [16, 39]. When hospitals are polled, a majority self-report the capacity to provide post-cardiac arrest care. However, many of these institutions do not provide this type of care on a routine basis (Martin-Gill: unpublished data). Even when an institution has a post-cardiac arrest care system in place, treatment is often delayed until admission, because of the perception that such care is too time and resource intensive for the ED [12].

Indications and contraindications

There are a number of potential barriers to the use of post-cardiac arrest care in the ED. As a result, a majority of emergency physicians report that they do not provide post-cardiac arrest care routinely [12]. Yet, just as early treatment of other critical illnesses, such as stroke, myocardial infarction, or trauma, in the ED improves patient outcomes, emergent treatment of post-cardiac arrest patients can improve survival to hospital discharge [11]. Reperfusion injury of the brain begins at the moment of return of spontaneous circulation; the earlier that treatment is begun, the more the potential benefit for improved neurological outcome [11]. Therefore, post-cardiac arrest care should be initiated in the ED for all out-of-hospital cardiac arrest patients without contraindications detailed in Table 2.1.

Although no one has reported on specific barriers to post-cardiac arrest care in the ED, research has identified the barriers to the use of ITH—the most novel component of post-cardiac arrest care. A survey of North American and European physicians identified the most common barriers

Table 2.1 Contraindications to induced therapeutic hypothermia and post-cardiac arrest care

---

Absolute contraindications
- Active uncontrolled or noncompressible hemorrhage
- Do not resuscitate/do not intubate status
- Rapid neurologic improvement (i.e., following commands with 60 minutes of return of spontaneous circulation)

Relative contraindications
- Multisystem trauma
- Shock from GI bleed or sepsis
- Intracranial hemorrhage (unless cleared by neurosurgery)

---

to the use of ITH in the ED [12]. Reasons for not using ITH include the following: "not enough data" (49% of North American physicians and 41% of European physicians), "too technically difficult" (35% North American physicians and 32% European physicians), and "have not considered it" (34% North American physicians and 23% European physicians) [12].

However, new data address these concerns of emergency physicians. For example, respondents in the Merchant study indicating "not enough data" pointed to the fact that studies only demonstrated a benefit to ITH only after out-of-hospital cardiac arrest due to ventricular fibrillation or pulseless ventricular tachycardia [12]. However, there is no evidence that the pathophysiology of CNS injury from out-of-hospital ventricular fibrillation arrest is different from that of any other type of cardiac arrest. A number of case series have found a benefit to the use of ITH in all cardiac arrest patients (in-hospital and out-of-hospital) and with all initial rhythms [40–43]. Large registries have shown that ITH provides outcome benefit to patients after cardiac arrests because of non-cardiac causes, such as asphyxiation or drug overdose [36, 40, 44]. Therefore, presently, there is sufficient data to support the use of ITH, and in association, post-cardiac arrest care, after all types of cardiac arrest.

Another frequent reason why physicians do not provide ITH is that they "have not considered it" [12]. This is despite these physicians understanding the benefit of ITH after out-of-hospital cardiac arrest; 34% of North American respondents felt that the data for ITH was compelling enough to make a trial randomizing some patients to normothermia unethical. The reason for this disparity may lie in the fact that emergency physicians provide care in a scarce resource model. They attempt to provide the best care possible to the most number of patients with the available time and resources. Consequently, emergency physicians may not consider the use of hypothermia in contrast to other lifesaving interventions such as intravenous thrombolytics for acute stroke or immediate coronary intervention in the setting of ST-segment elevation myocardial infarction. In short, many emergency physicians may feel that, despite the proven benefit of ITH after cardiac arrest, the magnitude of this benefit does not outweigh the risk incurred to other patients when ITH is initiated for cardiac arrest.

Pessimism about the survivability from cardiac arrest may bias physicians into believing that aggressive post-cardiac arrest care is rarely useful. One study demonstrated that a majority (63%) of in-hospital cardiac arrest patients after return of spontaneous circulation were placed in "do not resuscitate" status. Of these patients, 43% had mechanical support actively discontinued during the hospitalization [45]. The fact that many patients after return of spontaneous circulation seem neurologically devastated may contribute to this pessimism. However, neurological assessment in the ED is not predictive of final neurological outcome after cardiac arrest [46–49]. Many patients receive medications during cardiac arrest that may make neurological assessment invalid. Atropine, for instance, will cause pupillary dilation because of its anticholinergic effect, in the absence of brain injury. Additionally, all patients after cardiac arrest suffer some degree of neurological stunning. The depth of this stunning is likely proportional to the ischemic injury suffered during the arrest. A patient with very little injury, such as one rapidly defibrillated in the field, may seem almost neurologically normal in the ED. However, even patients who demonstrate no neurological function shortly after a prolonged cardiac arrest will improve neurologically during the next 48–72 hours [49]. Because of this initial inability to predict final neurological outcome of out-of-hospital cardiac arrest patients, the benefit of post-cardiac arrest care may be less obvious to the emergency physician than the benefit from interventions for ST-segment elevation myocardial infarction or stroke.

The final barrier to care identified—that ITH is "too technically difficult"—probably has two components. First, many physicians may not feel comfortable with the mechanical steps needed to implement ITH. Additionally, physicians may be concerned about the possible side effects of ITH that could lead to worse patient outcomes. As with any new therapy or medication, there is a learning curve to the implementation of post-cardiac arrest care. Providing an algorithm for emergency physicians to manage patients after cardiac arrest may clarify both how post-cardiac arrest care can be integrated into the patient's ED care as well as for which patients such care is contraindicated.

The algorithm we recommend is the "ABCs" of resuscitation—already well known to all emergency physicians. After return of spontaneous circulation, the emergency physician should return back to the beginning of the ABCs and ensure that the patient's airway is secured, followed by assessments of oxygenation, ventilation, perfusion, and focal neurological disability. This algorithm helps the physician provide post-cardiac arrest care using a well-known pathway. In addition, by following this pathway, those few patients in whom post-cardiac arrest care is contraindicated will be evident. For instance, patients in shock due to multisystem trauma, hemorrhage, or sepsis should have their ED resuscitation focused on correction of these illnesses or injuries processes prior to specialized post-cardiac arrest care. However, the presence of one of these medical problems is only a relative contraindication to treatment with post-cardiac arrest care. Similarly, a brief focused neurological assessment, with the addition of neuroimaging via CT, should identify patients with intracranial hemorrhage. If cleared by neurosurgery, these patients may still be treated with post-cardiac arrest care. Initial resuscitation may focus on correction of the intracranial hemorrhage first. Previously accepted contraindications to post-cardiac arrest care, such as pregnancy or under-18 age, do not have physiologic bases. There have been published case reports detailing successful use of ITH in these settings [50–52].

It is true that despite optimal care, a patient's final neurological status can only be maximized to the level of functioning prior to the recent cardiac arrest. In an ED setting, therefore, it may be reasonable to withhold aggressive post-cardiac arrest care for a patient whose neurological status prior to cardiac arrest is poor. Some patients, in addition, have made their decision on the use of lifesaving technology clear prior to their event in the form of an advanced directive. As post-cardiac arrest care is a therapy that may take days to accomplish, it is reasonable for the emergency physician to not aggressively treat a post-cardiac arrest patient who has specifically declined intensive care therapy. However, in other cases, aggressive post-cardiac arrest care in the ED can make a profound difference in patients' final neurological outcome.

Nuts and bolts

The application of post-cardiac arrest care in the ED is straightforward and requires resources that are already available in most institutions. However, some preparation is needed to ensure that the needed equipment is resourced to the ED to minimize time delay from return of spontaneous circulation to the beginning of neuroresuscitation. It is also imperative that the care provided in the ED not be labor or resource intensive. This will ensure that providers, even in a chaotic ED environment, are able to provide maximum care to the post-arrest patient without compromising care to other patients. The familiar "ABCs" algorithm is a useful framework for defining the care to be provided with some modification (Table 2.2).

Airway
The beginning of post-cardiac arrest care in the ED is an assessment of the patient's airway. If, after return of spontaneous circulation, the patient is alert and protecting his or her own airway, further interventions may not be necessary. However, most survivors of cardiac arrest will be neurologically injured and require placement of an artificial airway. Recent

Table 2.2 Recommended emergency department post-cardiac arrest care protocol

- A (airway)
  - ○ Replace rescue airway with endotracheal tube
- B (pulmonary function)
  - ○ Arterial blood gas
  - ○ Continuous pulse oximetry
    - □ Avoid hypoxia OR hyperoxia (O_2 sat—94%–98%)
  - ○ Continuous end-tidal capnography
    - □ Maintain eucapnia ($PaCO_2$ 35–45 mm Hg)
- C (systemic and cerebral perfusion)
  - ○ Frequent or continuous blood pressure evaluation (continuous arterial line monitoring is preferred)
    - □ Maintain central venous pressure (12–15 mm Hg adjusting for any positive-end expiratory pressure)
      - Use intravenous fluid boluses
    - □ Maintain mean arterial pressure (80–100 mm Hg)
      - Use ionotropes or vasopressors
  - ○ Obtain ECG
    - □ Percutaneous coronary intervention based on standard criteria
    - □ Maintain low threshold for cardiac catheterization with evidence of ischemia or cardiogenic shock
- D (neuroresuscitation)
  - ○ Induced therapeutic hypothermia
    - □ Continuous temperature monitoring with esophageal, rectal, or bladder probe
    - □ Goal temperature of 32–34°C within 6 hours of return of spontaneous circulation
    - □ Infusion cooling
      - 30 mL/kg 4°C crystalloid infusion (bolus)
      - Gastric/bladder cold irrigation
    - □ Surface cooling
      - Application of ice packs to head, neck, axilla and groin
      - Cooling blanket
    - □ Prevention of motion
      - Neuromuscular paralysis (short term)
      - Sedation with benzodiazapine/barbiturate
      - Shivering control with narcotic
- Other possible therapies per local protocols (discuss with admitting physician)
  - ○ Control of hyperglycemia
    - □ Low-dose insulin infusion
  - ○ Anticoagulation
  - ○ Antimicrobial use

data on patients in cardiac arrest has demonstrated a significant association between the amount of time chest compressions were performed and survival [53, 54]. Endotracheal intubation often requires lengthy interruption in chest compressions [55]. Supraglottic airways, in contrast, can be more easily placed without an interruption of chest compressions [56]. For this reason, some local protocols have begun using these airways for rescue when endotracheal intubation cannot be accomplished or favoring immediate supraglottic airway placement over standard intubation [57, 58]. If a rescue airway or primary supraglottic airway was placed during resuscitation, it should be converted to a standard endotracheal tube in the ED, as most patients will require mechanical ventilation for at least 24 hours. Additionally, a common complication of out-of-hospital cardiac arrest is aspiration; therefore, intubation should be accomplished with an endotracheal tube large enough to allow for frequent suctioning [24, 25].

Pulmonary function

The next step in post-cardiac arrest care is an evaluation and management of pulmonary function. The patient should be placed on continuous pulse oximetry. An arterial blood gas (ABG) should be assessed to evaluate the partial pressure of oxygen (PaO_2) and carbon dioxide ($PaCO_2$). If possible, a continuous end-tidal carbon dioxide detector may be used as well. Immediately after return of spontaneous circulation, the CNS is extremely vulnerable to hypoxia. Therefore, ED care should ensure that adequate oxygenation is maintained throughout [32]. In addition, early hyperoxia is also associated with poorer final neurologic outcomes. Patients with initial PaO_2 less than 60 or greater than 300 had worse outcomes than those with PaO_2 between 61 and 299 [59]. Therefore, the emergency physician should titrate supplemental oxygen to avoid these extremes of blood oxygenation. To avoid repetitive ABG sampling, continuous pulse oximetry can be used to reduce oxygen levels to the lowest possible to maintain saturations >94%.

Management of ventilation is also an important component of post-cardiac arrest care. Hypocapnia decreases cerebral blood flow. Therefore, maintenance of normal $PaCO_2$ (between 35–45 mm Hg) is useful in preventing a secondary reduction in CNS perfusion. Initial management can be done on the basis of the ABG, with subsequent changes being performed using the end-tidal carbon dioxide monitor.

Systemic and cerebral perfusion

Thirdly, the emergency physician should continually evaluate the adequacy of circulation and CNS perfusion after return of spontaneous circulation. In the first 24 hours after return of spontaneous circulation, myocardial dysfunction is common, likely due to primary cardiac disease or coronary reperfusion injury. This cellular damage results in decreased cardiac stroke volume and decreased cardiac output and cerebral blood flow [60]. Also, during initial resuscitation, vasopressors, such as epinephrine, are often used, which artificially increase systemic blood pressure. The effect of these vasopressors is quite transient; as their effect wanes, hemodynamic compromise may occur. Without an adequate mean arterial pressure, CNS perfusion will not be maintained [11]. After reperfusion, autoregulation of the cerebral circulation causes further decrease in cerebral blood flow due to cerebral vasoconstriction. Due to this, mean arterial pressures after return of spontaneous circulation should be kept on the higher end of normal (80–100 mm Hg) to avoid secondary CNS injury [61]. One study demonstrated that even transient hypotension in the first 2 hours following return of spontaneous circulation was associated with poor neurologic recovery [33]. Therefore, emergency care of the post-cardiac arrest patient should include frequent assessments of global perfusion. At a minimum, measurement of blood pressure should be made frequently (every 5 minutes) using noninvasive measures. Ideally, arterial cannulation should be performed to measure blood pressure continuously. Adequate fluid resuscitation is needed to maintain adequate cardiac filling pressures. Either inotropes, such as dopamine, or vasopressors, such as norepinephrine, may be needed to ensure adequate perfusion.

Other cardiac therapy within post-cardiac arrest care must include an evaluation of the need for coronary intervention. All patients after out-of-hospital cardiac arrest should have a 12-lead ECG obtained. The presence of ischemia should be aggressively managed including a low threshold for percutaneous coronary intervention. Routine cardiac catheterization may lead to increased survival from cardiac arrest, and standard criteria for direct coronary intervention, such as the presence of ST-segment elevations, should prompt immediate intervention [62, 63]. One series showed that 48% of patients with return of spontaneous circulation after cardiac arrest had some coronary artery occlusion [64]. Another study showed that 51% of resuscitated patients had either cardiac enzyme elevation or electrocardiographic evidence of acute myocardial infarction [65]. Multiple studies have shown that emergent coronary intervention with angioplasty or coronary stenting is safe in patients during ITH [66, 67]. Patients in cardiogenic shock, even without ST-segment elevation, may also benefit from coronary intervention or the placement of an intra-aortic balloon pump, although the evidence for this benefit is more from correlation rather than clinical trials [63]. ITH has been used with concomitant fibrinolytic therapy after cardiac arrest and stroke, with no more bleeding than usually expected after fibrinolysis [68, 69]. Therefore, ITH should be considered for patients regardless of the reperfusion strategy selected. From the standpoint of the emergency physician, the data supports that a strong partnership with cardiology and an ability to carry out immediate coronary intervention are needed to care for post-cardiac arrest patients.

Neuroresuscitation

The most novel portion of post-cardiac arrest care is the focus on neuroresuscitation. The major component of this is ITH. However, other therapies, such as the use of benzodiazapine or barbiturate sedation and control of hyperglycemia, may be useful as well. As described above, ITH has many effects on the CNS that may contribute to its effectiveness in improving survival from out-of-hospital cardiac arrest. Interestingly, many different treatment protocols for ITH have been tested, and all have demonstrated similar benefits [30, 31, 70]. The techniques for ITH can be grossly divided into three categories: (1) surface cooling, (2) infusion cooling, and (3) endovascular cooling. The use of the first two types of cooling requires minimal preparation and no special equipment. Endovascular cooling, in contrast, requires the purchase of specialized equipment. All three methods have similar effectiveness for induction of hypothermia. However, because of the ease of use of surface and infusion cooling, we recommend the use of these methods in the ED.

Many of the parameters of ITH, such as the optimal temperature, optimal rate of temperature change, and the maximum time delay to beginning therapy, are unknown. Current recommendations are, therefore, adapted from successful clinical trials. It is reasonable to attempt to induce hypothermia to between 32°C and 34°C within 6 hours of return of spontaneous circulation. The optimal rate of cooling is unknown, but no ill effects have been noted with rapid reduction of temperature [71]. Many patients after return of spontaneous circulation are mildly hypothermic with temperatures ranging from 35°C to 35.5°C [25,72]. However, if the induction of hypothermia is delayed, spontaneous rewarming occurs within 1 to 2 hours [73, 74]. Therefore, prompt temperature control after return of spontaneous circulation may reduce the amount of effort required to provide ITH.

Surface cooling is performed using ice packs and cooling blankets. We have found that true ice packs should be used, as opposed to chemical cooling packs, which lack the thermal mass and duration of action to be effective. These ice packs are placed about the patient's head, neck, axilla, and groin with adequate padding to minimize the chance of frost injury. Additionally, a cooling blanket can be placed to help lower core temperature. Initial experience with surface cooling showed it to be slow—needing between 4 and 6 hours to reach goal temperature [24,25,75]. More advanced protocols have added neuromuscular blockade and sedation to minimize motion and shivering and have successfully cooled most patients below 34°C within 4 hours [71]. The only preparations to use surface cooling are having a source of ice and a readily available cooling blanket.

Infusion cooling is performed by the administration of cold fluids, either intravenously or via gastric and/or bladder lavage. The most effective of these interventions is a rapid infusion of cold (4°C) crystalloid intravenous fluids [74]. The recommended dose is 30 mL/kg of crystalloid administered as a bolus via central line or pressure infuser peripherally [76]. Minimal preparation is needed for the use of infusion cooling. Standard 1 L bags of crystalloid fluid can be placed within a refrigerator and infused when needed. Some institutions require that these bags be rotated or replaced in a standard fashion, although no study has evaluated this requirement. Cold crystalloid infusion may be contraindicated in patients with pulmonary edema or others who cannot tolerate such a volume load. In these patients, gastric and bladder irrigation with cold (4°C) fluids may be used as an alternative.

Although infusion of cold fluids is effective at induction of hypothermia, it is not an effective method for hypothermia maintenance [77]. Another method must be used to maintain hypothermia once the patient reaches goal temperature. Most protocols provide simultaneous infusion cooling with surface or endovascular cooling. Sedation and short-term paralysis are essential to ensure that the patient does not generate body heat and rewarm prematurely during induction. One important caveat is that, due to a high incidence of seizures in post-cardiac arrest patients, care must be taken to ensure that neuromuscular blockade does not mask seizure activity. Our recommendation is to discontinue paralysis once goal temperature is reached and to control movement of shivering with sedation and narcotic pain medications. For example, one regimen might consist of sedation with a propofol infusion and analgesia with fentanyl. If the patient's blood pressure does not tolerate propofol, then a midazolam infusion might be substituted. Figure 2.1 shows a model patient receiving ITH.

Other therapies for neuroresuscitation are more controversial than those detailed above. Such treatments include control of hyperglycemia, anticoagulation, and antimicrobial treatment of suspected infection. However, each of these strategies has not shown significant benefit when added to

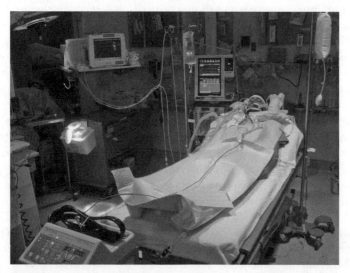

Figure 2.1 Model patient receiving induced therapeutic hypothermia.

ITH [78–80]. Therefore, although these therapies are reasonable and may become part of local protocol [81], we do not recommend their use in the ED without coordination with the intensive care unit.

Appropriate admission

The final aspect of post-cardiac arrest care that should be discussed is appropriate disposition from the ED. Obviously, the use of post-cardiac arrest care requires institutional buy-in and support, in addition to being a focus of ED care. Any patients undergoing post-cardiac arrest care in the ED should be managed in a center with the ability to continue this care in the intensive care setting. With the possibility of deterioration of cardiac function, an admitting facility must have the ability to perform immediate percutaneous coronary intervention. Finally, some research indicates that post-cardiac arrest care may have fewer complications when performed in specific referral centers [16, 39, 80].

Overall, initiation of post-cardiac arrest care in the ED is straightforward when done in an algorithmic fashion. Focusing on airway (A), pulmonary function (B), systemic and brain perfusion (C), neuroresuscitation (D), and appropriate disposition in a stepwise approach makes the induction of this therapy more practical in a busy ED. However, a typical patient requires and deserves 1 hour or more of critical care time while still in the ED with potential for more depending on the procedures performed. A close relationship with intensivists or partners in the ED to provide this coverage should be considered. In many ways, the resource requirements of the post-cardiac arrest patient are similar to those of a high-acuity trauma patient.

Special situations

Emergency medical services

Many emergency physicians, as medical directors, play a significant role in their local emergency medical services agency. A recent focus in prehospital medicine is on "best practices" cardiac arrest care. For instance, by implementing multiple small changes in how paramedics provide care to out-of-hospital cardiac arrest patients, survival to hospital discharge can triple [57, 58]. Similarly, research is being done on the implementation of post-cardiac arrest care, specifically ITH, prior to arrival at the hospital. Theoretically, treatment with ITH in the field could provide additional neurological benefit because of minimization of the time delay from return of spontaneous circulation to neuroresuscitation. Intravenous crystalloid in portable coolers can be easily maintained at the appropriate temperature [82]. Furthermore, infusion of cold intravenous fluids can lower body temperature prior to a patient's arrival at the hospital [74]. However, no study has shown a significant neurological outcome difference between patients cooled in the field and those cooled in the ED [44]. However, a number of prehospital systems have implemented protocols encouraging ITH in the field. Importantly, data from patients in the intensive care unit shows that those patients with high variability in their temperature (i.e., those who fluctuate from goal temperature to either overcooling or under-cooling) have a poorer neurologic outcome than those whose temperature is less labile [83,84]. Therefore, patients who have ITH initiated in the field should be transported to institutions where ITH can be continued. Patients that arrive in the ED after undergoing ITH in the field should have ITH continued without interruption.

Ethics

Ethical concerns regarding ITH and post-cardiac arrest care are often expressed by physicians and patients' family members. For instance, there exists a worry that the use of aggressive post-cardiac arrest care will result in more patients surviving cardiac arrest, but in a neurologically devastated state. Prior to the widespread use of ITH, of the 8% of patients who survived cardiac arrest, most had a high quality of life [18,85]. This is likely due to the fact that a majority of resuscitated cardiac arrest patients are given "do not resuscitate" status while in the hospital and, therefore, do not survive if severely debilitated [86]. After the implementation of standardized use of ITH, the relative proportion of patients with good neurologic survival, when compared with those who survive with severe neurologic injury, has not changed [87]. Another group found that the use of ITH has decreased the number of neurologically injured survivors [88].

Another concern deals with termination of care, i.e., when can care be ethically withdrawn after the initiation of post-cardiac arrest care? For instance, if post-cardiac arrest care is begun in the ED prior to the arrival of the patient's family, it is possible that the family may provide evidence of the patient's wishes for end-of-life care to not have intensive care level interventions. Unfortunately, the benefits of ITH and post-cardiac arrest care are not necessarily evident in the first 24 hours. If the emergency physician feels that the cardiac arrest can be survivable with aggressive therapy, it may be reasonable to delay discussions about withdrawal of care until the treatment protocol is completed, i.e., after the first 24 hours. In the event that the provider and the family have very different views on continuing care, a consult to the hospital ethics service may be useful to clarify both sides' positions and develop a coordinated plan of care.

Finally, emergency physicians may be concerned with the need for families to provide informed consent for post-cardiac arrest care, and any potential liability from the initiation of post-cardiac arrest care. No specific case law on post-cardiac arrest care exists. The use of ITH and other post-cardiac arrest care interventions has been supported by the AHA and

ILCOR as standard of care after out-of-hospital cardiac arrest. For this reason, we do not believe that informed consent is needed to provide post-cardiac arrest care. However, our institutional practice is to inform the patient's nearest relative of the plan of care if possible.

The next five years

The future may bring a further specialization in institutions that care for post-cardiac arrest patients. Some centers may self-designate themselves as "cardiac arrest centers" analogous to "trauma centers" or "stroke centers" and provide comprehensive post-cardiac arrest care from ITH to neurological rehabilitation [11, 39]. These centers will likely be staffed by in-house neurointensivists and interventional cardiologists, who are prepared to care for post-cardiac arrest patients at all times [11,39].

Not all patients would benefit from this level of care, however. For example, some patients after return of spontaneous circulation are awake and without complaint. These patients usually have received rapid defibrillation for ventricular fibrillation or pulseless ventricular tachycardia. Patients presenting with these initial rhythms are more likely to have coronary disease amenable to percutaneous coronary intervention [64, 66]. Therefore, even in the absence of obvious criteria for cardiac catheterization, such patients should be managed in a center capable of immediate percutaneous coronary intervention, though they may not require all the features of a full cardiac arrest center. At the other extreme, certain patients have severe cardiac and neurologic damage even prior to their cardiac arrest. These patients may require aggressive ventilator support, vasopressor management, and pharmacologic control of seizures to survive. However, despite maximal therapy, it is impossible for such a patient to improve beyond their baseline severely debilitated state. In this circumstance, supportive care might be managed in any center. In fact, the risk of transfer of such patients may far outweigh any potential benefits. Additionally, transfer of these patients may make it more difficult for family to be involved in their care due to distance and transportation issues. Patients who fall between these extreme categories will probably benefit most from treatment by a cardiac arrest center. These centers would be best equipped to identify and manage complications of care and provide the intensive rehabilitation and coordinated effort needed to maximize survival with good neurologic outcome. From a medical standpoint, the potential direct benefit to the patient from specialized care should outweigh any administrative concerns about losing business. Therefore, in the case of an ED without tertiary care abilities, post-cardiac arrest care should be initiated prior to the patient being transferred to a higher level of care—including a cardiac arrest center.

Conclusion

A focus on post-cardiac arrest care has shown uniform and absolute improvement in patients' survival to hospital discharge with good neurological outcome of greater than 15% [24, 25, 70]. Although recommended by the AHA and ILCOR, most EDs presently do not provide post-cardiac arrest care [2, 3]. Those centers that have implemented post-cardiac arrest care protocols continue to show an improvement in patient survival [43, 87]. Post-cardiac arrest care can be accomplished in any ED using a well-known algorithm and readily available resources once logistical and attitudinal barriers are addressed in the care of this challenging patient population.

References

1. A report from the American Heart Association. Heart disease and stroke statistics—2010 update. *Circulation* 2010; 121(7): e46–e215.
2. ECC Committee, Subcommittees and Task Forces of the American Heart Association. 2005 American heart association guidelines for cardiopulmonary resuscitation and emergency cardiovascular care. *Circulation* 2005; 112(24 Suppl.): 1–203.
3. Nolan JP, Morley PT, Vanden Hoek TL, Hickey RW. Therapeutic hypothermia after cardiac arrest: an advisory statement by the advance life support task force of the International Liaison Committee on Resuscitation. *Circulation* 2003; 108(1): 118–121.
4. Nichol G, Thomas E, Callaway CW, et al. Regional variation in out-of-hospital cardiac arrest incidence and outcome. *JAMA* 2008; 300(12): 1423–1431.
5. Callaway CW, Hostler D, Doshi AA, et al. Usefulness of vasopressin administered with epinephrine during out-of-hospital cardiac arrest. *Am J Cardio* 2006; 98(10): 1316–1321.
6. Kudenchuk PJ, Cobb LA, Copass MK, et al. Amiodarone for resuscitation after out-of-hospital cardiac arrest due to ventricular fibrillation. *N Engl J Med* 1999; 341(12): 871–878.
7. Dorian P, Cass D, Schwartz B, Cooper R, Gelaznikas R, Barr A. Amiodarone as compared with lidocaine for shock-resistant ventricular fibrillation. *N Engl J Med* 2002; 346(12): 884–890.
8. Stratton S, Niemann JT. Effects of adding links to the chain of survival for prehospital cardiac arrest: a contrast in outcomes in 1975 and 1995 at a single institution. *Ann Emerg Med* 1998; 31(4): 471–477.
9. Callaham M, Madsen C, Barton C, Saunders C, Daley M, Pointer J. A randomized clinical trial of high-dose epinephrine and norepinephrine versus standard-dose epinephrine in prehospital cardiac arrest. *JAMA* 1992; 268(19): 2667–2672.
10. Stiell IG, Hebert PC, Weitzman BN, et al. High-dose epinephrine in adult cardiac arrest. *N Engl J Med* 1992; 327(15): 1045–1050.
11. Neumar RW, Nolan JP, Adrie C, et al. Post-cardiac arrest syndrome: epidemiology, pathophysiology, treatment, and prognostication. A consensus statement from the International Liaison Committee on Resuscitation; (American Heart

Association, Australian and New Zealand Council on Resuscitation, European Resuscitation Council, Heart and Stroke Foundation of Canada, InterAmerican Heart Foundation, Resuscitation Council of Asia, and the Resuscitation Council of Southern Africa); the American Heart Association Emergency Cardiovascular Care Committee; the Council on Cardiovascular Surgery and Anesthesia; the Council on Cardiopulmonary, Perioperative, and Critical Care; the Council on Clinical Cardiology; and the Stroke Council. *Circulation* 2008; 118(23): 2452–2483.

12. Merchant RM, Soar J, Skrifvars MB, et al. Therapeutic hypothermia utilization among physicians after resuscitation from cardiac arrest. *Crit Care Med* 2006; 34(7): 1935–1940.

13. Marma AK, Berry JD, Ning H, Persell SD, Lloyd-Jones DM. Distribution of 10-year and lifetime predicted risks for cardiovascular disease in US adults. Findings from the National Health and Nutrition Survey 2003 to 2006. *Circ Cardiovasc Qual Outcomes* 2010; 3(1): 8–14.

14. Cobb LA, Fahrenbruch CE, Olsufka M, Copass MK. Changing incidence of out-of-hospital ventricular fibrillation 1980–2000. *JAMA* 2002; 288(23): 3008–3013.

15. Zheng, ZJ, Croft JB, Giles WH, Mensah GA. Sudden cardiac death in the United States, 1989–1998. *Circulation* 2001; 104(18): 2158–2163.

16. Callaway CW, Schmicker R, Kampmeyer M, et al.; Resuscitation Outcomes Consortium (ROC) Investigators. Receiving hospital characteristics associated with survival after out-of-hospital cardiac arrest. *Resuscitation* 2010; 81(5): 524–529.

17. American Heart Association. Guidelines 2000 for cardiopulmonary resuscitation and emergency cardiovascular care: an international consensus on science. *Circulation* 2000; 102(8 Suppl.): s1–s370.

18. de Vos R, de Haes HC, Koster RW, de Hann RJ. Quality of survival after cardiopulmonary resuscitation. *Arch Intern Med* 1999; 159(3): 249–254.

19. Laver S, Farrow C, Turner D, Nolan J. Mode of death after admission to an intensive care unit following cardiac arrest. *Intensive Care Med* 2004; 30(11): 2126–2128.

20. Brain Resuscitation Clinical Trial I Study Group. A randomized clinical study of cardiopulmonary-cerebral resuscitation: design, methods, and patient characteristics. *Am J Emerg Med* 1986; 4(1): 72–86.

21. Brain Resuscitation Clinical Trial II Study Group. A randomized clinical trial of calcium entry blocker administration to comatose survivors of cardiac arrest. Design, method, and patient characteristics. *Control Clin Trials* 1991; 12(4): 525–545.

22. Longsteth WT, Fahrenbruch CE, Olsufka M, Walsh TR, Copass MK, Cobb LA. Randomized clinical trial of magnesium, diazepam, or both after out-of-hospital cardiac arrest. *Neurology* 2002; 59(4): 506–514.

23. Hachimi-Idrissi S, Corne L, Ebinger G, Michotte Y, Huyghens L. Mild hypothermia induced by a helmet device: a clinical feasibility study. *Resuscitation* 2001; 51(3): 275–281.

24. HACA – Hypothermia after Cardiac Arrest Study Group. Mild therapeutic hypothermia to improve the neurologic outcome after cardiac arrest. *N Engl J Med* 2002; 346(8): 549–556.

25. Bernard SA, Gray TW, Buist MD, et al. Treatment of comatose survivors of out-of-hospital cardiac arrest with induced hypothermia. *N Engl J Med* 2002; 346(8): 557–563.

26. Bernard SA, Buist M. Induced hypothermia in critical care medicine: a review. *Crit Care Med* 2003; 31(7): 2041–2051.

27. Bigelow WG, Lindsay WK, Greenwood WF. Hypothermia, its possible role in cardiac surgery: an investigation of factors governing survival in dogs at low body temperatures. *Ann Surg* 1950; 132(5): 849–866.

28. Belsey RH, Dowlatshahi K, Keen G, Skinner DB. Profound hypothermia in cardiac surgery. *J Thorac Cardiovasc Surg* 1968; 56(4): 497–509.

29. Holzer M, Bernard SA, Hachimi-Idrissi S, Roine RO, Sterz F, Mullner M. Hypothermia for neuroprotection after cardiac arrest: systemic review and individual patient data meta-analysis. *Crit Care Med* 2005; 33(2): 414–418.

30. Arrich J, Holzer M, Herkner H, Mullner M. Hypothermia for neuroprotection in adults after cardiopulmonary resuscitation. *Cochrane Database Syst Rev* 2009; (4): CD004128.

31. Sagalyn E, Band RA, Gaieski DF, Abella BS. Therapeutic hypothermia after cardiac arrest in clinical practice: review and compilation of recent experiences. *Crit Care Med* 2009; 37(7 Suppl.): s223–s226.

32. Wright WL, Geocadin RG. Post resuscitative intensive care: neuroprotective strategies after cardiac arrest. *Semin Neurol* 2006; 26(4): 396–402.

33. Mullner M, Sterz F, Binder M, et al. Arterial blood pressure after human cardiac arrest and neurologic recovery. *Stroke* 1996; 27(1): 59–62.

34. Mullner M, Sterz F, Binder M, Schreiber W, Deimel A, Laggner AN. Blood glucose concentration after cardiopulmonary resuscitation influences functional neurological recovery in human cardiac arrest survivors. *J Cereb Blood Flow Metab* 1997; 17(4): 430–436.

35. Langhelle A, Tyvold SS, Lexow K, Hapnes SA, Sunde K, Steen PA. In-hospital factors associated with improved outcome after out-of-hospital cardiac arrest. A comparison between four regions in Norway. *Resuscitation* 2003; 56(3): 247–263.

36. Oddo M, Schaller M, Feihl F, Ribordy V, Liaudet L. From evidence to clinical practice: effective implementation of therapeutic hypothermia to improve patient outcome after cardiac arrest. *Crit Care Med* 2006; 34(7): 1865–1873.

37. Holzer M, Mullner M, Sterz F, et al. Efficacy and safety of endovascular cooling after cardiac arrest: Cohort study and Bayesian approach. *Stroke* 2006; 37(7): 1792–1797.

38. Engdahl J, Abrahamsson P, Bang A, Lindquist J, Karlsson T, Herlitz J. Is hospital care of major importance for outcome after out-of-hospital cardiac arrest? Resuscitation 2000; 43(3): 201–211.

39. Nichol G, Aufderheide TP, Eigel B, et al. Regional systems of care for out-of-hospital cardiac arrest: a policy statement from the American Heart Association. *Circulation* 2010; 121(5): 709–729.

40. Arrich J (European Resuscitation Council Hypothermia after Cardiac Arrest Registry Study Group). Clinical application of mild therapeutic hypothermia after cardiac arrest. *Crit Care Med* 2007; 35(4): 1041–1047.

41. Don CW, Longstreth WT, Maynard C, et al. Active surface cooling protocol to induce mild therapeutic hypothermia after out-of-hospital cardiac arrest: a

retrospective before-and-after comparison in a single hospital. *Crit Care Med* 2009; 37(12): 3062–2069.

42. Nolan JP, Soar J. Post resuscitation care: entering a new era. *Curr Opin Crit Care* 2010; 16(3): 216–222.

43. Sunde K, Pytte M, Jacobsen D, et al. Implementation of a standardised treatment protocol for post resuscitation care after out-of-hospital cardiac arrest. *Resuscitation* 2007; 73(1): 29–39.

44. Bernard S. Hypothermia after cardiac arrest: expanding the therapeutic scope. *Crit Care Med* 2009; 37(7 Suppl.): s227–s233.

45. Peberdy MA, Kaye W, Ornato JP, et al. Cardiopulmonary resuscitation of adults in the hospital: a report of 14,720 cardiac arrests from the National Registry of Cardiopulmonary Resuscitation. *Resuscitation* 2003; 58(3): 297–308.

46. Levy DE, Caronna JJ, Singer BH, Lapinski RH, Frydman H, Plum F. Predicting outcome from hypoxic-ischemic coma. *JAMA* 1985; 253(10): 1420–1426.

47. Booth CM, Boone RH, Tonlinson G, Detsky AS. Is this patient dead, vegetative, or severely neurologically impaired? Assessing outcome for comatose survivors of cardiac arrest. *JAMA* 2004; 291(7): 870–879.

48. Adrie C, Cariou A, Mourvillier B, et al. Predicting survival with good neurological recovery at hospital admission after successful resuscitation of out-of-hospital cardiac arrest: the OHCA score. *Eur Heart J* 2006; 27(23): 2840–2845.

49. Wijdicks EF, Hijdra A, Young GB, Bassetti CL, Wiebe S. Practice parameter: prediction of outcome in comatose survivors after cardiopulmonary resuscitation (an evidence-based review). *Neurology* 2006; 67(2): 203–210.

50. Rittenberger JC, Kelly E, Jang D, Greer K, Heffner A. Successful outcome utilizing hypothermia after cardiac arrest in pregnancy: a case report. *Crit Care Med* 2008b; 36(4): 1354–1356.

51. Fink EL, Kochanek PM, Clark RS, Bell MJ. How I cool children in neurocritical care. *Neurocrit Care* 2010; 12(3): 414–420.

52. Wible EF, Kass JS, Lopez GA. A report of fetal demise during therapeutic hypothermia after cardiac arrest. *Neurocrit Care* 2010; 13(2): 239–242.

53. Berg RA, Sanders AB, Kern KB, et al. Adverse hemodynamic effects of interrupting chest compressions for rescue breathing during cardiopulmonary resuscitation for ventricular fibrillation cardiac arrest. *Circulation* 2001; 104(20): 2465–2470.

54. Christenson J, Andrusiek D, Everson-Stewart S, et al. (Resuscitation Outcomes Consortium Investigators). Chest compression fraction determines survival in patients with out-of-hospital ventricular fibrillation. *Circulation* 2009; 120(13): 1241–1247.

55. Wang HE, Simeone SJ, Weaver MD, Callaway CW. Interruptions in cardiopulmonary resuscitation from paramedic endotracheal intubation. *Ann Emerg Med* 2009; 54(5): 645–652.

56. Gabrielli A, Layon AJ, Wenzel V, Dorges V, Idris AH. Alternative ventilation strategies in cardiopulmonary resuscitation. *Curr Opin Crit Care* 2002; 8(3): 199–211.

57. Bobrow BJ, Clark LL, Ewy GA, et al. Minimally interrupted cardiac resuscitation by emergency medical services for out-of-hospital cardiac arrest. *JAMA* 2008; 229(10): 1158–1165.

58. Kellum MJ, Kennedy KW, Barney R, et al. Cardiocerebral resuscitation improves neurologically intact survival of patients with out-of-hospital cardiac arrest. *Ann Emerg Med* 2008; 52(3): 244–252.

59. Kilgannon JH, Jones AE, Shapiro NI, et al. Association between arterial hyperoxia following resuscitation from cardiac arrest and in-hospital mortality. *JAMA* 2010; 303(21): 2165–2171.

60. Angelos MA, Menegazzi JJ, Callaway CW. Resuscitation from prolonged ventricular fibrillation bench-to-bedside. *Acad Emerg Med* 2001; 8(9): 909–924.

61. Sundgreen C, Larsen FS, Herzog TM, Knudsen GM, Boesgaard S, Aldershville J. Autoregulation of cerebral blood flow in patients resuscitated from cardiac arrest. *Stroke* 2001; 32(1): 128–132.

62. Keelan PC, Bunch TJ, White RD, Packer DL, Holmes DR. Early direct coronary angioplasty in survivors of out-of-hospital cardiac arrest. *Am J Cardiol* 2003; 91(12): 1461–1463.

63. Reynolds JC, Callaway CW, El Khoudary SR, Moore CG, Alvarez RJ, Rittenberger JC. Coronary angiography predicts improved outcome following cardiac arrest: propensity-adjusted analysis. *J Intensive Care Med* 2009; 24(3): 179–186.

64. Spaulding CM, Joly LM, Rosenberg A, et al. Immediate coronary angiography in survivors of out-of-hospital cardiac arrest. *N Engl J Med* 1997; 336(23): 1629–1633.

65. Bulut S, Aengevaeren WRM, Luijten HJE, Verheugt FWA. Successful out-of-hospital cardiopulmonary resuscitation: what is the optimal in-hospital treatment strategy? *Resuscitation* 2000; 47(2): 155–161.

66. Knafelj R, Radsel P, Ploj T, Noc M. Primary percutaneous coronary intervention and mild induced hypothermia in comatose survivors on ventricular fibrillation with ST-elevation acute myocardial infarction. *Resuscitation* 2007; 74(2): 227–234.

67. Wolfrum S, Pierau C, Radke PW, Schunkert H, Kurowski V. Mild therapeutic hypothermia in patients after out-of-hospital cardiac arrest due to acute ST-segment elevation myocardial infarction undergoing immediate percutaneous coronary intervention. *Crit Care Med* 2008; 36(6): 1780–1786.

68. Hovland A, Bjørnstad H, Hallstensen RF, et al. Massive pulmonary embolism with cardiac arrest treated with continuous thrombolysis and concomitant hypothermia. *Emerg Med J* 2008; 25(5): 310–311.

69. Hemmen TM, Raman R, Guluma KZ, et al.; ICTuS-L Investigators. Intravenous thrombolysis plus hypothermia for acute treatment of ischemic stroke (ICTuS-L): final results. *Stroke* 2010; 41(10): 2265–2270.

70. Holzer M. Targeted temperature management for comatose survivors of cardiac arrest. *N Engl J Med* 2010; 363(13): 1256–1264.

71. Heard KJ, Peberdy MA, Sayre MR, et al. A randomized controlled trial comparing the Arctic Sun to standard cooling for induction of hypothermia after cardiac arrest. Resuscitation. 2010; 81(1): 9–14.

72. Callaway CW, Tadler SC, Lipinski CL, Latz LM, Brader E. Feasibility of external cranial cooling during resuscitation. *Resuscitation* 2002; 52(2): 159–165.

73. Zeiner A, Holzer M, Sterz F, et al. Hyperthermia after cardiac arrest is associated with unfavorable neurologic outcome. *Arch Intern Med* 2001; 161(16): 2007–2012.

74. Kim F, Olsufka M, Longstreth WT, et al. Pilot randomized clinical trial of pre-hospital induction of mild hypothermia in out-of-hospital cardiac arrest patients with a rapid infusion of 4°C normal saline. *Circulation* 2007; 115(24): 3064–3070.

75. Marion DW, Penrod LE, Kelsey SF et al. Treatment of traumatic brain injury with moderate hypothermia. *N Engl J Med* 1997; 336(8): 540–546.

76. Bernard S, Buist M, Monteiro O, Smith K. Induced hypothermia using large volume, ice-cold intravenous fluid in comatose survivors of out-of-hospital cardiac arrest: a preliminary report. *Resuscitation* 2003; 56(1): 9–13.

77. Kliegel A, Janata A, Wandallar C, et al. Cold infusions alone are effective for induction of therapeutic hypothermia but do not keep patients cool after cardiac arrest. *Resuscitation* 2007; 73(1): 46–53.

78. Skrifvars MB, Pettila V, Rosenberg PH, Castren M. A multiple logistic regression analysis of in-hospital factors related to survival at six months in patients resuscitated from out-of-hospital ventricular fibrillation. *Resuscitation* 2003; 59(3): 319–328.

79. Oksanen T, Skrifvars MB, Varpula T, et al. Strict versus moderate glucose control after resuscitation from ventricular fibrillation. *Intensive Care Med* 2007; 33(12): 2093–2100.

80. Nielsen N, Hovdenes J, Nilsson F, et al. Outcome, timing, and adverse events in therapeutic hypothermia after out-of-hospital cardiac arrest. *Acta Anaesthesiol Scand* 2009; 53(7): 926–934.

81. Gaieski DF, Band RA, Abella BS, et al. Early goal-directed hemodynamic optimization combined with therapeutic hypothermia in comatose survivors of out-of-hospital cardiac arrest. *Resuscitation* 2009; 80(4): 418–424.

82. Kampmeyer M, Callaway C. Method of cold saline storage for prehospital induced hypothermia. *Prehospital Emerg Care* 2009; 13(1): 81–84.

83. Merchant RM, Abella BS, Peberdy MA, et al. Therapeutic hypothermia after cardiac arrest: unintentional overcooling is common using ice packs and conventional cooling blankets. *Crit Care Med* 2006; 34(12 Suppl.): s490–s494.

84. Suffoletto B, Peberdy MA, Vanden Hoek T, Callaway C. Body temperature changes are associated with outcomes following in-hospital cardiac arrest and return of spontaneous circulation. *Resuscitation* 2009; 80(12): 1365–1370.

85. Nichol G, Stiell IG, Herbert P, Wells GA, Vandembeen K, Laupacis A. What is the quality of life for survivors of cardiac arrest? A prospective study. *Acad Emerg Med* 1999; 6(2): 95–102.

86. Niemann JT, Stratton SJ. The Utstein template and the effect of in-hospital decisions: the impact of do-not-attempt resuscitation status on survival to discharge statistics. *Resuscitation* 2001; 51(3): 233–237.

87. Rittenberger JC, Guyette FX, Tisherman SA, DeVita MA, Alvarez RJ, Callaway CW. Outcomes of a hospital-wide plan to improve care of comatose survivors of cardiac arrest. *Resuscitation* 2008; 79(2): 198–204.

88. Martinell L, Larsson M, Bang A, et al. Survival in out-of-hospital cardiac arrest before and after use of advanced post resuscitation care: a survey focusing on incidence, patient characteristics, survival, and estimated cerebral function after post resuscitation care. *Am J Emerg Med* 2010; 28(5): 543–551.

CHAPTER 3

Adults with congenital heart disease

Kara M. Iskyan[1] and Craig R. Cohen[2]
[1]Maricopa Medical Center, Phoenix, AZ, USA
[2]Arizona Pediatric Cardiology Consultants, Phoenix, AZ, USA

Introduction and epidemiology

Congenital heart disease (CHD) is defined as cardiac abnormalities present at birth. In the 1950s, the surgical mortality of children with CHD was greater than 50% [1]. With the improvement of diagnostic techniques, surgical interventions, and specialized care, more than 85% of children with CHD now reach adulthood [2, 3]. There are now more than 1 million adult congenital heart disease (ACHD) patients [3]. As of today, there are more adults than children with CHD [1]. As a result, outpatient cardiac care of ACHD patients has rapidly increased. In Canada, for example, the outpatient ACHD workload has increased by 400% [2].

With the increasing number of ACHD patients, emergency physicians are likely to encounter this population. Most of these patients will already carry a diagnosis of CHD. However, 10% of congenital heart defects are not discovered until adulthood [1]. ACHD patients seek care for both cardiac and non-cardiac emergencies. European studies have shown that the most common reasons ACHD patients visit the emergency department (ED) are related to cardiovascular dysfunction (specifically arrhythmias and heart failure) and infection (such as endocarditis) [4, 5].

ACHD patients who seek emergency care are often quite ill. A prospective study of 126 emergent admissions of ACHD patients showed that 20% of urgent admissions resulted in mortality or transplant within 3 years of the initial admission [5]. Additionally, those who experienced a lapse in routine care for CHD are three times more likely to require urgent cardiac intervention [6]. Overall, ACHD patients have an admission rate 2–3 times the general population [7].

Challenging and Emerging Conditions in Emergency Medicine, First Edition. Edited by Arvind Venkat.
© 2011 by John Wiley & Sons, Ltd. Published 2011 by Blackwell Publishing Ltd.

Table 3.1 Symptoms and findings frequently missed or inadequately treated in adults with CHD (As per author experience)

Rapid increase in heart rate
New widening of the QRS complex
Atrial flutter
New onset supraventricular tachycardia
Syncope
Rapid increase in hypoxia
Hemoptysis
Extracardiac conditions due to disease, medications, and alcohol

---

General considerations for adult congenital heart disease patients in the emergency department

With the exception of uncomplicated bicuspid aortic valve, most ACHD patients will have required treatment during childhood and have had subsequent follow-up with a cardiologist. Based on recommendations from the American Heart Association and the American College of Cardiology, most patients will carry with them specific details of their cardiac history. It behooves emergency physicians to contact the treating cardiologist early in the patient encounter to avoid complications that can arise from not having access to a detailed medical history. In addition, ED patients requiring either cardiac or surgical intervention, even if not cardiac-related, should be transferred to a center with expertise in managing congenital heart disease [8]. Emergency physicians can find the nearest referral center by accessing the website of the Adult Congenital Heart Association (http://www.achaheart.org).

There are a number of common mistakes made by physicians with limited CHD experience. Table 3.1 outlines symptoms and findings that are frequently missed or inadequately treated. Table 3.2 describes common mistakes made during the treatment of ACHD patients.

Table 3.2 Common mistakes made while treating adults with CHD (As per author experience)

Late or no referral to congenital cardiologist
Extracardiac surgery or endoscopy without referral to or discussion with a Regional Congenital Heart Disease Center

Injudicious use of medications (such as NSAIDs)
Poor arrhythmia management
Use of proarrhythmic medications
Lack of aggressive treatment of arrhythmias
Poorly managed anticoagulation
Not measuring electrolytes

Clinical implications of non-cyanotic congenital heart conditions

Table 3.3 outlines the presenting symptoms/signs, findings on physical exam, ECG and chest radiograph, and long-term complications of adults with each non-cyanotic congenital heart condition.

Atrial septal defect

Atrial septal defect (ASD) is one of the most common adult congenital heart defects. Nearly 4 of every 100,000 newborns are found to have an ASD [3]. An ASD is a persistent communication between the right and left atria [8]. There are three types of ASDs. The most common type (70%–80%) of ASD is the secundum ASD. The primum ASD accounts for 15%–20% of all ASDs. It is a deficiency in the endocardial cushion tissue and commonly associated with Trisomy 21. The sinus venous ASD is rare, accounting for only 5%–10% of all ASDs [3]. About 30% of ASDs are associated with additional malformations, most commonly mitral valve prolapse or valvular pulmonic stenosis [8].

Given the higher pressure on the left side of the heart, the shunt across the ASD is predominantly left to right. Over time, however, the chronic overload of the right ventricle causes hypertrophy and pulmonary overcirculation. Right-sided heart failure, frequent pulmonary infections, fatigue, exercise intolerance, atrial arrhythmias, and pulmonary hypertension may bring these patients to the ED. Pulmonary hypertension and right ventricular hypertrophy can result in a right to left shunt [3, 8].

Large ASDs are repaired in childhood to avoid long-term complications. These patients are asymptomatic after repair. Small ASDs can remain asymptomatic until the fourth or fifth decade of life when coronary artery disease, acquired valvular disease, or hypertension decrease left ventricular compliance causing an increase in shunting [1, 8]. This physiology causes adults with ASDs to present in four distinct ways:

1. Progressive dyspnea on exertion from pulmonary overcirculation. These symptoms are not usually attributed to the ASD until a transthoracic echocardiography is done [9].
2. Atrial arrhythmia from dilated atria. This rarely occurs before the age of 40. If right atrial enlargement occurred prior to repair, the patient still has a high risk of atrial arrhythmias.
3. Transient ischemic attack, stroke, or other systemic ischemic event.
4. Incidentally during echocardiography for other reasons or to evaluate cardiomegaly on a chest X-ray [1, 3, 10].

Adults with unrepaired ASDs are usually candidates for closure although arrhythmias may persist after repair [9].

Examination of the adult with an ASD reveals a fixed splitting of the second heart sound with respirations. A systolic pulmonary flow murmur

Table 3.3 Description of non-cyanotic congenital heart defects

Condition	Adult presenting symptoms/signs	Physical exam findings (unrepaired)	ECG (unrepaired)	Chest X-ray (unrepaired)	Long-term complications (unrepaired)	Long-term complications (repaired)
Atrial septal defect (ASD)	Progressive dyspnea Atrial arrhythmia TIA/CVA Incidental finding on echocardiography	Fixed splitting of second heart sound Systolic pulmonary flow murmur (if large) Palpable RV lift (if RV overload present) Lateral retraction of apex (if RV overload present)	Normal sinus rhythm Right axis deviation RA enlargement rSR' pattern in V1	RA and RV enlargement Prominent pulmonary artery Increased pulmonary vascularity	Right-sided heart failure Frequent pulmonary infections Fatigue Exercise intolerance Atrial arrhythmia Pulmonary hypertension	None
Ventricular septal defect (VSD)	Infectious endocarditis Incidental finding on echocardiography	Blowing pansystolic murmur at LL sternal border (if small) Low-pitch diastolic murmur at apex (if large)	NSR Intraventricular conduction delay Biventricular hypertrophy RV hypertrophy	LA and LV enlargement Increased pulmonary vascularity	One functional ventricle Infectious endocarditis Cyanosis Arrhythmia	Arrhythmia (including PVCs, RBBB, and ventricular tachycardia)

(Continued)

Table 3.3 (*Continued*)

Condition	Adult presenting symptoms/signs	Physical exam findings (unrepaired)	ECG (unrepaired)	Chest X-ray (unrepaired)	Long-term complications (unrepaired)	Long-term complications (repaired)
Patent ductus arteriosus (PDA)	Cyanosis Angina Endarteritis Left heart failure Arrhythmia Pulmonary hypertension	Continuous machinery-like murmur at L upper sternal border	NSR LA enlargement (if large PDA) LV hypertrophy (if large PDA) RV hypertrophy (if pulmonary hypertension)	Cardiomegaly (if large) Increased pulmonary vascularity (if large) Calcified ductus	Coronary "steal" phenomenon Endarteritis Left heart failure Arrhythmia Pulmonary hypertension	Injury to recurrent laryngeal nerve, phrenic nerve or thoracic duct
Coarctation of aorta	Hypertension Exertional headache Leg claudication Epistaxis Cool extremities Fatigue	Hypertension Discrepant pulses in upper and lower extremities Systolic ejection murmur at left infrascapular area and over left scapula Strong apical impulse (if LV hypertrophy) Hyperdynamic carotid pulsations (if LV hypertrophy)	LV hypertrophy ST–T wave abnormalities RV conduction delay	Dilated ascending aorta "Figure of three" Notching on underside of ribs 3–9	Hypertension Coronary artery disease Recurrent stenosis Aortic aneurysm Cerebral aneurysm/CVA	Hypertension Coronary artery disease Recurrent stenosis Aortic aneurysm Cerebral aneurysm/CVA

is present if there is a significant left to right intra-cardiac shunt. Right ventricular volume overload will produce a palpable right ventricular lift (or a left parasternal heave) and lateral retraction of the apex [11]. An ECG and chest X-ray will reflect a volume overloaded right heart. The ECG usually shows a sinus rhythm with right axis deviation, right atrial enlargement and an rsR' pattern in lead V1. The chest X-ray will show right atrial and ventricular enlargement, prominent pulmonary artery segment, and increased pulmonary vascularity [12]. Echocardiography with color flow Doppler is the diagnostic test of choice [13].

The treatment for ASDs is closure. In the absence of pulmonary hypertension, early mortality for an ASD closure is less than 1% [8]. One week to a month after repair, an autoimmune disorder called post-pericardiotomy syndrome may occur. It presents with fever, fatigue, vomiting, chest pain, and abdominal pain. Physical exam will reveal a pericardial friction rub while a chest radiograph will show cardiomegaly and possible bilateral pleural effusions. Echocardiography may show a pericardial effusion. Unless there is cardiac tamponade, post-pericardiotomy syndrome can be treated with nonsteroidal anti-inflammatory drugs (NSAIDs) or steroids. Post-pericardiotomy syndrome usually responds to pharmacologic treatment, but may recur [14]. Many secundum ASDs are now amenable to catheter device closure, thus avoiding post-operative morbidity.

Ventricular septal defect

Ventricular septal defect (VSD), a persistent communication between the right and left ventricles, account for 20% of all cardiac malformations [3]. It is one of the most common congenital heart defects at birth with an incidence of 2%–5% [15]. Nearly 80% of small, isolated VSDs close spontaneously; so the incidence in older infants and children is lower [8]. Perimembranous VSDs account for 80% of all VSDs. The perimembranous VSD may create a pouch, or "aneurysm," that limits left to right shunting and can result in partial or full closure of the defect. The remaining 20% of VSDs are usually muscular. This muscular VSD may have multiple openings, but spontaneous closure is common. An inlet VSD exists as part of the endocardial cushion defect and usually occurs in patients with Down syndrome [3, 8].

The direction of the shunt created by a VSD is determined by the difference between the systemic and pulmonary pressures. If the defect is small, the systemic pressure is greater than the pulmonary pressure so the blood flow through the shunt is left to right. However, if the VSD is large, increased pulmonary resistance may result in a right to left shunt (Eisenmenger's syndrome) [3]. Large VSDs are usually closed before 2 years of age. Smaller, isolated VSDs may present in adulthood as infectious endocarditis or incidentally on evaluation for a murmur [8].

The physical exam of an adult with a small VSD includes a blowing pan-systolic murmur best heard at the left lower sternal border. Large VSDs have an additional low-pitched diastolic murmur at the apex [12]. The ECG is usually normal but may exhibit an intraventricular conduction delay, biventricular hypertrophy, or isolated RV hypertrophy [8, 16]. A significant left to right shunt may result in left atrial and ventricular enlargement and increased pulmonary vascular markings on chest x-ray [8]. Echocardiography is the best noninvasive form of definite diagnosis as it is extremely sensitive [16].

The treatment for VSDs is surgical closure. Most VSDs are not amenable to percutaneous device closure and require surgical closure with synthetic material. Early closure usually avoids the development of long-term pulmonary hypertension. Patients who undergo cardiac surgery for VSDs are at increased risk of arrhythmias [8, 16].

Patent ductus arteriosus

Patent Ductus Arteriosus (PDA) refers to a persistent communication between the pulmonary artery and aorta beyond the first post-natal week [3, 8]. The incidence is highest in pregnancies complicated by persistent perinatal hypoxemia and among infants born at high altitude or prematurely [13, 15]. The most common lesions associated with PDAs are VSDs and ASDs [8].

The pathophysiology of the PDA is based on the difference in resistance between the systemic and pulmonary circulations. As a result, a left to right shunt develops [3]. Most PDAs are diagnosed on physical exam (continuous murmur and wide pulse pressure) and treated in infancy or childhood. A patient with a large PDA has a 50% survival rate at 20 years and 10% survival rate at 50 years of age [17]. Without correction for size of the PDA, the mortality of an untreated adult with a PDA is 1.8% per year [18]. Adults with an undiagnosed PDA may present with consequences of a left to right shunt, angina from coronary "steal" phenomenon (in which the ductus competes for aortic diastolic flow), endarteritis (endocarditis of the artery), left heart failure, arrhythmia (mainly atrial tachycardias), and pulmonary hypertension [3, 19]. PDAs in adults may be well tolerated until combined with acquired heart conditions such as ischemic heart disease or calcific aortic stenosis.

The physical exam of an adult with an unrepaired PDA reveals a continuous machinery-like murmur best heard at the left upper sternal border [12]. With pulmonary hypertension, upper extremity oxygen saturation may be higher than the lower extremities [8]. The ECG may be normal if the PDA is small. If the PDA is large, the ECG may show left atrial enlargement and left ventricular hypertrophy [18]. If the disease has progressed to involve pulmonary hypertension, there will also be right ventricular hypertrophy. Chest X-ray findings, again, depend on the size of the shunt. A larger shunt may reveal cardiomegaly with increased pulmonary vascular markings and calcification in the area of the ductus [12]. Echocardiography is the procedure of choice to confirm diagnosis and further characterize the PDA and associated anomalies [19].

Definitive treatment for a PDA is percutaneous or surgical closure, but medical therapy may be required in order to prepare for an operation. If the PDA is isolated, device closure or coils have a high success rate with few complications. If the PDA is not amenable to a percutaneous approach, the surgical approach through a left lateral thoracotomy is often successful with low early mortality. Complications of the surgical approach include injury to the recurrent laryngeal nerve, phrenic nerve, or thoracic duct. Once treated, recannulization of the PDA is rare [8].

Coarctation of the aorta

Coarctation of the aorta is a discrete narrowing of the aorta in the region of the ligamentum arteriosum. There is usually a discrete narrowing distal to the left subclavian artery or, less commonly, at the aortic arch or isthmus [8]. Coarctation of the aorta accounts for about 5% to 8% of all congenital heart disease [20]. Other cardiac lesions, such as bicuspid aortic valve, subaortic stenosis, and VSDs, are commonly associated with coarctation of the aorta. There is a small incidence of associated berry aneurysms of the Circle of Willis [8].

The vast majority of coarctations are recognized and repaired in the neonatal period [1]. The average age of survival for untreated patients with coarctation is only 35 years with 90% of these patients dying before the age of 50 [21]. Hypertension develops quickly as the diminished pressure to the lower portions of the body, including the juxtaglomerular apparatus of the kidney, perceives low blood flow and modulates vascular tone and intravascular volume in an attempt to restore perfusion pressure to the distal aorta [20].

Adults with unrepaired coarctation of the aorta may present with exertional headache or leg claudication, epistaxis, cool extremities, or fatigue [8, 20]. The patient will have a history of hypertension and, if started on antihypertensive medication, may have worsening claudication or prerenal azotemia [20]. Physical exam of an adult with unrepaired coarctation of the aorta will show upper extremity hypertension with discrepant pulses between the upper and lower extremities. A systolic ejection murmur loudest in the left infrascapular position is due to the coarctation or collateral vessels. There may be signs of left ventricular hypertrophy with a forceful, pressure-load apical impulse and hyperdynamic carotid pulsations [11]. The ECG will show left ventricular hypertrophy, secondary ST–T wave abnormalities and, possibly, right ventricular conduction delay [8]. The chest X-ray can have the following three distinct findings [20, 22]:

1. Prominent curvilinear shadow along the right sternal border indicating a dilated ascending aorta
2. A "figure of three" sign at the upper left mediastinal border from the indentation of the aorta with post-stenotic dilation, left subclavian artery dilation, or aortic knob dilation
3. Notching on the underside of ribs 3 through 9 from collateral vessels

Beyond treatment for hypertension, there is a controversy as to whether surgical or interventional therapy should be the preferred treatment of native coarctation of the aorta in adults [23]. Surgical repair is accomplished by excision of the narrowed segment with extended end-to-end anastomosis or with a subclavian flap angioplasty [1, 20]. Interventional therapy consists of a stent and possibly balloon angioplasty [21]. Early mortality after a coarctation repair in an adult is less than 1% [8].

Coarctation of the aorta involves a structural defect that diminishes arterial wall compliance and increases rigidity. Even after repair, long-term survival is still reduced with 91% of the patients alive at 20 years and 80% alive at 40 years after surgery [21]. The main complications after repair of aortic coarctation include hypertension, coronary artery disease, restenosis, aneurysm, and stroke. Around one-third to one-half of patients still have hypertension after late aortic coarctation repair [21]. Aggressive management of hypertension and other cardiovascular risk factors is important to prevent or decrease the impact of coronary artery disease [24], which accounts for about a fourth of deaths in patients with a repaired coarctation of the aorta [21]. Recurrent coarctation, usually found on routine follow-up exam or imaging [21], occurs because the graft does not grow with the patient, poor growth of the repaired segment, or from surgical scarring [20, 24]. Recurrence of coarctation occurs in less than 10% of patients who are repaired as adults [21]. Treatment for restenosis is usually catheter-based with a balloon or stent [2]. In most circumstances, it is the preferred alternative to surgery. Aortic aneurysm occurs in about 10% of patients after repair of coarctation [21]. Older patients with a prosthetic repair may present to the ED with an aneurysm at the graft site resulting in an aortobronchial fistula [1]. Other factors, such as intrinsic aortic wall abnormalities, transverse aortic arch hypoplasia, chronic hypertension, and pregnancy, also increase the risk of aneurysm formation. Aneurysm rupture is rare but devastating [21]. Lastly, strokes from Circle of Willis aneurysm rupture occurs in 3%–5% of both unrepaired and repaired coarctation of the aorta patients. Hypertension is not the only precondition for this complication as normotensive patients who are many years from their repair also experience cerebral aneurysms [21, 24].

Clinical implications of cyanotic congenital heart conditions

Compared to the lesions previously described, cyanotic defects result in the delivery of blood to the body that is only partially oxygenated. As a result, the anatomic and physiologic complications of both the disease and the repair are more complex than those of non-cyanotic lesions. Most cyanotic CHD is diagnosed and treated in infancy or childhood. In order to evaluate and treat patients with a history of cyanotic CHD lesions, the emergency physician must be knowledgeable about the surgical anatomy of the repair and its physiological consequences as outlined in Table 3.4. Adults with unrepaired cyanotic CHD usually have a mild defect or arrive from a country where diagnosis and treatment are not feasible.

Late complications of cyanotic lesions

The body compensates for long-standing cyanotic CHD. Chronic hypoxemia from unrepaired lesions not only alters the hematologic and renal systems most prominently, but is also manifested in the gastrointestinal and musculoskeletal systems.

The main hematologic complications of chronic hypoxemia are erythrocytosis, thrombosis, iron deficiency, and bleeding. When the tissues do not receive adequate oxygenation, the bone marrow responds by increasing the amount of red blood cells (RBCs) transporting oxygen. This erythrocytosis increases blood viscosity. Given the chronic nature of the hypoxemia, most patients with cyanotic CHD have a normal compensatory hemoglobin that is high. The expected value of hemoglobin for a given degree of hypoxemia is not known; however, the elevated level often does not require any intervention. Although thrombosis is possible, the most common complication from erythrocytosis is inappropriate, aggressive phlebotomy or blood loss. Therapeutic phlebotomy is indicated if the hemoglobin is greater than 20 g/dL and hematocrit greater than 65% with symptoms of hyperviscosity (headache, increasing fatigue) and no evidence of dehydration. One unit of blood is replaced with an equal volume of dextrose containing intravenous fluid or saline. Repetitive phlebotomies, recurrent hemoptysis, epistaxis, and menorrhagia cause iron-deficiency anemia. Erythrocytosis with iron deficiency reduces oxygen-carrying capacity even further, deforms RBCs, increases the risk of stroke, and leads to symptoms of hyperviscosity at much lower levels. Symptoms with a hematocrit of less than 65% are usually due to iron-deficiency anemia. Iron repletion, not phlebotomy, will improve symptoms. Lastly, 20% of cyanotic CHD patients have other hematologic abnormalities including thrombocytopenia, disseminated intravascular coagulation, primary fibrinolysis, impaired production of coagulation factors,

Table 3.4 Description of cyanotic congenital heart defects

Condition	Defect	Repair	Physical exam findings (repaired)	ECG (repaired)	Chest X-ray (repaired)	Long-term complications (repaired)
Tetralogy of Fallot	RV obstruction VSD Overriding aorta RV hypertrophy	Relief of RV outflow obstruction VSD closure	Systolic ejection murmur Diastolic murmur of pulmonary insufficiency	Prolonged QRS Complete RBBB	Right-sided aortic arch	Pulmonary regurgitation Atrial and ventricular tachycardias Sudden death
Complete transposition of the great arteries	Atrio-ventricular concordance Ventriculo–arterial discordance	Mustard and Senning procedures (or Atrial Baffle; RV is systemic pump) Arterial-switch operation (ASO; LV is systemic pump)	*Atrial Baffle* RV enlargement Tricuspid regurgitation *ASO* Systolic murmur (if arterial obstruction)	*Atrial Baffle* Right axis deviation RV hypertrophy *ASO* NSR	Narrow mediastinal shadow	*Atrial Baffle* Obstruction Heart failure Atrial and ventricular arrhythmias *ASO* Coronary insufficiency Restenosis Aortic root dilation Valvular regurgitation

Lesion	Anatomy	Treatment	Examination	ECG	Imaging	Complications
Congenitally corrected transposition of the great arteries	Atrio-ventricular discordance; Ventricular-arterial discordance	Replacement of systemic atrial-ventricular valve (if needed)	RV parasternal lift; Palpable second heart sound	Prolonged PR interval; Complete heart block; Intraventricular conduction delay; No Q waves in precordial leads; Q waves in II, aVF, and V1	Straight left heart border	Atrial tachycardia; Complete heart block
Ebstein's anomaly	Abnormal tricuspid valve; RV "atrialized"	Biventricular repair; Conversion to single ventricle; Tricuspid valve repair or replacement	(Unrepaired) Multiple systolic clicks	(Unrepaired) Ventricular pre-excitation; Atrial enlargement; Complete or incomplete RBBB; Small R waves in V1 and V2	(Unrepaired) Normal; "Globular" with prominent RA	Congestive heart failure; Atrial tachycardias
Tricuspid atresia	Absent or imperforated tricuspid valve; Hypoplastic RV	Fontan	(Unrepaired) Cyanosis; Clubbing; Various murmurs	(Unrepaired) RA or LA enlargement; RV and LV hypertrophy	(Unrepaired) Cardiomegaly; RA or LA enlargement	Atrial tachycardias; Protein losing enteropathy; Ventricular failure; Pulmonary AV malformations or fistulas; Iatrogenic (e.g., failed catheter placement)

and platelet dysfunction. Treatment for all these hematologic abnormalities focuses on risk reduction. Vaccines are given to decrease infectious complications. Routine use of anticoagulants, NSAIDs, and phlebotomy, as well as conditions such as anemia and dehydration, should be avoided [25–27].

Chronic hypoxemia also results in hypercellular renal glomeruli. With years of congestion, the glomeruli become sclerotic causing a reduced glomerular filtration rate, increased creatinine and proteinuria. Even with normal renal function there should be judicious use of intravenous contrast and medications that affect renal function [8]. As renal function worsens, so does urate clearance. Despite decreased urate excretion, acute gouty arthritis is relatively infrequent. Treatment for gout is difficult as colchicine can cause dehydration through the side effects of vomiting and diarrhea and NSAIDs worsen intrinsic hemostatic abnormalities and renal function [27].

The gastrointestinal and musculoskeletal systems are affected by chronic hypoxemia. Calcium bilirubinate gallstones occur more frequently with the increased RBC turnover from erythrocytosis. Similar to cholelithiasis in the patient without CHD, treatment is not warranted until the patient becomes symptomatic. Hypertrophic osteoarthropathy is the irregular thickening of the periosteum. It presents with aching and tenderness of the long bones [8]. A final important consideration for emergency physicians caring for adults with a history of cyanotic congenital heart disease is the possibility of causing systemic air embolism with the use of standard intravenous infusion equipment. When providing intravenous fluid or medications to this population, it is important to include an air filter in the system to prevent this complication.

Tetralogy of Fallot

Tetralogy of Fallot (TOF) is the most common cyanotic congenital heart defect. The four particular structural abnormalities of TOF are as follows:
1. Subpulmonary infundibular stenosis
2. VSD
3. Overriding aorta
4. Right ventricular hypertrophy

Like other forms of CHD, there are varying forms of severity with the most extreme form of TOF being pulmonary atresia with a VSD [8]. The most common associated anomaly is a right-sided aortic arch [8]. About 15% of patients with TOF also have the chromosome 22q11.2 deletion commonly manifested as DiGeorge syndrome (which is described as impairment in social function, schizophrenia, mental disability, deafness, immune deficiencies, endocrinopathies, and clubbed feet) [8]. Prior to effective treatment, patients with TOF had a 95% mortality by the age of 40 [1].

The severe cyanosis associated with TOF means nearly all cases are identified and repaired at a very young age. Two rare circumstances in which an adult with TOF may present are if the patient has "pink tetralogy," a form with mild pulmonary obstruction and mild cyanosis often mistaken for a small VSD or in a patient that has had extremely limited medical care [8].

Most infants undergo complete repair of TOF during the first year of life. Without surgical intervention, only 10% of these patients would survive beyond 21 years of age [12]. The repair consists of relief of the right ventricular outflow obstruction and VSD closure. If an anomalous coronary artery crosses the obstructed right ventricle outflow tract, an extracardiac conduit from the right ventricle to the pulmonary artery may be required [8].

On physical examination, the patient with a repaired TOF usually has a systolic ejection murmur from residual right ventricular outflow obstruction and a diastolic murmur of pulmonary insufficiency. A pansystolic murmur from a residual VSD is less common. The ECG of a patient with a repaired TOF may have a prolonged QRS from right ventricular dilation. If that patient underwent a transventricular repair, there may also be a complete right bundle branch block on the ECG [8].

Despite the success of TOF repair, there are serious long-term complications. Adult patients with repaired TOF are at risk for residual pulmonary stenosis, arrhythmias, and valvular insufficiency. Pulmonary regurgitation is the most common valvular complication and results from valvotomy or transannular patch repair. In the long term, this causes right ventricular volume overload and failure [2]. The strain placed on the right heart contributes to the high risk of arrhythmias and sudden death. Nearly 33% of patients with repaired TOF will develop symptomatic atrial tachycardias, while 10% develop high-grade ventricular arrhythmias by adulthood. In several large series, TOF patients have a 2.5% risk of sudden death per decade of follow-up. While most of the sudden deaths are attributed to ventricular tachycardia, the culprit can also be an atrial–ventricular block or intra-atrial reentrant tachycardia [28]. The immediate treatment of arrhythmias in patients with repaired TOF does not vary from standard Advanced Cardiac Life Support protocols. β-blockers, amiodarone, and Class Ib agents (such as phenytoin and mexiletine) are effective [29]. In the long term, however, pulmonary valve replacement with surgical ablation and implantable defibrillators may be needed [30]. Clearly, patients who have experienced significant arrhythmias require an electrophysiology evaluation and treatment. Given the long-term complications, patients with a repaired TOF who present with hypoxia, palpitations, arrhythmias, dizziness, chest pain, syncope, exercise limitations, or heart failure require prompt, detailed evaluation and admission [8].

Complete transposition of the great arteries
Complete Transposition of the Great Arteries (TGA) is atrio–ventricular concordance with ventriculo–arterial discordance. The nomenclature

"d-TGA" means the aorta arises from the right ventricle and the pulmonary artery from the left ventricle. Nearly two-thirds of patients with d-TGA do not have any other associated cardiac anomalies [1]. In those who do have associated defects, the most common conditions are VSD, left ventricular outflow tract obstruction, and coarctation of the aorta [8].

Infants born with d-TGA present with severe cyanosis and, if unrepaired, mortality is 90% in the first year of life. In order to survive, there must be a communication between the pulmonary and systemic circuits. Two-thirds of patients rely on the ductus arteriosus and foramen ovale while the rest may have a VSD to allow for some mixing of oxygenated with deoxygenated blood [31]. Unrepaired d-TGA is rarely found in an adult [1, 8, 22].

Adults with d-TGA usually have had neonatal or early childhood surgical repairs and should have regular follow-up with cardiology. The surgical options for uncomplicated d-TGA treatment have changed in the past 40 years. Prior to the 1980s, the primary repair options for d-TGA were the Mustard and Senning procedures. As shown in Figure 3.1, these procedures involve the creation of an atrial baffle (a surgically created

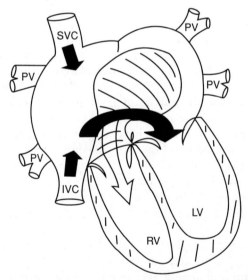

Figure 3.1 Atrial switch operation (Mustard/Senning) for d-TGA. A "chamber" is created along the back wall of the atria, such that pulmonary venous (PV) return is redirected to the tricuspid valve, to flow to the right ventricle (RV) and aorta (white arrow). Systemic venous blood from superior vena cava (SVC) and inferior vena cava (IVC) (black arrows) is excluded from the tricuspid valve and must flow over the baffle to the mitral valve, then to the left ventricle (LV) and lungs. (Reprinted with permission: Sommer et al. Pathophysiology of congenital heart disease in the adult part III: complex congenital heart disease. *Circulation* 2008 Mar 11; 117: 1340–1350. (http://lww.com))

connection) that redirects deoxygenated blood to the mitral valve and left ventricle, which empties into the pulmonary artery. At the same time, oxygenated blood is redirected to the tricuspid valve and right ventricle, which empties into the aorta. As a result, the morphologic right ventricle acts as the systemic ventricle [31]. An adult who has undergone a previous Mustard or Senning procedure has a relatively normal physical exam with the exception of right ventricular enlargement and tricuspid regurgitation. The ECG shows right axis deviation and right ventricular hypertrophy. The chest X-ray has a narrow mediastinal shadow due to the parallel relationship between the great arteries [8].

The most common late complications of atrial baffle procedures are obstruction, heart failure, and arrhythmias. Baffle obstruction, occurring in nearly one-fourth of atrial baffle patients, usually affects the superior limb resulting in superior vena cava syndrome (plethora, truncal venous engorgement). Inferior vena cava obstruction, on the other hand, causes hepatic congestion and eventual cirrhosis [8]. Heart failure occurs because the right ventricle is not structured to withstand years of systemic pressure and is a major factor for morbidity and mortality in d-TGA patients [2]. Atrial arrhythmias occur from the extensive suture lines created during the atrial baffle procedure and sinus node dysfunction. In the ED, the care of tachyarrhythmias does not deviate from the standard pharmacologic or electrical treatments. Eventually, the patient will require chronic pharmacologic management, ablation and/or pacemaker therapy. Ventricular tachycardia and ventricular fibrillation account for many sudden deaths, which usually occur during exercise [8].

Surgical repair for uncomplicated d-TGA changed from atrial baffle repairs to arterial-switch operations (ASO) in the 1980s. In the ASO, the pulmonary artery and ascending aorta are transected and switched so the aorta is connected to the neoaortic valve arising from the left ventricle and the pulmonary artery is connected to the neopulmonary valve arising from the right ventricle. The coronary arteries are transected and relocated to the neoaorta to restore normal coronary circulation [31]. Knowing which procedure a patient has undergone is fundamental for treatment in the ED.

The ASO is superior to the atrial baffle in terms of late morbidity and mortality. Teenagers with an ASO have similar quality of life and health status as children without CHD. Survival at 10 years is greater than 90%. Physical exam of adults who had an ASO will reveal a systolic murmur if there is arterial obstruction at the anastomosis site. The ECG is usually normal. Long-term concerns of ASO include right ventricular outflow obstruction, neopulmonary valvular stenosis, and aortic root dilation. The coronary arteries are reimplanted during ASO. Ischemic injury is possible in the early post-operative period from coronary artery kinking or ostial stenosis. Late coronary mortality and myocardial infarction have a prevalence of less than 2% [8, 33].

L-transposition of the great arteries/congenitally corrected transposition of the great arteries

Congenitally Corrected Transposition of the Great Arteries (CCTGA) encompasses a wide spectrum of morphological features and clinical profiles, but the underlying abnormalities are atrio–ventricular and ventricular–arterial discordances. In other words, the right atrium connects to the left ventricle which gives rise to the pulmonary artery. The left atrium connects to the right ventricle that connects to the aorta. As a result, the morphological right ventricle acts as the systemic ventricle while the left ventricle functions as part of the pulmonary system. The tricuspid and mitral valves maintain their relationships with their "normal" ventricles. Thus, the tricuspid valve is the systemic atrio–ventricular valve (SAVV) [8]. The nomenclature can be tricky. "Corrected" means the direction of the blood flow through the pulmonary and systemic circulations is physiologic. Another name for CCTGA is l-Transposition of the Great Arteries.

Many patients with CCTGA have other congenital cardiac lesions. The most common is a perimembranous VSD, but subvalvular pulmonary stenosis and abnormality of the SAVV are also seen. Most patients are diagnosed with CCTGA in childhood but, if the lesion is not hemodynamically significant, surgery may not be necessary until adulthood. Associated lesions may require intervention in the early childhood [8].

A common complication associated with both repaired and unrepaired CCTGA is arrhythmia. During the embryonic development of CCTGA, the AV node is displaced away from Koch's triangle to a position more anterior and superior within the right atrium resulting in accessory pathways or sinus node dysfunction. Patients with CCTGA, repaired and unrepaired, have a 2% chance of spontaneous complete heart block per year. Treatment of arrhythmias must take these important issues into consideration to avoid complete AV block [8].

Systemic (right ventricular) failure is common and may be associated with SAVV (tricuspid) insufficiency. In one series, systemic ventricular failure was a major cause of morbidity and mortality in 50% of unrepaired patients. In addition to heart failure, there is also a high incidence of coronary perfusion mismatch causing myocardial perfusion defects and impaired ventricular contractility [8].

The physical exam of a patient with unrepaired CCTGA reveals an abnormal ventricular impulse with a right ventricular parasternal lift and a palpable second heart sound that relates to the anterior aorta. The ECG of the patient with unrepaired CCTGA may show a prolonged PR interval or complete heart block. The septum is activated from right to left resulting in absent Q waves in the left precordial leads but present in III, aVF, and V1. This ECG pattern can be mistaken for an inferior infarct. The chest X-ray shows a straightened left heart border from the abnormal relationship between the aorta and pulmonary artery [8]. Medical treatment of systemic right ventricular failure is controversial. Afterload reduction with angiotensin-converting enzyme inhibitors and angiotensin receptor blockers may be less successful than when used for the morphologic left ventricle [34]. Surgery is usually related to repair of associated defects (VSD, pulmonary stenosis) or SAVV insufficiency. Surgical strategies to restore "normal" atrio–ventricular and ventriculo–arterial relationships (double switch repair) are more complex, but may offer improved long-term survival if performed at an early age [8].

Ebstein's anomaly

Ebstein's anomaly accounts for 1% of all congenital defects. It involves the atrialization of the right ventricle with inferior displacement of the tricuspid valve. Over half of patients with Ebstein's anomaly have an atrial septal defect that may produce cyanosis. Other common abnormalities with Ebstein's anomaly are VSDs, accessory conduction pathways (such as Wolff–Parkinson–White syndrome) and right ventricular outflow obstructions. Nearly half of patients with CCTGA have an Ebstenoid left AV valve. Ultimately, the impact and clinical presentation of Ebstein's anomaly depends on the severity of the tricupsid insufficiency and hemodynamics of the shunts [8, 35]. Severe Ebstein's anomaly presents in neonates as congestive heart failure and cyanosis. As peripheral vascular resistance drops over the first weeks of life, symptoms may improve and may not require immediate surgery [8].

Asymptomatic Ebstein's anomaly patients who reach late adolescence and adulthood may not require surgical repair [8]. Twenty percent of Ebstein's anomaly cases are complicated by atrial or ventricular arrhythmias. Atrial dilation and Wolff–Parkinson–White syndrome are associated with Ebstein's anomaly and increase the likelihood of recurrent atrial arrhythmias [32]. Arrhythmias may also precipitate congestive heart failure [8].

The physical exam of a patient with unrepaired Ebstein's anomaly varies depending on the severity of the defect and the resulting hemodynamics. On exam, multiple systolic clicks are common [8, 35]. The ECG may show ventricular preexcitation. The P waves are often tall and peaked from atrial enlargement. There is a complete or incomplete right bundle branch block with small R waves in lead V1 and V2. The chest X-ray again varies depending on the severity of the disease. It may be normal or have cardiomegaly with a "globular" contour of the prominent right atrium [8, 32].

Two of the most common causes of death in adults with Ebstein's anomaly are congestive heart failure and arrhythmia [36]. Treatment for right-sided heart failure should be directed toward decreasing right-sided preload and diminishing tricuspid valve regurgitation [32]. Arrhythmias may be amenable to catheter ablation. Unfortunately, success rates are low and recurrence rates are high as many Ebstein's anomaly patients have multiple accessory pathways and landmarks for the procedure are distorted

[8, 32]. Chronic or recurrent arrhythmias require anticoagulation. Surgery is considered in Ebstein's anomaly for uncontrolled tachyarrhythmias, severe tricuspid regurgitation, or associated lesions.

Tricuspid atresia/single ventricle

Tricuspid atresia is the prototypical single ventricle defect. Other single ventricle defects include double inlet left ventricle, double outlet right ventricle, and hypoplastic left heart syndrome [36]. Tricuspid atresia involves an absent or imperforate tricuspid valve with a hypoplastic right ventricle. As a result, there is only one ventricle [8].

Given the severity of single ventricle defects and tricuspid atresia, adult survival without intervention is rare. Surgery involves a staged approach that ultimately provides a pathway from the systemic venous return to the pulmonary artery in the absence of a pulmonary ventricle. The Fontan operation has evolved to become the preferred "palliative" treatment for functional or anatomical single ventricles and complex anomalies considered unsuitable for biventricular repair.

The classic Fontan involved a direct connection from the right atrium or atrial appendage to the pulmonary arteries. Suboptimal systemic venous flow characteristics resulted in right atrial dilation. This increases the risk of atrial arrhythmias and thrombus formation. The current single ventricle strategy involves a staged repair. Neonatal palliation involves an initial aortopulmonary shunt. Next, the bidirectional Glenn (or bidirectional cavopulmonary anastomosis) connects the superior vena cava to the confluent pulmonary artery. It provides a stable source of pulmonary blood flow without overloading the systemic ventricle. It is usually performed in infancy or early childhood as a stepping-stone to Fontan completion. The last step creates a lateral tunnel or extracardiac conduit connection from the inferior vena cava to the pulmonary artery, thus separating the oxygenated and unoxygenated blood [8]. Compared to older Fontan procedures, the lateral tunnel or extracardiac conduit connections eliminate atrial suture lines, improves flow dynamics, and may reduce atrial arrhythmias [36]. Figure 3.2 shows the cardiac anatomy after an extraconduit Fontan procedure.

Although survival after the Fontan has improved, complications are common. Nearly 50% of patients with the older-style Fontan develop atrial tachycardia within a decade of surgery. With lateral tunnel or extracardiac conduit connections, fewer than 10% of patients suffer from recurrent atrial arrhythmias. Atrial tachycardia results in significant hemodynamic compromise and may be associated with thrombus formation or Fontan obstruction. Uniform anticoagulation of the Fontan patient is a source of controversy as this may not eliminate the risk of cardiac thrombus. Drug dosing for antiarrhythmic medications should be carefully calculated as sinus node dysfunction is common and venous pacing is not

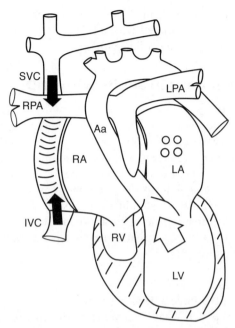

Figure 3.2 External conduit-type Fontan operation in a patient with a hypoplastic right ventricle. The superior vena cava (SVC) is disconnected from the right atrium (RA) and connected directly to the pulmonary artery (PA) (bidirectional Glenn shunt), and the inferior vena cava (IVC) flow is rerouted through the external conduit to the PA. Systemic venous blood (black arrows) flows to the lungs; only pulmonary venous blood is pumped to the aorta (Ao; white arrow). RPA, right pulmonary artery; LPA, left pulmonary artery; RA, right atrium; LA, left atrium; RV, right ventricle; LV, left ventricle. (Reprinted with permission: Sommer et al. Pathophysiology of congenital heart disease in the adult part III: complex congenital heart disease. *Circulation* 2008 Mar 11;117: 1340–1350. (http://lww.com))

always possible due to the complex Fontan anatomy [2, 8]. Another serious but less common complication of the Fontan procedure is protein losing enteropathy (PLE). It occurs in 10% of patients and presents as ascites, peripheral edema, chronic diarrhea, and pleural and pericardial effusions. PLE is a poor prognostic sign [1, 8]. Also with time, cyanosis can worsen. New right to left shunts, worsening ventricular function, and pulmonary arteriovenous malformations or fistulas can form. Attempts at central lines or Swans by physician unfamiliar with the complex venous anatomy of Fontan patients can result in thrombus or vascular obstruction [8].

"Failed" Fontan procedures may result in ventricular dysfunction, intractable arrhythmias, or PLE. As a result, Fontan revision carries an operative mortality ranging from 5% to 25%. Heart transplantation remains an option but is associated with a relatively higher operative mortality than in non-congenital cardiac patients.

Other considerations in adults with CHD

Non-cardiac surgery

Unless operative intervention is an absolute emergency, guidelines suggest that patients with high-risk CHD (defined as prior Fontan, severe pulmonary arterial hypertension, cyanotic CHD, complex CHD with residual heart failure, valvular disease, or malignant arrhythmias) have operative interventions at a regional adult CHD center. In an urgent intervention, basic preoperative evaluation should include systemic arterial oximetry, ECG, chest X-ray, transthoracic echocardiography, and complete blood count and coagulation studies. Involvement of a congenital heart specialist is highly recommended [8].

Psychiatric illness

Most adults with CHD have a life-long condition. A pilot study suggested 33% of adult CHD patients have a psychiatric disorder, compared to 20% of the general population. The majority of psychiatric disorders suffered by adults with CHD are anxiety and depression. While medications have been proven to be effective, a Cochrane Review showed there are no non-pharmacologic treatments that have randomized controlled clinical studies. When a depressed or anxious CHD patient presents to the ED, consider the patient's support system, sense of fear, overall physical health, and current relationship with a psychologist, psychiatrist, or cardiologist to help guide treatment [8, 37, 38].

Endocarditis

Infectious endocarditis accounts for about 4% of admissions to an adult CHD service [39]. The most identified causes for endocarditis are dental manipulation, cardiovascular surgery, pneumonia, and cutaneous infection. TOF, TGA, unrepaired VSD, PDA, coarctation of the aorta, and the presence of prosthetic materials or conduit or unexplained febrile illness should prompt a complete cardiac evaluation including multiple blood cultures prior to initiating antibiotics. Early consultation with a surgeon or cardiologist experienced in adults with CHD should occur as these patients have the potential for rapid deterioration. One study showed a mortality of 8% with medical treatment alone and 11% for those who required surgery. Antibiotic prophylaxis in adults with CHD is recommended for dental procedures involving manipulation of gingival tissue or the periapical region of teeth or perforation of the oral mucosa when a prosthetic valve or prosthetic material, previous infectious endocarditis, unrepaired CHD lesion, CHD repair, or catheter intervention in the past 6 months and repaired CHD with residual defects near prosthetic material are present [8].

The next five years

Ever evolving technology will continue to improve the care of pediatric and adult patients with CHD. The future will also have many new issues created by an aging CHD population such as health care needs, complexity of disease, repeat surgical intervention, ischemic heart disease, heart transplantation and others that can not be envisioned yet.

As more children with CHD survive to adulthood, the health care system will have to provide adequate and appropriate resources to serve these patients. Current areas of concern include the small number of specialty clinics, regional centers and health care providers, adequate health insurance, transition from pediatric to adult care, and infrastructure for case management [7, 8]. Additionally, the nature of adult CHD will change as survivors of complex CHD surgery age. There will be an increasing numbers of adults with multiple interventions for univentricular hearts, complex pulmonary atresia, and common arterial trunk [11].

As CHD patients age, they will require additional interventions for associated co-morbidities. For instance, patients with repaired TOF may require several pulmonary valve replacements in a lifetime [30]. Repeat surgeries result in increased bleeding from adhesions and further complicated anatomy. Additionally, ACHD patients may suffer from ischemic heart disease [40]. Vascular access for cardiac catheterization may be difficult due to multiple previous catheterizations and surgeries.

Heart transplantation as a treatment for CHD continues to be evaluated. Currently only 3% of cardiac transplants involve adult CHD patients [41]. Although adults with CHD have a higher 1-year mortality compared to other groups who undergo heart transplantation, they also have a comparable or improved 10-year survival rate (with the exception of patients with a previous Fontan) [42]. The increase in HLA antibodies from previous transfusions and reconstructions makes matching a donor less likely [41]. Next, despite surgical ingenuity to overcome anatomical complications, dense adhesions, cardiomegaly, and abnormal positioning of native and collateral vessels can produce substantial hemorrhage [41, 42]. The rate of infections and wound dehiscence is also higher in CHD patients [42].

ACHD patients will continue to age and present with new issues that may not have emerged yet. The current changes in pediatric and adult CHD treatment will produce new complications down the road.

Conclusion

With improvements in medical and surgical management, adults with a history of CHD are more likely to present to the ED. Careful understanding of the anatomic and physiologic changes that result from treatment of CHD and close communication with a congenital cardiologist will aid the emergency physician in caring for this challenging and emerging patient population.

References

1. Mettler BA, Peeler BB. Congenital heart disease surgery in the adult. *Surg Clin North Am* 2009 Aug; 89(4): 1021–1032, xi.
2. Bhat AH, Sahn DJ. Congenital heart disease never goes away, even when it has been 'treated': the adult with congenital heart disease. *Curr Opin Pediatr* 2004 Oct; 16(5): 500–507.
3. Sommer RJ, Hijazi ZM, Rhodes JF, Jr. Pathophysiology of congenital heart disease in the adult: part I: shunt lesions. *Circulation* 2008 Feb 26; 117(8): 1090–1099.
4. Kaemmerer H, Bauer U, Pensl U, et al. Management of emergencies in adults with congenital cardiac disease. *Am J Cardiol*. 2008 Feb 15; 101(4): 521–525.
5. Kaemmerer H, Fratz S, Bauer U, et al. Emergency hospital admissions and three-year survival of adults with and without cardiovascular surgery for congenital cardiac disease. *J Thorac Cardiovasc Surg* 2003 Oct; 126(4): 1048–1052.
6. Yeung E, Kay J, Roosevelt GE, Brandon M, Yetman AT. Lapse of care as a predictor for morbidity in adults with congenital heart disease. *Int J Cardiol* 2008 Mar 28; 125(1): 62–65.
7. Verheugt CL, Uiterwaal CS, van der Velde ET, et al. The emerging burden of hospital admissions of adults with congenital heart disease. *Heart* 2010 Jun; 96(11): 872–878.
8. Warnes CA, Williams RG, Bashore TM, et al. ACC/AHA 2008 guidelines for the management of adults with congenital heart disease: a report of the American College of Cardiology/American Heart Association Task Force on Practice Guidelines (Writing Committee to Develop Guidelines on the Management of Adults With Congenital Heart Disease). Developed in Collaboration With the American Society of Echocardiography, Heart Rhythm Society, International Society for Adult Congenital Heart Disease, Society for Cardiovascular Angiography and Interventions, and Society of Thoracic Surgeons. *J Am Coll Cardiol* 2008 Dec 2; 52(23): e1–e121.
9. Lindsey JB, Hillis LD. Clinical update: atrial septal defect in adults. *Lancet* 2007 Apr 14; 369(9569): 1244–1246.
10. Webb G, Gatzoulis MA. Atrial septal defects in the adult: recent progress and overview. *Circulation* 2006 Oct 10; 114(15): 1645–1653.
11. Alvarez N, Prieur T, Connelly M. The ten most commonly asked questions about management of congenital heart disease in adults. *Cardiol Rev* 2002 Mar–Apr; 10(2): 77–81.

12. Moodie DS. Diagnosis and management of congenital heart disease in the adult. *Cardiol Rev* 2001 Sept–Oct; 9(5): 276–281.
13. Brickner ME, Hillis LD, Lange RA. Congenital heart disease in adults. First of two parts. *N Engl J Med* 2000 Jan 27; 342(4): 256–263.
14. Prince SE, Cunha BA. Post-pericardiotomy syndrome. *Heart Lung* 1997 Mar–Apr; 26(2): 165–168.
15. Hoffman JI, Kaplan S. The incidence of congenital heart disease. *J Am Coll Cardiol* 2002 Jun 19; 39(12): 1890–1900.
16. Ammash NM, Warnes CA. Ventricular septal defects in adults. *Ann Intern Med* 2001 Nov 6; 135(9): 812–824.
17. Hoffman JI, Kaplan S, Liberthson RR. Prevalence of congenital heart disease. *Am Heart J* 2004 Mar; 147(3): 425–439.
18. Wiyono SA, Witsenburg M, de Jaegere PP, Roos-Hesselink JW. Patent ductus arteriosus in adults: case report and review illustrating the spectrum of the disease. *Neth Heart J* 2008 Aug; 16(7–8): 255–259.
19. Schneider DJ, Moore JW. Patent ductus arteriosus. *Circulation* 2006 Oct 24; 114(17): 1873–1882.
20. Rhodes JF, Hijazi ZM, Sommer RJ. Pathophysiology of congenital heart disease in the adult, part II. Simple obstructive lesions. *Circulation* 2008 Mar 4; 117(9): 1228–1237.
21. Vriend JW, Mulder BJ. Late complications in patients after repair of aortic coarctation: implications for management. *Int J Cardiol* 2005 Jun 8; 101(3): 399–406.
22. Baron MG, Book WM. Congenital heart disease in the adult: 2004. *Radiol Clin North Am* 2004 May; 42(3): 675–690, vii.
23. Webb G. Treatment of coarctation and late complications in the adult. *Semin Thorac Cardiovasc Surg* 2005 Summer; 17(2): 139–142.
24. Ramnarine I. Role of surgery in the management of the adult patient with coarctation of the aorta. *Postgrad Med J* 2005 Apr; 81(954): 243–247.
25. Tempe DK, Virmani S. Coagulation abnormalities in patients with cyanotic congenital heart disease. *J Cardiothorac Vasc Anesth* 2002 Dec; 16(6): 752–765.
26. Oechslin E. Hematological management of the cyanotic adult with congenital heart disease. *Int J Cardiol* 2004 Dec; 97(1 Suppl.): 109–115.
27. Perloff JK, Rosove MH, Child JS, Wright GB. Adults with cyanotic congenital heart disease: hematologic management. *Ann Intern Med* 1988 Sept 1; 109(5): 406–413.
28. Apitz C, Webb GD, Redington AN. Tetralogy of Fallot. *Lancet* 2009 Oct 24; 374(9699): 1462–1471.
29. Papagiannis JK. Post-operative arrhythmias in Tetralogy of Fallot. *Hellenic J Cardiol* 2005 Nov–Dec; 46(6): 402–407.
30. Huehnergarth KV, Gurvitz M, Stout KK, Otto CM. Repaired Tetralogy of Fallot in the adult: monitoring and management. *Heart* 2008 Dec; 94(12): 1663–1669.
31. Brickner ME, Hillis LD, Lange RA. Congenital heart disease in adults. Second of two parts. *N Engl J Med* 2000 Feb 3; 342(5): 334–342.
32. Walsh EP, Cecchin F. Arrhythmias in adult patients with congenital heart disease. *Circulation* 2007 Jan 30; 115(4): 534–545.
33. Raja SG, Shauq A, Kaarne M. Outcomes after arterial switch operation for simple transposition. *Asian Cardiovasc Thorac Ann* 2005 Jun; 13(2): 190–198.

34. Hornung TS, Calder L. Congenitally corrected transposition of the great arteries. *Heart* 2010 Jul; 96(14): 1154–1161.
35. Attenhofer Jost CH, Connolly HM, Dearani JA, Edwards WD, Danielson GK. Ebstein's anomaly. *Circulation* 2007 Jan 16; 115(2): 277–285.
36. Ellis CR, Graham TP, Jr, Byrd BF, 3rd. Clinical presentations of unoperated and operated adults with congenital heart disease. *Curr Cardiol Rep* 2005 Jul; 7(4): 291–298.
37. Horner T, Liberthson R, Jellinek MS. Psychosocial profile of adults with complex congenital heart disease. *Mayo Clin Proc* 2000 Jan; 75(1): 31–36.
38. Lip GY, Lane DA, Millane TA, Tayebjee MH. Psychological interventions for depression in adolescent and adult congenital heart disease. *Cochrane Database Syst Rev* 2003; (3): CD004394.
39. Niwa K, Perloff JK, Webb GD, et al. Survey of specialized tertiary care facilities for adults with congenital heart disease. *Int J Cardiol* 2004 Aug; 96(2): 211–216.
40. Deanfield J, Thaulow E, Warnes C, et al. Management of grown up congenital heart disease. *Eur Heart J* 2003 Jun; 24(11): 1035–1084.
41. Irving C, Parry G, O'Sullivan J, et al. Cardiac transplantation in adults with congenital heart disease. *Heart* 2010 Aug; 96(15): 1217–1222.
42. Simmonds J, Burch M, Dawkins H, Tsang V. Heart transplantation after congenital heart surgery: improving results and future goals. *Eur J Cardiothorac Surg* 2008 Aug; 34(2): 313–317.

CHAPTER 4

The renal transplant patient

Joseph B. Miller[1,2] and K. K. Venkat[1,2]
[1]Henry Ford Hospital, Detroit, MI, USA
[2]Wayne State University School of Medicine, Detroit, MI, USA

Introduction and epidemiology

End-stage renal disease (ESRD) is a major and growing global public health problem. Renal transplantation is the preferred treatment option for ESRD because it confers improved quality of life and longevity compared to dialysis. Currently in the United States, approximately 160,000 ESRD patients have their lives sustained by a functioning kidney transplant, and worldwide, the number of renal transplant recipients is approximately three times this number [1].

Renal transplant recipients are prone to a variety of serious medical problems that cause them to seek care in the emergency department (ED). Over the past 2 decades, the risk of developing such emergent medical problems has increased significantly in the transplant population for a variety of reasons. There is an increasing acceptance for transplantation of older patients with a number of serious co-morbidities such as diabetes and cardiovascular disease. There is also an increasing length of time spent on dialysis awaiting a deceased-donor transplant (up to 4 to 5 years in many patients) that adds dialysis-related co-morbidities. Finally, the availability of more potent immunosuppressive drugs has reduced the risk of acute rejection, but increased the risk of drug-related adverse effects including opportunistic infections and malignancies [2].

The emergency physician must be aware of a number of unique considerations in evaluating and managing the renal transplant patient. These patients may present with disorders that are uncommon in the general patient population. They may also present with blunted symptoms of common disorders as a results of immunosuppressive drugs, especially corticosteroids. The presenting complaint of renal transplant recipients may be due to the adverse effect of drugs unique to the transplant population

Challenging and Emerging Conditions in Emergency Medicine, First Edition. Edited by Arvind Venkat.
© 2011 by John Wiley & Sons, Ltd. Published 2011 by Blackwell Publishing Ltd.

with which emergency physicians may be unfamiliar. There are multiple serious drug interactions with immunosuppressive medications, and the possibility that the patient's symptoms may be the result of such an interaction must always be entertained. Care should be exercised while prescribing new medications or altering the renal transplant patient's current medications as this may lead to serious drug interactions and alterations in the blood level of immunosuppressive drugs [2].

This chapter presents a review of background aspects of renal transplantation pertinent to emergency physicians followed by an organ system-based discussion of the medical problems that might result in presentation of the renal transplant recipient to the ED.

Surgical aspects of renal transplantation

Knowledge of the surgical anatomy of the kidney transplant (allograft) is essential for the proper evaluation of the renal transplant patient. The allograft is usually placed extraperitoneally in the right or left lower abdominal quadrant. Occasionally, for technical reasons, the transplanted organ is placed intra-peritoneally. The operation involves three anastomoses (Figure 4.1): renal artery and vein of the allograft to the recipient's ipsilateral internal or external iliac artery and vein, respectively, and the ureter of the allograft to the recipient's bladder (ureteroneocystostomy) [3].

A single kidney is transplanted into most recipients. Occasionally, because of the concern of inadequate nephron mass in a small kidney, both kidneys from a pediatric donor (placed en bloc in one or other lower abdominal quadrant) or both kidneys from an older donor with age-related loss of nephron mass (placed one on each side) are transplanted [3]. Because of a shorter period of ischemic preservation after removal from the donor prior to transplantation, most living-donor transplants function immediately with no need for post-operative dialysis. However, up to one-third of cadaveric donor transplants do not function immediately (due to the longer period of ischemic preservation), and dialysis may be required until transplant kidney function is established—a condition referred to as delayed graft function (DGF) [4, 5]. A well-functioning kidney transplant usually results in a post-transplant nadir serum creatinine (SCr) level lower than 1.5 to 2.0 mg/dL.

Post-transplant immunosuppression regimens

With the exception of the very rare recipient of a kidney from an identical twin donor, renal transplant recipients require lifelong maintenance antirejection therapy. In the immediate post-transplant period with its attendant risk of acute rejection, a combination of three drugs ("triple therapy") is used for immunosuppression: a calcineurin inhibitor

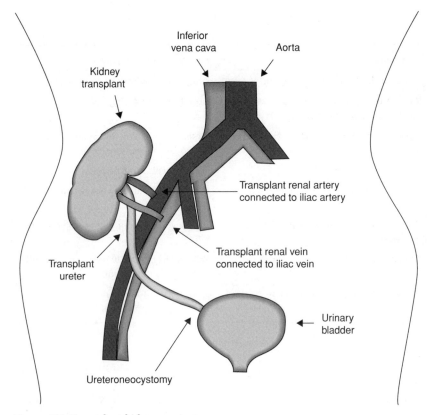

Figure 4.1 Transplant kidney anatomy.

(CNI—cyclosporine or tacrolimus) plus an antilymphocyte proliferative agent (mycophenolate mofetil, mycophenolate sodium, or azathioprine) plus a corticosteroid (prednisone, prednisolone, or methylprednisolone) [6, 7]. Mycophenolate has largely replaced the less potent azathioprine in current clinical practice except in patients with serious adverse reactions to the former. Sirolimus (or the related drug everolimus) is generally not used in the early post-transplant period.

In renal transplant patients with good renal function, one of the three drugs in the initial triple therapy regimen may be discontinued post-transplant in order to minimize its long-term adverse effects [6, 7]. Thus, a patient presenting to the ED may be on only two antirejection medications. Corticosteroid is the most commonly withdrawn antirejection medication. In patients with chronically impaired allograft function, the nephrotoxic CNI may have been stopped and replaced with sirolimus or everolimus [6]. Rarely, one might encounter a renal transplant patient in whom all immunosuppressive medications have been discontinued due to severe

Table 4.1 Commonly used maintenance immunosuppressive medications in current clinical practice

Medication	Recommended drug level
Azathioprine (Imuran® or generic)	Drug level monitoring not recommended
Corticosteroids (Prednisone, Prednisolone or Methylprednisolone)	Drug level monitoring not recommended
Cyclosporine (Sandimmune®, Neoral™ or generic)	*Trough level:* 250 to 400 ng/mL (initial) and 125 to 200 ng/mL (long term)
Everolimus (Zortress®)	*Trough level:* 3 to 8 ng/mL
Mycophenolate Mofetil (CellCept® or generic)	Drug level monitoring not recommended
Mycophenolate Sodium (Myfortic® or generic)	Drug level monitoring not recommended
Sirolimus (Rapamune® or generic)	*Trough level:* 10 to 20 ng/mL (initial) and 5 to 15 ng/mL (long term)
Tacrolimus (Prograf® or generic)	*Trough level:* 10 to 15 ng/mL (early) and 5 to 10 ng/mL (long term)

infection or malignancy. The currently approved maintenance immuno-suppressive drugs are shown in Table 4.1.

In addition to the above-mentioned maintenance drugs, antilympho-cyte antibodies are used immediately after transplantation as induction therapy to prevent rejection (currently in >70% of renal transplant re-cipients in the United States), or as treatment of acute rejection unre-sponsive to initial therapy with high-dose intravenous methylprednisolone for 3 to 5 days [8]. If the renal transplant team requests the adminis-tration of intravenous methylprednisolone (250 to 1000 mg per dose) in the ED for presumed acute rejection, it should be remembered that such doses should be given over 30 to 60 minutes because fatal cardiac arrhythmia has been reported with rapid bolus administration [9]. Cur-rently available antilymphocyte agents for induction therapy are rabbit an-tilymphocyte globulin (Thymoglobulin®), horse antilymphocyte globulin (ATGAM®), muromonab (OKT3®), alemtuzumab (Campath®), basilix-imab (Simulect®), and daclizumab (Zenapax®) [8]. The first four of these drugs can also be used for treatment of corticosteroid-resistant rejection.

The commonly encountered adverse effects of maintenance immuno-suppressive medications are shown in Table 4.2 [6].

The emergency physician should also be aware of the clinically im-portant drug interactions involving antirejection medications which are shown in Table 4.3 [6].

Table 4.2 Adverse effects of maintenance immunosuppressive medications

Medication	Adverse effects
Azathioprine	Macrocytic anemia, leukopenia, thrombocytopenia, hepatotoxicity, pancreatitis
Corticosteroids	Obesity, mooning of the face, diabetes mellitus, cataracts, acne, thinning of skin, bruising, gastro-duodenal ulceration/bleeding, hyperlipidemia, psychosis, osteoporosis/fracture, avascular necrosis of bone
Cyclosporine	Reversible (dose and level-related) acute nephrotoxicity, chronic/progressive/irreversible nephrotoxicity, hyperkalemia, hypomagnesemia, hemolytic–uremic syndrome, hypertension, hyperlipidemia, diabetes mellitus, increased uric acid level $\pm$ gout, abnormal liver function tests, neurotoxicity (tremor, paresthesiae, cramps, headache, insomnia, seizure), hirsutism, gingival hyperplasia
Mycophenolate mofetil	Nausea, vomiting, esophageal ulceration/dysphagia, heartburn, abdominal pain, loss of appetite/weight loss, upper gastrointestinal ulceration/bleeding, colitis/diarrhea/lower gastrointestinal bleeding, anemia, leukopenia, thrombocytopenia
Mycophenolate sodium	Similar to mycophenolate mofetil (see above); gastrointestinal adverse effects may be less severe
Sirolimus/everolimus	Anemia, leukopenia, thrombocytopenia, diarrhea, hyperlipidemia, oral ulcers, skin rash, localized /asymmetric edema, proteinuria, interstitial pneumonitis, delayed wound healing, increased incidence of lymphocele, increased incidence/duration of delayed graft function
Tacrolimus	Generally similar to cyclosporine (see above) with the following differences: more diabetogenic and neurotoxic, causes alopecia rather than hirsutism, does not cause gingival hyperplasia

Approach to acute and chronic renal and urinary tract disorders in renal transplant recipients

The allograft and the urinary tract of the renal transplant patient can be affected by any of the disorders that occur in their native counterparts [5]. Thus, the emergency physician may encounter renal transplant recipients presenting with acute kidney injury (AKI, previously referred to as acute renal failure), chronic kidney disease (CKD, previously referred to as chronic renal failure), proteinuria/nephrotic syndrome, hematuria, urinary tract obstruction, or urinary tract infection (UTI). Rejection

Table 4.3 Clinically important drug interactions with immunosuppressive drugs

Immunosuppressive drug(s)	Drug(s) causing interaction	Mechanism and result(s) of interaction
Azathioprine	Allopurinol	Azathioprine is metabolized by xanthine oxidase, the enzyme inhibited by allopurinol. Allopurinol, therefore increases azathioprine blood levels with an increased risk of azathioprine induced bone marrow suppression.
Cyclosporine, tacrolimus, sirolimus or everolimus	Phenobarbital, Phenytoin, Carbamazepine, Rifampin, or Isoniazid	Potentiation of hepatic cytochrome P-450 enzyme system with increased metabolism and decreased blood level of immunosuppressive drug and resultant increased risk of rejection.
	Diltiazem, Verapamil, Amiodarone, Azole antifungals*, Macrolide antibiotics[†]	Inhibition of cytochrome P-450 decreases metabolism, causing increased blood levels and a higher incidence of known adverse drug effects, particularly a higher risk of cyclosporine or tacrolimus nephro- and neurotoxicity
Cyclosporine or tacrolimus	Aminoglycosides, iodinated radiocontrast, Amphotericin, nonsteroidal anti-inflammatory drug	These nephrotoxic drugs may potentiate cyclosporine or tacrolimus nephrotoxicity. No change in metabolism or blood level of the immunosuppressive drug
Cyclosporine	HMG CoA-reductase inhibitors	Statin blood level increased by cyclosporine: increased risk of statin-induced rhabdomyolysis $\pm$ acute kidney injury

*Keto-, Flu-, Vori- or Itroconazole.
[†]Erythromycin and Clarithromycin. Azithromycin has only minimal drug interaction.

is, of course, a unique disorder affecting only the kidney transplant. Renal dysfunction due to BK-polyomavirus-associated nephropathy affects 5%–10% of renal transplant patients but is very rare in native kidneys [10].

The same differential diagnostic approach traditionally used when evaluating AKI affecting the native kidneys is also applicable to the renal transplant patient: pre-renal, post-renal and intra-renal causes [5]. The diagnosis of AKI requires an acute increase in the serum creatinine level of

$\geq$0.3 mg/dL over the most recently documented baseline level; smaller increases may be the result of random laboratory variation. After the exclusion of pre- and post-renal causes, the two common diagnostic considerations in the renal transplant patients with AKI are acute rejection and acute CNI-nephrotoxicity. Elevation in SCr associated with a higher than therapeutic blood level of cyclosporine or tacrolimus favors the diagnosis of CNI-nephrotoxicity. A key point for the emergency physician to remember is that it is the trough level of cyclosporine or tacrolimus that is used in therapeutic monitoring. These drugs are administered every 12 hours and the trough level should be obtained in the 1 to 3 hour period immediately preceding the drug dose. Since the renal transplant recipient may come to the ED after having already taken the medication, the random level obtained on arrival in the ED may be elevated because it was drawn prior to the trough period. A low fractional excretion of sodium (FENa) in the urine supports the diagnosis of pre-renal azotemia in native kidney AKI. However, acute rejection and acute CNI-nephrotoxicity may also be associated with a low FENa, making this test less useful in the evaluation of post-transplant AKI [2]. To decrease the risk of AKI, the intrinsically nephrotoxic drugs shown in Table 4.3 and iodinated radiocontrast should be avoided in renal transplant patients.

Evaluation of the allograft by ultrasonography is especially useful in the renal transplant patient presenting with AKI [11]. Demonstration of new onset hydronephrosis suggests obstructive uropathy. Doppler ultrasonography helps in diagnosing renal arterial or venous occlusion as the cause of AKI.

The most common cause (65% to 70% of cases) of CKD in the renal transplant recipient is the entity previously referred to as chronic rejection and currently called chronic allograft nephropathy (CAN) or interstitial fibrosis/tubular atrophy [12]. This syndrome is characterized by a gradually increasing SCr level and proteinuria over months to years. Recurrence of the original disease that caused ESRD and the uncommon development of de novo renal disease in the allograft account for the remainder of the cases of CKD in renal transplant patients [13].

It is important to remember that microscopic or gross hematuria and UTI in the renal transplant patient may originate from the lower urinary tract, the native kidneys, or the allograft [14, 15]. Thus, it is necessary to include both the native kidneys and the allograft when performing imaging studies to evaluate these disorders. Although the microbial spectrum causing UTI in this patient population is similar to that in the native urinary tract, the clinical presentation of UTI may be more severe post-transplant, especially during the first post-transplant year due to the higher dose of immunosuppressive medications during this period [15]. It should also be remembered that besides UTI, acute rejection may also cause pyuria in renal transplant recipients [2]. The current incidence of UTI in the first post-transplant year

Table 4.4 Special considerations in the evaluation and initial treatment of acute kidney injury (AKI) in renal transplant recipients

---

1. Any disorder (pre-renal, intra-renal and post-renal) that can cause AKI in the native kidneys can affect the transplant kidney.
2. After exclusion of other causes of AKI, acute rejection and acute calcineurin inhibitor (CNI) nephrotoxicity are the major diagnostic considerations.
3. Elevated CNI (cyclosporine or tacrolimus) trough level in association with AKI supports the diagnosis of acute CNI nephrotoxicity.
4. Random CNI blood level drawn upon arrival in the ED may not be a trough level. Time of last intake of CNI should be ascertained.
5. Fractional excretion of sodium (FENa) in the urine has limitations when used in this patient population. Urinalysis, including microscopy of urinary sediment, is more useful.
6. Doppler ultrasonography of the kidney transplant is a very useful test in evaluating AKI. It helps to identify obstructive uropathy, peritransplant fluid collection (urinoma, lymphocele, seroma/hematoma) and renal arterial or venous occlusion.
7. Unless unavoidable, prescription of nephrotoxic drugs (Table 4.3) and use of iodinated radiocontrast is not advisable.
8. When prescribing new drugs or changing the dose of existing drugs, the possibility of drug interactions involving immunosuppressive medications should always be considered (Table 4.3).

---

is 10% to15%. Pyelonephritis affecting the allograft can cause severe AKI, and may be complicated by gas formation in the renal collecting system and urinary tract (emphysematous pyelonephritis, best demonstrated by a CT) [16]. In the initial treatment of severe UTI in a renal transplant recipient, a combination of two potent antibiotics intravenously (for example, vancomycin and a third-generation cephalosporin) should be used. Unless unavoidable, nephrotoxic drugs such as aminoglycosides and high-dose trimethoprim–sulfamethoxazole should not be used.

Table 4.4 summarizes the special considerations when evaluating a renal transplant patient with AKI.

Surgical complications related to the kidney transplant operation

A variety of surgical complications, most of them requiring prompt consultation with the transplant surgery team, may be encountered in the renal transplant patient [3,17].

1. *Generic post-operative complications:* Disorders that can complicate any type of surgery can also occur in the renal transplant patient. These include pulmonary atelectasis and pneumonia following general

anesthesia, surgical wound infection, abdominal ileus, post-operative bleeding, and venous thrombosis/pulmonary embolism, among others.

2. *Acute vascular occlusion:* Occlusion of the transplant renal artery or vein occurs in up to 8% of renal transplant patients [3, 17]. This catastrophe usually occurs in the first few weeks post-transplant and results in sudden onset oligoanuric AKI. Doppler ultrasonography is the most expeditious method of confirming the diagnosis, and prompt surgical intervention offers the only (albeit small) chance of salvaging the kidney transplant.

3. *Transplant renal artery stenosis:* Significant (>50% to 70%) narrowing of the allograft renal artery has to be considered in the differential diagnosis of post-transplant hypertension and/or acute or chronic renal dysfunction. It has been reported in up to 10% of renal transplant recipients [3].

4. *Bleeding from or near the kidney transplant:* This complication has been reported in 2%–3% of renal transplant patients, usually in the early post-transplant period [3,5]. Failure to achieve adequate hemostasis intra-operatively, initiation of anticoagulation for any indication post-operatively, bleeding following biopsy of the allograft, and (rarely) severe acute rejection resulting in marked swelling/rupture of the allograft are contributory factors. Presenting symptoms of allograft rupture include tenderness over the allograft, sudden hypotension, a drop in the hemoglobin level, AKI of the kidney transplant, and/or difficult to control hyperkalemia due to red cell lysis in the peritransplant hematoma. Noncontrast CT is the best diagnostic test, and significant peritransplant bleeding requires prompt surgical intervention.

5. *Urine leak (urinoma):* Disruption of the ureteroneocystostomy anastomosis leads to urine leak into the pelvis [17, 18]. Urea, creatinine, and water in the extravasated urine will be reabsorbed into the blood stream with resultant oliguria and azotemia. This complication usually occurs within the first month post-transplant with a reported incidence of 2% to 5%. The resultant peritransplant fluid collection can be detected by ultrasonography. Percutaneous, ultrasound-guided aspiration of the fluid with demonstration of a markedly higher creatinine level in the aspirate compared to a simultaneously measured SCr level confirms the diagnosis of urinoma, and differentiates it from other peritransplant fluid collections such as lymphocele (see below), hematoma, or seroma. Unlike a urinoma, the aspirate creatinine level in these other types of fluid collections is nearly the same as the SCr level. Another method of confirming a urinary leak is isotopic renography with demonstration of persistent radioactivity over several hours in the peritransplant fluid collection due to extravasation of urine containing the intravenously injected radioisotope.

6. *Peritransplant lymph collection (lymphocele):* This complication occurs in 5% to 15% of renal transplant patients usually within the first 3 months post-transplant [3,19]. It results from persistent leakage from pelvic lymphatics severed during the transplant operation. Small lymphoceles may be asymptomatic and detected incidentally by ultrasonography. Larger lymphoceles may cause local pain and/or fullness, increase in the SCr level by extrinsic pressure on the transplant ureter, pressure on the bladder with urinary frequency, and lower extremity edema on the side of the kidney transplant due to pressure on the iliac veins. Compression by lymphocele may cause iliac venous thrombosis and, very rarely, partial or complete renal arterial occlusion. Percutaneous, ultrasound-guided external drainage is the initial treatment for patients with symptomatic lymphoceles.

7. *Urinary tract obstruction in the renal transplant recipient:* Obstructive uropathy occurs in 3% to 6% of renal transplant patients [3]. During the first 3 post-transplant months, this complication is usually caused by either technical problems at the ureteroneocystostomy, extrinsic compression of the ureter by a lymphocele, occlusion of the ureter, or Foley catheter by blood clots in patients with gross hematuria or inability to empty the bladder (caused by the prostate or neurogenic bladder). Beyond the first 3 months, obstruction is the result of ureteric stenosis due to ischemia or scarring following episodes of rejection, or inability to empty the bladder because of the disorders mentioned above. Elevation of SCr associated with ultrasonographic demonstration of new onset or worsening of pre-existing hydronephrosis is strongly suggestive of obstructive uropathy. Percutaneous nephrostomy with external drainage of urine is the preferred initial step in treating obstructive uropathy in this patient population.

8. *Bleeding following biopsy of the kidney transplant:* Biopsy of the kidney transplant for evaluation of renal dysfunction is performed mostly as an ambulatory procedure in which the patient is sent home after a few hours of observation. Although uncommon, this procedure may be complicated by bleeding [20]. Such a patient may return to the ED with pain overlying the renal allograft, gross hematuria, hypotension, fall in the hemoglobin level, and/or AKI. CT identifies peritransplant bleeding better than ultrasonography. Blood transfusions and embolization of the bleeding vessel by allograft angiography may be required.

9. *Lower quadrant abdominal pain at the site of the kidney transplant:* This is a common complaint in this patient population. Common causes of this complaint are shown in Table 4.5. It is important to remember that the pain may be unrelated to the allograft and causes of right or left lower quadrant abdominal pain in the general population should also be considered in the differential diagnosis.

Table 4.5 Causes of lower quadrant abdominal pain at the site of the kidney transplant

Transplant-related causes	Transplant-unrelated causes
1. Severe acute rejection	1. Acute appendicitis
2. Transplant pyelonephritis	2. Diverticulitis
3. Pressure from large lymphocele, urinoma or peritransplant hematoma	3. Ischemic colitis
4. Transplant wound infection/peritransplant infection	4. Infectious or inflammatory bowel disease
5. Chronic, recurrent incisional pain*	5. Ovarian and pelvic inflammatory disorders

*Experienced by some patients and likely the result of injury to cutaneous nerves during surgery.

The febrile renal transplant patient in the ED

Fever is a challenging complaint that frequently leads renal transplant recipients to seek evaluation in the ED. Signs and symptoms of infection may be partially masked by immunosuppression. Additionally, the risk of opportunistic infections and the potential for a fulminant course complicate the diagnostic and therapeutic approach to fever in these patients. It should be remembered that these patients are more susceptible to severe sepsis, multilobar pneumonia, and meningitis compared to the general population. It is useful to consider the time elapsed after transplantation when a renal transplant patient presents with fever (Table 4.6).

These patients carry the highest risk of opportunistic infections during the second through the sixth month following transplant. During the first month after transplant, nosocomial and post-operative infections such as wound infection, line-sepsis, and UTIs may occur, but are infrequent. Early opportunistic infections are rare since the full effect of immunosuppression is not yet present. Also encountered in the first month (though rarely) are donor-derived (transmitted through the allograft) infections such as Hepatitis C virus or West Nile virus. Between 30 days and 6 months post-transplant, a wide spectrum of opportunistic infections reach their highest incidence in this patient population [21]. The prevalence of specific opportunistic pathogens varies geographically, and consultation with the transplant team can aid emergency physicians to narrow down the diagnostic possibilities in patients they encounter.

Cytomegalovirus (CMV) is a significant opportunistic pathogen in all types of transplant recipients. Despite universal prophylaxis with ganciclovir or valganciclovir, symptomatic CMV infection still occurs in 10% to 25% of renal transplant patients [22]. CMV infection may present as

Table 4.6 Infectious risk based on time post-transplant

0–1 Month	1–6 Months	>6 Months
Nosocomial	**Bacterial**	**Community-acquired**
C. difficile colitis	Pneumococcus, Staphylococcus,	Pneumonia
VRE, MRSA	Gram-negatives, Legionella	Urinary tract infections
Candida		Influenza, adenovrius
	Fungal	
Post-surgical	Cryptococcus, Aspergillus, PCP	**Fungal**
Wound infections		Aspergillus, Nocardia
Anastamotic leaks	**Viral**	Atypical molds
	Influenza, CMV, EBV, VZV	
Donor-derived	BK virus, HCV, HBV	**Latent viral**
West Nile virus		CMV colitis/retinitis
HSV, HIV, HCV	**Other**	HBV, HCV, HSV, EBV
	Toxoplasmosis, Mycobacterial,	
	C. difficile colitis, Strongyloides	

Source: Adapted from Fishman [21].
VRE, Vancomycin resistant Enterococcus faecalis; MRSA, Methicillin resistant Staphylococcus aureus; HSV, Herpes simplex virus; HIV, Human immunodeficiency virus; HCV, Hepatitis C virus; PCP, Pneumocystis jiroveci (carinii); CMV, Cytomegalovirus; EBV, Epstein-Barr virus; VZV, Varicella zoster virus; HBV, Hepatitis B virus.

CMV disease, characterized by high fever, elevated liver enzymes, and pancytopenia. Tissue-invasive CMV infection (pulmonary, gastrointestinal, or central nervous) represents the more severe spectrum of CMV disease. The most expeditious method to confirm the diagnosis within 24 to 48 hours is the polymerase chain reaction (PCR) assay for CMV DNA in the blood. Use of routine antimicrobial prophylaxis has decreased but not eliminated the chance of Pneumocystis or CMV infection.

The ED evaluation of the febrile renal transplant patient should include complete blood count and differential, serum creatinine, urinalysis, urine and blood cultures, and chest radiograph. Additional tests (especially CMV-PCR and liver function tests) may be necessary in the appropriate clinical setting. Consideration of non-infectious causes of fever is also warranted in these patients, particularly severe acute rejection, administration of antilymphocyte antibodies, and post-transplant lymphoma [21]. Post-transplant lymphoma may initially present as an infectious mononucleosis-like illness [23].

Past the first 6 months, community-acquired infections predominate in renal transplant recipients. By this time, in the majority of patients the immunosuppressive regimen has been tapered to maintenance doses, thus decreasing the risk of opportunistic infections. However, opportunistic infections may still occur, especially if a recent rejection episode has required intensified antirejection therapy.

In the first year post-transplant, most febrile renal transplant patients will require hospitalization due to the potential for a fulminant course, and the risk of nosocomial or opportunistic infections and rejection. A lower threshold for admission and observation is still warranted in more long-term patients, but outpatient management of milder infectious processes may be possible in consultation with the transplant team.

Cardiovascular and hypertension-related disorders in renal transplant recipients

Atherosclerotic cardiovascular disease is the leading cause of death in renal transplant patients, accounting for approximately 40% of post-transplant mortality [24]. In comparison to an age-matched general population, these patients carry a three- to fivefold higher risk of cardiovascular disease [25]. Even prior to transplantation, chronic kidney disease is associated with accelerated atherogenesis. High prevalence of diabetes (40% to 50%), hypertension (up to 90%) and hyperlipidemia (50% to 60%) are major contributors to the increased cardiovascular risk [26]. No matter how atypical the presentation and even in patients younger than 40 years, a high index of suspicion for an acute coronary syndrome is justified in the transplant population.

The diagnostic and therapeutic approach to cardiovascular disorders in renal transplant recipients is the same as in the general population. There are no unique contraindications to anticoagulation or the use of any parenteral or oral antihypertensive agents in these patients. However, diltiazem, verapamil, and amiodarone inhibit the hepatic cytochrome P-450 enzyme system and can lead to cyclosporine or tacrolimus nephrotoxicity due to decreased metabolism of these immunosuppressants [27]. Brief use of these agents as an emergent antiarrhythmic agent is acceptable, but continuing long-term outpatient use requires coordination with the transplant team to monitor immunosuppressive drug levels and adjust dosing downward as necessary.

Renal transplant recipients presenting with respiratory complaints

When evaluating respiratory symptoms, the risk of an opportunistic pneumonia, and the possibility of a more fulminant course, separates the renal transplant patient from the general population. Factors that influence their evaluation and treatment in the ED include the time period since transplantation, severity of illness, and radiographic appearance.

Post-operative, non-opportunistic pneumonia may occur in the first post-transplant month. Opportunistic infections become a significant problem past the first month and must be considered in the evaluation of respiratory symptoms. The pattern of pulmonary infiltrate can offer clues to possible etiology. Lobar consolidation is suggestive of bacterial pneumonias caused by organisms such as *Pneumococcus* or *Legionella*. A bilateral interstitial pattern points to *Pneumocystis* or CMV pneumonia [28]. Additionally, interstitial pneumonitis associated with sirolimus therapy should be considered [29]. Nodular or cavitating lesions suggest fungal infections such as *Aspergillus*, *Cryptococcus*, or *Histoplasma*. Even in the setting of mild symptoms, findings suggestive of fungal infection require aggressive investigation due to the risk of significant morbidity [30].

CT is frequently necessary in evaluating pulmonary complaints in transplant patients. Nondiagnostic radiographs do not rule out the early stages of bacterial pneumonia. Tuberculous, fungal, *Pneumocystis*, and CMV pneumonias can present with subacute symptoms and unimpressive radiographs [31]. The risk of these pathogens is greatest in months 1 through 6 post-transplant and during periods of intensified immunosuppression. Pneumocystis may present with hypoxemia, dyspnea, and cough with subtle or absent physical and radiographic findings. There should be a high index of suspicion for the diagnosis of tuberculosis because its incidence is increased in immunosuppressed patients [21].

The threshold for hospital admission of renal transplant patients with suspected pulmonary infection should be low due to the potential for a rapidly deteriorating course. Unless tuberculosis is suspected, strict isolation precautions are not required. Nevertheless, many institutions elect to place hospitalized transplant patients in private rooms for the first 6 to 12 months post-transplant to decrease the risk of nosocomial infections.

Because of the risk of unusual opportunistic and resistant pathogens, every attempt should be made to obtain adequate blood and sputum culture specimens before initiating empiric antimicrobial therapy. Nevertheless, empiric therapy should be initiated promptly, particularly during the first 6 months post-transplant, due to the risk of rapid deterioration. Treatment for a community-acquired pneumonia or healthcare-associated pneumonia should be initiated according to established guidelines [32, 33]. Patients within the first 6 months of transplant require this same treatment but warrant additional consideration for antimicrobials targeted at opportunistic organisms in consultation with the transplant team.

The macrolide antibiotics are commonly used to treat respiratory infections, but can have significant pharmacological interaction in transplant patients. The majority of macrolides inhibit the hepatic enzymes that metabolize cyclosporine, tacrolimus, and sirolimus. Therefore, it is important to monitor the blood level and reduce the dose of these immunosuppressants if a macrolide antibiotic is selected. Azithromycin is preferred because it is the macrolide least likely to affect the metabolism of these immunosuppressants [27].

Renal transplant recipients presenting with gastrointestinal complaints

Just as immunosuppressants blunt the immune system's response to various microbes, these medications (corticosteroids in particular) may also mask the peritoneal response to significant intra-abdominal pathology. The clinical presentation of serious abdominal conditions such as acute cholecystitis, visceral perforation, diverticulitis, and bowel infarction may be muted [34]. An intra-abdominal catastrophe cannot be excluded because abdominal pain is mild and guarding and/or rebound tenderness are absent. The care of renal transplant patients with abdominal pain requires a low threshold for ultrasound or CT imaging and surgical consultation.

There are a broad range of gastrointestinal/hepatobiliary/pancreatic problems that are encountered in transplant patients. The two major causes of these disorders are direct adverse effects of immunosuppressants and a variety of infections that occur in immunosuppressed patients. Table 4.7 summarizes these disorders.

Renal transplant recipients presenting with neurological or psychiatric problems

New onset headache, seizure, or change in mental status in a renal transplant patient may be the result of very serious disorders such as meningitis, encephalitis, or neoplasm. Such symptoms warrant prompt

Table 4.7 Gastrointestinal disorders in renal transplant recipients due to infectious or drug-related complications

Disorder	Infectious	Drug-related complications
Oral ulcers, plaques	*Candida*, HSV	Sirolimus
Esophagitis	*Candida*, HSV, CMV	Mycophenolate mofetil
Gastroduodenitis, upper gastrointestinal ulceration/bleeding	CMV infection, EBV-related gastrointestinal lymphoma	Mycophenolate mofetil, corticosteroids
Diarrhea, lower gastrointestinal ulceration/bleeding	CMV infection, Microsporidium, Cryptosporidium, EBV-related intestinal lymphoma	Mycophenolate mofetil, sirolimus
Hepatic dysfunction	CMV, EBV, Hepatitis C and B	Cyclosporine, tacrolimus
Pancreatitis	CMV	Azathioprine

HSV, *Herpes simplex* virus; CMV, Cytomegalovirus; EBV, Epstein-Barr virus.

imaging and lumbar puncture. The incidence of an opportunistic central nervous system (CNS) infection approaches 10% in this population, particularly within the first 6 months post-transplant. Common pathogens include *Cryptococcus neoformans*, *Mycobacterium tuberculosis*, and *Listeria monocytogenes* [35–37]. Additional pathogens to consider are CMV, *Herpes simplex*, JC-Polyoma and West Nile viruses, and *Toxoplasma gondii*. Because of the masking effect of immunosuppression, fever, leukocytosis, and meningismus may be absent in these patients. Hence, the threshold for cerebrospinal fluid (CSF) analysis in these patients should be low. It should also be remembered that despite severe meningoencephalitis, CSF chemical abnormalities and pleocytosis may be equivocal. The most common CNS neoplasm in renal transplant recipients is post-transplant lymphoma [38].

Immunosuppressant medications are also associated with neurological adverse effects. CNIs are known to cause headache, insomnia, tremors, paresthesiae affecting the hands/feet, seizures, and global encephalopathy [39]. Tacrolimus is more neurotoxic than cyclosporine. Severe encephalopathy may also be due to neurological toxicity of drugs such as acyclovir, penicillins, and cephalosporins, especially when given to patients with impaired allograft function.

Corticosteroid psychosis may also underlie alterations in mood in transplant recipients. Lastly, the prevalence of depression and risk of suicide are higher among renal transplant patients compared to the general population [40].

Hematologic disorders in renal transplant recipients

Medication-associated cytopenias are common in renal transplant recipients [41]. Additionally, chronic transplant dysfunction may cause anemia of chronic kidney disease. The prevalence of anemia approaches 21% at 1 year and 36% at 3 years following transplantation [42]. Opportunistic viral infections, particularly CMV and *Parvovirus*, are also associated with cytopenias. Lastly, common prophylactic medications such as trimethoprim–sulfamethoxazole, ganciclovir, and valgancyclovir can all be associated with cytopenias. When blood product transfusions are required for symptomatic anemia, the use of leukocyte-poor blood is recommended for transplant patients to decrease the risk of sensitization to HLA-antigens [22].

Hemolytic-uremic syndrome (HUS) is an emergent condition to consider when a renal transplant patient presents with the triad of anemia, thrombocytopenia, and AKI. History of ESRD secondary to native kidney HUS, cyclosporine, tacrolimus or sirolimus therapy, severe acute vascular rejection, and CMV infection are the risk factors for post-transplant HUS [43].

Table 4.8 Common hematologic disorders and special considerations in renal transplant recipients

Disorder	Special considerations
Cytopenias	CMV or *Parvovirus* infection *Drug effects:* Mycophenolate mofetil, sirolimus, everolimus, azathioprine, ganciclovir, valgancyclovir, trimethoprim–sulfamethoxazole
Hemolytic–uremic syndrome (HUS)	Recurrence of native kidney HUS, severe vascular rejection, CMV infection *Drug effects:* Cyclosporine, tacrolimus, sirolimus
Leukocytosis	Corticosteroids (conversely, discontinuation of corticosteroids may result in leukopenia)
Erythrocytosis	Endogenous erythropoietin (*source:* native kidney more so than the allograft) and other factors

Diagnostic clues include elevated lactate dehydrogenase, low haptoglobin levels, and the presence of schistocytes on a peripheral blood smear.

Leukocytosis and erythrocytosis can also occur in renal transplant patients. The primary cause of non-infectious leukocystosis is demargination of leukocytes by corticosteroids. Band forms should be absent with demargination, and their presence suggests infection. Up to 20% of renal transplant recipients will have erythrocytosis in the first year following transplant, and in half of these patients, erythrocytosis may persist long term [44]. Erythrocytosis predisposes post-transplant patients to thromboembolic events, and may cause chronic dizziness and headaches.

Table 4.8 summarizes the common hematological disorders encountered in renal transplant recipients.

Renal transplant recipients presenting with musculoskeletal and articular complaints

Renal transplant recipients are at increased risk for a number of musculoskeletal and articular emergencies. Corticosteroids accelerate osteoporosis resulting in an increased risk of fractures. For unclear reasons, the most common site of fractures in renal transplant recipients is the foot [45]. Unexplained foot pain with or without trauma may well be the result of a fracture. Avascular necrosis with hip and/or knee pain occurs in up to 3.5% of renal transplant recipients and may require MRI for diagnosis in its early stages [46]. Pending imaging, immobilization for presumed fracture may be appropriate.

Table 4.9 Special considerations in evaluating musculoskeletal complaints in renal transplant recipients

Complaint	Special considerations
Foot pain	Foot fractures are common and history of trauma may be lacking
Hip pain	Increased risk of avascular necrosis due to corticosteroid use
Acute arthritis	Increased risk of gout on CNI, but care should be taken to rule out a septic joint. NSAIDs and colchicine use not advisable
Quadriceps or achilles tendon pain	Corticosteroid and quinolone use and tendon calcification cause increased risk of tendon rupture

Acute gout is common in renal transplant patients on CNIs. These medications reduce renal uric acid excretion and cause hyperuricemia. In the diagnostic evaluation of arthritis in renal transplant recipients, arthrocentesis is important to differentiate septic arthritis from gout. The therapeutic approach also has a few caveats: nonsteroidal anti-inflammatory drugs may cause AKI/ARF, and colchicine can interact with cyclosporine and cause leukopenia, hepatic dysfunction, and rhabdomyolysis [47]. In this population, corticosteroids and alternative analgesics are better therapeutic choices for gout.

Long-term corticosteroid use may cause proximal muscle weakness of the limbs secondary to steroid myopathy. Corticosteroids and tendon calcification secondary to hyperparathyroidism contribute to increased risk of tendon rupture in this patient population [48]. Quinolone antibiotic use may further increase this risk [2]. Pain and swelling over common sites of rupture such as the Achilles or quadriceps tendon should prompt soft-tissue ultrasonography or MRI for rupture even in the setting of minor trauma. Following complete discontinuation of corticosteroids, renal transplant patients may present with polymyalgia and polyarthralgia that may respond to reinstitution of a small dose of corticosteroid [2].

Table 4.9 shows the special considerations in the evaluation of musculoskeletal and articular problems in renal transplant recipients.

Common electrolyte disorders encountered in renal transplant recipients

Potassium and magnesium abnormalities are common among renal transplant recipients. Patients on cyclosporine and tacrolimus frequently require magnesium replacement secondary to chronic renal magnesium wasting [49]. The CNIs also reduce urinary potassium excretion, resulting in hyperkalemia. Additional medications that contribute to hyperkalemia in these patients are trimethoprim–sulfamethoxazole, ACE-inhibitors, and angiotensin II receptor blockers [2].

Hypercalcemia and hypophosphatemia occur in 5% to 10% of renal transplant patients due to persistence of secondary hyperparathyroidism in the setting of good allograft function [2]. Lastly, normal anion gap renal tubular acidosis may be noted in patients with allograft dysfunction [2].

Endocrine complications in renal transplant recipients

New-onset diabetes mellitus occurs in approximately 25% of patients within 3 years of renal transplantation [50]. Both corticosteroid and CNI (particularly tacrolimus) use contribute to this increased risk of diabetes. Symptoms of polyuria, polydipsia, and weight loss should prompt testing for diabetic emergencies in renal transplant recipients. Diabetic ketoacidosis occurs in approximately 8% and hyperosmolaity in 3% of renal transplant patients who develop post-transplant diabetes mellitus [51]. The treatment of these diabetic complications is not different from that of non-transplant patients.

Acute adrenal insufficiency is a significant concern in critically ill renal transplant recipients. The majority of these patients receive corticosteroids for some period of time for immunosuppression with resultant suppression of their pituitary–adrenal axis. Stress-dose corticosteroid coverage (intravenous hydrocortisone 100 mg every 8 hours) is required in the critically ill renal transplant patient unless steroid therapy had been discontinued more than 6 to 12 months earlier [52].

The next five years

Currently, there are approximately 90,000 patients wait-listed for kidney transplantation in the United States [1]. With the increasing global incidence/prevalence of ESRD due to a combination of aging of the population and the epidemic of obesity and diabetes, the demand for kidney transplantation is bound to increase. If the availability of organs for transplantation increases, the number of renal transplant recipients and ED visits by these patients will likewise rise. HIV infection was, until recently, considered an absolute contraindication to kidney transplantation. Nevertheless, the increasing success of antiretroviral therapy has cleared the way for carefully selected HIV-positive ESRD patients to be accepted for transplantation [53]. This high-risk population will be more likely to seek care in the ED.

Several new and potent immunosuppressive medications and monoclonal antibodies are likely to be approved in the coming years (e.g., belatacept) and may result in a higher incidence of emergent adverse effects, including drug interactions, infection, and malignancy. The pattern of post-transplant infections for which a renal transplant patient may seek care in the ED may subsequently change with time as new immunosuppressant medications are introduced and patients with more co-morbidities become renal transplant recipients. Finally, transplant tourism (patients traveling to countries where commercial transplantation using paid live donors is practiced) is increasing [54]. These patients may present to the ED with uncommon infections acquired abroad.

Conclusion

Renal transplant patients represent a growing and challenging ED patient population. Careful consideration of the time since transplantation and broad differential diagnosis can aid the emergency physician in the evaluation and management of these individuals when presenting for acute care. Early consultation with the transplant team can be invaluable in assuring that renal transplant recipients receive quality care in the emergency department.

References

1. United States Renal Data System - 2009 annual data report. Atlas of chronic kidney disease and end-stage renal disease in the United States, Chapter 4: treatment Modalities. *Am J Kidney Dis* 2010 Jan; 55(1 Suppl.): S249–S258.
2. Venkat K, Venkat A. Care of the renal transplant recipient in the emergency department. *Ann Emerg Med* 2004 Oct; 44(4): 330–41.
3. Veale J, Singer J, Gritsch H. The transplant operation and its surgical complications. In: Danovitch GM (ed.) *Handbook of Kidney Transplantation*. 5th ed. Philadelphia: Lippincott Williams and Wilkins; 2009.
4. Peeters P, Terryn W, Vanholder R, Lameire N. Delayed graft function in renal transplantation. *Curr Opin Crit Care* 2004 Dec; 10(6): 489–498.
5. Wilkinson A. The "first quarter". The first three months after transplant. In: Danovitch GM (ed.) *Handbook of Kidney Transplantation*. 5th ed. Philadelphia: Williams and Wilkins; 2009: pp. 198–216.
6. Halloran P. Immunosuppressive drugs for kidney transplantation. *N Engl J Med* 2004 Dec; 351(26): 2715–2729.
7. Kidney Disease: Improving Global Outcomes (KDIGO) Group. KDIGO clinical practice guideline for the care of kidney transplant recipients. *Am J Transplant* 2009 Nov; 9(3 Suppl.): S1–S155.
8. Padiyar A, Augustine J, Hricik D. Induction antibody therapy in kidney transplantation. *Am J Kidney Dis* 2009 Nov; 54(5): 935–944.
9. McDougal B, Whittier F, Cross D. Sudden death after bolus steroid therapy for acute rejection. *Transplant Proc* 1976 Sep; 8(3): 493–496.
10. Wiseman A. Polyomavirus nephropathy: a current perspective and clinical considerations. *Am J Kidney Dis* 2009 Jul; 54(1): 131–142.
11. Irshad A, Ackerman S, Campbell A, Anis M. An overview of renal transplantation: current practice and use of ultrasound. *Semin Ultrasound CT MR* 2009 Aug; 30(4): 298–314.

12. Birnbaum L, Lipman M, Paraskevas S, et al. Management of chronic allograft nephropathy: a systematic review. *Clin J Am Soc Nephrol* 2009 Apr; 4(4): 860–865.

13. Ivanyi B. A primer on recurrent and de novo glomerulonephritis in renal allografts. *Nat Clin Pract Nephrol* 2008 Aug; 4(8): 446–457.

14. Kim D, Abouljoud M, Parasuraman R. The role of microscopic hematuria in the evaluation of urologic malignancy in renal transplant recipients. *Transplant Proc* 2010 Jun; 42(5): 1641–1642.

15. de Souza R, Olsburgh J. Urinary tract infection in the renal transplant patient. *Nat Clin Pract Nephrol* 2008 May; 4(5): 252–264.

16. Fujita S, Watanabe J, Reed A, et al. Case of emphysematous pyelonephritis in a renal allograft. *Clin Transplant* 2005 Aug; 19(4): 559–562.

17. Humar A, Matas A. Surgical complications after kidney transplantation. *Semin Dial* 2005 Nov–Dec; 18(6): 505–510.

18. Englesbe M, Dubay D, Gillespie B, et al. Risk factors for urinary complications after renal transplantation. *Am J Transplant* 2007 Jun; 7(6): 1536–1541.

19. Zietek Z, Sulikowski T, Tejchman K, et al. Lymphocele after kidney transplantation. *Transplant Proc* 2007 Nov; 39(9): 2744–2747.

20. Nast CC, Cohen AH. Pathology of kidney transplantation. In: Danovitch GM (ed.) *Handbook of Kidney Transplantation*. Philadelphia: Lippincott Williams and Wilkins; 2009: pp. 311–329.

21. Fishman J. Infection in solid-organ transplant recipients. *N Engl J Med* 2007 Dec; 357(25): 2601–2614.

22. Schnitzler M, Lowell J, Hmiel S, et al. Cytomegalovirus disease after prophylaxis with oral ganciclovir in renal transplantation: the importance of HLA-DR matching. *J Am Soc Nephrol* 2003 Mar; 14(3): 780–785.

23. Gross T, Savoldo B, Punnett A. Post-transplant lymphoproliferative diseases. *Pediatr Clin North Am* 2010 Apr; 57(2): 481–503, table of contents.

24. Ojo A. Cardiovascular complications after renal transplantation and their prevention. *Transplantation* 2006 Sep; 82(5): 603–611.

25. Rigatto C. Clinical epidemiology of cardiac disease in renal transplant recipients. *Semin Dial* 2003 Mar–Apr; 16(2): 106–110.

26. Tedla F, Hayashi R, McFarlane S, Salifu M. Hypertension after renal transplant. *J Clin Hypertens (Greenwich)* 2007 Jul; 9(7): 538–545.

27. Mignat C. Clinically significant drug interactions with new immunosuppressive agents. *Drug Saf* 1997 Apr; 16(4): 267–278.

28. Johnson P, Hogg K, Sarosi G. The rapid diagnosis of pulmonary infections in solid organ transplant recipients. *Semin Respir Infect* 1990 Mar; 5(1): 2–9.

29. Feagans J, Victor D, Moehlen M, et al. Interstitial pneumonitis in the transplant patient: consider sirolimus-associated pulmonary toxicity. *J La State Med Soc* 2009 May–Jun; 161(3): 166, 168–172.

30. Mueller N, Fishman J. Asymptomatic pulmonary cryptococcosis in solid organ transplantation: report of four cases and review of the literature. *Transpl Infect Dis* 2003 Sep; 5(3): 140–143.

31. Fishman J. Pneumocystis carinii and parasitic infections in transplantation. *Infect Dis Clin North Am* 1995 Dec; 9(4): 1005–1044.

32. American Thoracic Society and Infectious Disease Society of America. Guidelines for the management of adults with hospital-acquired, ventilator-associated, and healthcare-associated pneumonia. *Am J Respir Crit Care Med* 2005 Feb; 171(4): 388–416.

33. Mandell L, Wunderink R, Anzueto A, et al. Infectious Diseases Society of America/American Thoracic Society consensus guidelines on the management of community-acquired pneumonia in adults. *Clin Infect Dis* 2007 Mar; 44(2 Suppl.): S27–S72.

34. Uchida H, Morioka H, Ogawa N, et al. Biliary tract complications in renal allograft recipients: two case reports. *Transplant Proc* 2000 Nov; 32(7): 1898–1900.

35. Ponticelli C, Campise M. Neurological complications in kidney transplant recipients. *J Nephrol* 2005 Sep–Oct; 18(5): 521–528.

36. Wu G, Vilchez R, Eidelman B, Fung J, Kormos R, Kusne S. Cryptococcal meningitis: an analysis among 5,521 consecutive organ transplant recipients. *Transpl Infect Dis* 2002 Dec; 4(4): 183–188.

37. Holden F, Kaczmer J, Kinahan C. Listerial meningitis and renal allografts: a life-threatening affinity. *Postgrad Med* 1980 Dec; 68(6): 69–74.

38. Loren A, Porter D, Stadtmauer E, Tsai D. Post-transplant lymphoproliferative disorder: a review. *Bone Marrow Transplant* 2003 Feb; 31(3): 145–155.

39. Bechstein W. Neurotoxicity of calcineurin inhibitors: impact and clinical management. *Transpl Int* 2000; 13(5): 313–326.

40. Fukunishi I, Aikawa A, Ohara T, Hasegawa A. Psychiatric problems among recipients of kidney transplants: a 10-year follow-up. *Transplant Proc* 2002 Nov; 34(7): 2766.

41. Hong J, Kahan B. Sirolimus-induced thrombocytopenia and leukopenia in renal transplant recipients: risk factors, incidence, progression, and management. *Transplantation* 2000 May; 69(10): 2085–2090.

42. Mix T, Kazmi W, Khan S, et al. Anemia: a continuing problem following kidney transplantation. *Am J Transplant* 2003 Nov; 3(11): 1426–1433.

43. Reynolds J, Agodoa L, Yuan C, Abbott K. Thrombotic microangiopathy after renal transplantation in the United States. *Am J Kidney Dis* 2003 Nov; 42(5): 1058–1068.

44. Vlahakos D, Marathias K, Agroyannis B, Madias N. Post-transplant erythrocytosis. *Kidney Int* 2003 Apr; 63(4): 1187–1194.

45. O'Shaughnessy E, Dahl D, Smith C, Kasiske B. Risk factors for fractures in kidney transplantation. *Transplantation* 2002 Aug; 74(3): 362–366.

46. Abbott K, Koff J, Bohen E, et al. Maintenance immunosuppression use and the associated risk of avascular necrosis after kidney transplantation in the United States. *Transplantation* 2005 Feb; 79(3): 330–336.

47. Colchicine. Serious interactions. *Prescrire Int* 2008 Aug; 17(96): 151–153.

48. Basic-Jukic N, Juric I, Racki S, Kes P. Spontaneous tendon ruptures in patients with end-stage renal disease. *Kidney Blood Press Res* 2009; 32(1): 32–36.

49. Ahmadi F, Naseri R, Lessan-Pezeshki M. Relation of magnesium level to cyclosporine and metabolic complications in renal transplant recipients. *Saudi J Kidney Dis Transpl* 2009 Sep; 20(5): 766–769.

50. Bodziak K, Hricik D. New-onset diabetes mellitus after solid organ transplantation. *Transpl Int* 2009 May; 22(5): 519–530.

51. Burroughs T, Swindle J, Takemoto S, et al. Diabetic complications associated with new-onset diabetes mellitus in renal transplant recipients. *Transplantation* 2007 Apr; 83(8): 1027–1034.
52. Coursin D, Wood K. Corticosteroid supplementation for adrenal insufficiency. *JAMA* 2002 Jan; 287(2): 236–240.
53. Reese P, Blumberg E, Bloom R. Kidney transplantation in patients with HIV infection. *Adv Chronic Kidney Dis* 2010 Jan; 17(1): 94–101.
54. Schiano T, Rhodes R. Transplant tourism. *Curr Opin Organ Transplant* 2010 Apr; 15(2): 245–248.

CHAPTER 5

The end-stage renal disease patient on dialysis

K. K. Venkat[1,2] and Arvind Venkat[3,4]
[1]Henry Ford Hospital, Detroit, MI, USA
[2]Wayne State University School of Medicine, Detroit, MI, USA
[3]Allegheny General Hospital, Pittsburgh, PA, USA
[4]Drexel University College of Medicine, Philadelphia, PA, USA

Introduction and epidemiology

During the last 30 years, the incidence and prevalence of end-stage renal disease (ESRD) have increased significantly worldwide. The major factors contributing to this increase are the aging of the population, and the global epidemic of obesity and diabetes mellitus. Currently in the USA, approximately 370,000 patients are on maintenance dialysis for ESRD. Of these, more than 90% receive in-center hemodialysis (HD) at hospital-based or free-standing dialysis centers, and less than 10% dialyze at home. The vast majority of home-dialysis patients receive peritoneal dialysis (PD) [1]. The number of dialysis patients worldwide is estimated to be approximately 2 million. The distribution of patients between in-center and home-dialysis varies widely between different countries [2].

Dialysis patients are prone to a variety of medical problems that frequently bring them to the emergency department (ED). There are several factors that contribute to the ESRD patient's susceptibility to medical emergencies: the increasing age at incidence of ESRD, the susceptibility of the HD access and the PD catheter to infection, dialysis-induced rapid changes in blood chemistry and body fluid volume, greater prevalence of severe generalized vascular disease, incomplete correction of the uremic state by dialysis, and patient noncompliance with therapy [3].

This chapter presents an overview of dialysis techniques, a review of the medical problems that cause dialysis patients to present to the ED,

---

Challenging and Emerging Conditions in Emergency Medicine, First Edition. Edited by Arvind Venkat.
© 2011 by John Wiley & Sons, Ltd. Published 2011 by Blackwell Publishing Ltd.

and the special diagnostic and management considerations that emergency physicians must be aware of in caring for them.

Principles of dialysis therapy

In-center HD is generally performed three times a week on alternate days, with each session lasting 3–4 hours. Home-HD is performed more frequently (up to 6 days per week). During HD, blood is drawn into an extracorporeal circuit and passed through a dialyzer ("artificial kidney") made of a semipermeable membrane [4, 5]. During HD, the patient's blood is drawn into the dialysis circuit through a variety of vascular accesses (Figure 5.1) [6].

Nitrogenous uremic waste, potassium, magnesium, and phosphate leave the blood down the concentration gradient across the semipermeable dialyzer membrane into the dialysis fluid (dialysate) flowing on the other side of membrane, whereas calcium and bicarbonate (in higher concentration in the dialysate) move into the circulation in the reverse direction. These processes partially correct the ESRD-associated biochemical abnormalities. Simultaneously, HD corrects ESRD-associated fluid overload by removing salt and water from the patient, aiming to bring down the patient's weight to the clinically estimated "dry weight" (weight at which the patient is euvolemic) by the end of each HD session [4].

In PD, access to the peritoneal cavity is provided by an implanted catheter (Figure 5.2).

Continuous ambulatory PD (CAPD) is performed manually by the patient, usually four times (exchanges) per day. During each exchange,

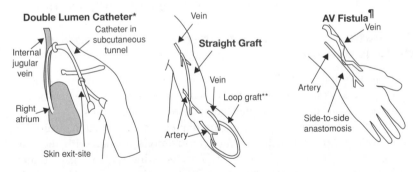

Figure 5.1 Accesses used for long-term hemodialysis. *Tunneled catheters can also be placed in the femoral vein or the inferior vena cava. **Forearm grafts can also be straight. Loop grafts can also be placed in the thigh. ¶AV fistula can also be created at the elbow. (Reprinted with permission from Venkat A, Kaufmann KR, Venkat K. Care of the end-stage renal disease patient on dialysis in the ED. *Am J Emerg Med* 2006; 24(7): 847–858.)

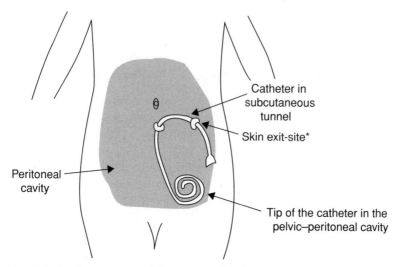

Figure 5.2 Surgical anatomy of the peritoneal dialysis catheter. *The skin exit site is usually in the right or left lower abdominal quadrant, but less commonly may be placed above the level of the umbilicus. (Reprinted with permission from Venkat A, Kaufmann KR, Venkat K. Care of the end-stage renal disease patient on dialysis in the ED. *Am J Emerg Med* 2006; 24(7): 847–858.)

dialysate (2 to 3 L) is infused through the catheter, allowed to dwell in the peritoneal cavity for several hours followed by draining out of the used dialysate. In the PD variant called "continuous cycling PD" (CCPD), a machine containing dialysate bags is connected to the PD catheter and multiple exchanges are completed as the patient sleeps, supplemented if necessary by one or two manual exchanges during the daytime [7].

Evaluation and initial management of the febrile dialysis patient

Fever in the dialysis patient may be due to any of the causes that apply to the general population with the caveat that HD access infection or PD-associated peritonitis are the major diagnostic considerations.

HD catheters are associated with the highest risk of infection, arteriovenous grafts with intermediate, and arteriovenous fistulae with the lowest risk. Local signs of infection (tenderness/redness/warmth/fluctuance over the access and/or purulent drainage from the cutaneous exit of the catheter spontaneously or after application of pressure along the catheter tunnel) should be sought in febrile HD patients, but the absence of these signs does not rule out access-related infection. Infection of the HD access is associated with the risk of hematogenous dissemination of infection potentially causing septic pulmonary emboli with multiple nodular and/or cavitary lung lesions, endocarditis, septic arthritis, vertebral osteomylitis,

Table 5.1 Microbiology of hemodialysis access infection and recommended initial antibiotic therapy

Organism (reported frequency in different series)	Initial presumptive antibiotic therapy
1. Coagulase-negative staphylococci and *Staphlococcus aureus* (40% to 80%)	Vancomycin 20 mg/kg intravenously over 30 to 60 minutes
2. *Enterococcus* species (2% to 20%)	*combined with*
3. Gram-negative bacilli (5% to 40%)	Gentamicin 1.0 to 2.0 mg/kg intravenously
4. Fungal and other organisms (rare)	*or*
(a) Single causative organism identified in 80% to 90% of patients	A third-generation cephalosporin (cefepime or ceftazidime 1 to 2 g intravenously)
(b) Polymicrobial infection identified in 10% to 20% of patients	

intervertebral diskitis and/or epidural abscess $\pm$ spinal cord compression. Evaluation of the febrile HD patient should include blood cultures, Gram's stain/culture of drainage at the exit site of the catheter and chest X-ray. Severely septic patients with hemodynamic compromise may require emergent removal of the catheter/graft/fistula by the access-surgery team. Echocardiography looking for vegetations, imaging studies to identify spine infection, and arthrocentesis to diagnose septic arthritis may be indicated in selected patients [8, 9].

The microbiological spectrum of HD-access infection and the recommended initial empiric therapy (after obtaining appropriate cultures) are shown in Table 5.1 [3, 10].

Less common HD-related causes of fever include lymphokine generation due to contact of blood with the dialyzer membrane, febrile reaction to blood products administered during dialysis, and endotoxemia from contaminated dialysis fluid [3]. However, these are diagnoses of exclusion, and fever should generally be assumed to be secondary to access-related infection. Febrile HD patients usually require hospitalization.

PD-associated peritonitis is usually due to spread of cutaneous organisms along the PD catheter. Less commonly, it may be caused by an intra-abdominal source such as diverticulitis, appendicitis, visceral perforation, or bowel infarction. It should be remembered that absence of fever does not rule out peritonitis since 40%–50% of such patients are afebrile. Diffuse abdominal pain/tenderness, cloudy dialysate, nausea, vomiting, diarrhea, and/or constipation are other presenting features. Severe peritonitis can cause paralytic ileus and/or septic shock. PD catheter cutaneous exit site or subcutaneous tunnel infection (suggested by purulent drainage from the exit site upon application of pressure along the tunnel) may predispose to peritonitis [11].

Table 5.2 Microbiology of peritoneal dialysis-associated peritonitis and recommended initial antibiotic therapy

Organism (reported frequency)	Initial presumptive antibiotic therapy
1. *Gram-positive organisms (50% to 60%):* Predominantly coagulase-negative staphylococci and *Staphylococcus aureus*, with a minority due to *Enterococcus* species, β-hemolytic streptococcus and *Corynebacterium* species	Intra-peritoneal vancomycin 2 g *combined with* Gentamicin 0.6 mg/kg *or* A third-generation cephalosporin (cefepime 1 g *or* ceftazidime 1 g) The two antibiotics are added to the same bag of peritoneal dialysis fluid. The
2. Gram-negative organisms (up to 20%)	antibiotic-containing dialysate is infused
3. Sterile/culture-negative (up to 20%)	intra-peritoneally over 15 to 30 min and
4. Polymicrobial—Gram-positive + Gram-negative + anerobes (up to 5%)	allowed to dwell in the peritoneal cavity for 6 h.
5. Fungal, mycobacterial, etc. (less than 2%)	

When PD-associated peritonitis is suspected, effluent dialysate should be sent for total and differential WBC count, Gram's stain, and aerobic and anaerobic cultures. Dialysate WBC count > 50 to 100 cells/mm^3 suggests peritonitis. In untreated bacterial peritonitis, dialysate WBC count is typically in thousands/mm^3 with neutrophilic predominance. Any drainage from the exit site should be submitted for Gram's stain and culture. Injecting dialysate into blood culture bottles increases the diagnostic yield. Polymicrobial peritonitis (mixture of Gram-positive and negative organisms) suggests and growth of anaerobes in dialysate culture is virtually diagnostic of an intra-abdominal source of peritonitis. Imaging studies should include plain abdominal X-rays and (in severe cases) CT [3, 11]. It should be remembered that small amounts of free air may be normally present in upright plain-abdominal X-rays in PD patients due to air entry during PD exchanges. However, if the height of the infradiaphragmatic air column is >5 mm, visceral perforation is more likely [12]. Initial management of PD-associated peritonitis includes parenteral narcotics for pain control and intra-peritoneal antibiotics (after obtaining dialysate cell count and cultures). The microbial spectrum of and the recommended initial empiric therapy for PD-associated peritonitis are shown in Table 5.2 [13].

Clinically severe peritonitis or suspected intra-abdominal source of infection should lead to prompt surgical consultation because emergent catheter removal and/or exploratory laparotomy may be required [3, 11]. Unless the peritonitis is mild (which can be managed as an outpatient in consultation with the nephrology team), the patient should be hospitalized.

Management of the dialysis patient presenting with cardiorespiratory and blood pressure-related problems

Chest pain

The very high prevalence of coronary artery disease in the dialysis patient should be remembered in evaluating chest pain in this population. Cardiovascular disorders account for approximately 50% of all mortality in dialysis patients. Compared to an age-matched general population, the cardiovascular risk is 10- to 100-fold higher in dialysis patients [14]. A high index of suspicion for an acute coronary event and a lower threshold for noninvasive testing and inpatient observation, however atypical the presentation, are appropriate in dialysis patients.

The interpretation of tests commonly used to evaluate acute coronary events is confounded in dialysis patients by the frequently present baseline EKG changes, due to left ventricular hypertrophy or electrolyte abnormalities, and elevated baseline cardiac troponin levels (due to the combination of cardiac hypertrophy and decreased renal excretion). Stress testing is limited by the inability of many dialysis patients to exercise. This frequently necessitates pharmacologic stress testing [14].

Several medications used in treating acute coronary syndromes may require dose modification in dialysis patients. Among the β-blockers, only atenolol requires dose reduction in ESRD patients. Enoxaparin is not recommended in this population because it is cleared by the kidneys. If used, it should be given at half the usual dose. Among the platelet glycoprotein IIb/IIIa inhibitors, eptifibatide is contraindicated in ESRD patients because of its renal excretion, tirofiban requires 50% dose reduction, and abciximab is preferred because no adjustment is required [15].

Uremic pericarditis should be considered in the differential diagnosis of retrosternal pain in the dialysis patient. Aggravation of pain by inspiration, and relief by sitting up and leaning forward are suggestive of pericardial pain. Pericarditis may cause fever. The presence of a pericardial rub supports the diagnosis. However, the rub may disappear once significant effusion develops. Pericardial effusion causes cardiac enlargement with a globular configuration on chest X-ray. The dreaded complication of pericardial effusion is cardiac tamponade. Relative or absolute hypotension, muffled heart sounds, elevated jugular venous pressure, and/or pulsus paradoxus are the manifestations of cardiac tamponade. However, the definitive test for tamponade is echocardiography, which should be performed urgently if this diagnosis is suspected. Patients with uremic pericarditis need hospitalization for intensive dialysis and close observation for development of tamponade. Patients presenting with tamponade require prompt cardiac surgery consultation for emergent surgical drainage by creation of a pericardial window, and should be admitted to an intensive care unit pending surgery. If emergent pericardiocentesis is required, the pericardial cavity should be continuously drained externally with a catheter, to prevent recurrence of tamponade secondary to intra-pericardial bleeding [16].

Dyspnea

The differential diagnostic approach to dyspnea in dialysis patients is similar to that in the general population with the caveat that fluid overload/pulmonary edema/acute left ventricular failure is a major cause. Most dialysis patients are oligo-anuric with markedly limited ability to excrete excess dietary salt and water. A number of factors may precipitate acute pulmonary edema in dialysis patients: excessive intake of salt and water especially over the weekend which involves an extra day without dialysis, missing HD sessions or PD exchanges, inadequate salt/water removal during HD and PD due to technical problems or overestimation of dry weight, and acute left ventricular dysfunction. Even in dialysis patients with dyspnea due to respiratory causes such as asthma, bronchitis, emphysema, pneumonia, or pulmonary embolism, fluid overload may be adding to the dyspnea caused by the primary pulmonary disorder [3, 17]. Brain natriuretic (BNP) level is unreliable as a diagnostic marker for heart failure/fluid overload in dialysis patients since other factors such as increased production secondary to cardiac hypertrophy and decreased renal excretion contribute to elevated BNP level in this population [18].

It should be remembered that even high-dose intravenous loop-diuretic therapy may be ineffective in relieving fluid overload in dialysis patients because most of them are oligo-anuric. Thus, the only effective treatment for the fluid-overloaded dialysis patient is urgent dialysis. Until dialysis can be started, therapy should consist of supplemental oxygen, hypertension control, treatment of arrhythmias and acute coronary event (if present), and preload reduction with intravenous or cutaneous nitrates [3]. Intubation and ventilatory support should be provided according to standard indications.

Despite the presence of uremia-associated qualitative platelet dysfunction, venous thrombosis and pulmonary embolism do occur in dialysis patients [3]. Pleural effusion of different etiologies (hydrothorax secondary to fluid overload, uremic pleurisy, infection, or malignancy) may cause dyspnea in dialysis patients. Fluid removal during dialysis is generally ineffective in decreasing the size of pleural effusions; thoracentesis may be required for relief of dyspnea [3]. In PD patients, transdiaphragmatic leakage of dialysate into the pleural cavity has been reported. The pleural fluid can be identified as dialysate by its much higher glucose concentration compared to the blood glucose level [19].

Fluid overload is less common in PD patients since fluid removal is continuous in this modality. However, noncompliance with PD exchanges or technical problems with fluid removal ("ultrafiltration failure") may result in fluid overload. Since fluid removal by PD is slow, a severely fluid overloaded PD patient may require temporary HD for rapid fluid removal [3].

Hypotension

Intra-dialytic hypotension during HD is a common problem occurring in 10% to 50% of patients. The major causative factor is rapid removal of salt and water during dialysis compounded by rapid changes in plasma osmolality, uremic and/or diabetic autonomic neuropathy, or intake of antihypertensive medications immediately before dialysis [20]. Intra-dialytic hypotension may result in the cessation of HD and transport of patient to the ED. The possibility of cardiac tamponade secondary to a pericardial effusion should be entertained in such patients. Other causes of hypotension such as acute myocardial infarction, and septic or anaphylactic shock also need to be excluded. The initial management of the hypotensive dialysis patient is the intravenous bolus administration of 250 to 500 mL of normal saline while watching for the development of fluid overload [3]. Acute hypotension is less common in PD patients since fluid removal is slow and continuous.

Severe hypotension in dialysis patients may necessitate the use of vasopressors. All currently available vasopressors can be used in ESRD patients. However, the greater risk of sympathomimetic pressor agents triggering arrhythmias in this population should be remembered [21].

Syncope

A common cause of syncope in dialysis patients is intra-dialytic hypotension [3]. Syncope ($\pm$ seizure) may occur during or upon standing up at the end of dialysis. Although less common, the possibility of syncope secondary to a potentially life-threatening arrhythmia such as transient ventricular tachycardia or fibrillation will have to be kept in mind given the high prevalence of coronary artery disease in ESRD patients [21]. Sudden cardiac death due to such an arrhythmia is not uncommon in dialysis patients [22]. Unless it is clear that transient hypotension caused syncope, hospitalization for cardiac monitoring is advisable.

Uncontrolled hypertension

Up to 85% of dialysis patients are chronically hypertensive, and hypertensive emergency/urgency is a commonly encountered problem in them. The major mechanism underlying hypertension in ESRD patients is salt and water excess. Thus, failure to achieve dry weight during and/or missing dialysis treatments as well as dietary salt/water excess are important contributors to hypertension in this population [23].

The treatment of hypertensive urgency/emergency in the dialysis patient is the same as in the general population, with no contraindication to the use of any of the antihypertensives used in the latter. However, the following points are worth remembering [24]:

1. Diuretics are not effective in lowering BP in oligo-anuric dialysis patients.
2. Risk of nitroprusside-associated cyanide toxicity is greater in patients with impaired renal function.
3. While sudden cessation of any antihypertensive agent might cause rebound hypertension, abrupt clonidine withdrawal is associated with the highest risk.
4. Sudden β-blocker withdrawal may precipitate arrhythmias and/or acute coronary events.

Emergent gastrointestinal problems in dialysis patients

Upper or lower gastrointestinal bleeding

The etiology of gastrointestinal hemorrhage in the ESRD patient is similar to that in the general population. However, bleeding tends to be more severe and transfusion requirements are greater in the dialysis patient because of uremic qualitative platelet dysfunction, heparin administration during dialysis, presence of uremic gastritis and colitis, and preexisting anemia of chronic kidney disease. When administering saline and/or blood to a dialysis patient with gastrointestinal bleeding, one should watch for volume overload and hyperkalemia (stored blood has high potassium content) [3]. Persistent bleeding may require rapid correction of uremic platelet dysfunction. Options include intravenous desmopressin/DDAVP, 0.3 to 0.4 mcg/kg over 20 to 30 minutes (the most commonly utilized treatment), and transfusion of fresh platelets or cryoprecipitate. Slower correction over days can be achieved by daily HD and/or administration of conjugated estrogens (0.6 mg/kg daily for 5 days) [25].

Abdominal pain

The differential diagnosis of abdominal in the dialysis patient is not different from that in the general population. However, the following points are worth emphasizing:

1. In PD patients, peritonitis is a major cause of abdominal pain.
2. As already discussed, subdiaphragmatic free air is not a reliable radiological sign of visceral perforation in PD patients.
3. Development of hernias due to increased intra-abdominal pressure is not uncommon in PD patients, and the possibility of abdominal pain due to an incarcerated hernia will have to considered [19].
4. The incidence and severity of acute pancreatitis are increased in ESRD patients [26]. Baseline serum amylase and lipase levels may be elevated in dialysis patients (due to their decreased urinary excretion) and a

greater than threefold elevation of these enzyme levels is required to definitively diagnose pancreatitis [3].

5. In patients with ESRD secondary to autosomal dominant polycystic kidney disease (ADPKD), there is increased prevalence of colonic diverticulosis with attendant risks of diverticulitis and colonic bleeding [27].

6. The combination of severe generalized vascular disease and intradialytic hypotension may cause bowel infarction and abdominal pain in dialysis patients [28].

Approach to worsening anemia in the dialysis patient

Chronic kidney disease-related anemia is present in most dialysis patients. Current erythropoietin-dose guidelines recommend only partial correction of this anemia (target hemoglobin level 11 to 12 g/dL) [29]. A common problem encountered in ED in the dialysis patient is a decreased hemoglobin level compared to recent values. The most common cause of this is blood loss. Uremic platelet dysfunction and heparinization during HD increase the risk of bleeding from different anatomical sites [3]. Two other sources of blood loss in ESRD patients are intra-dialytic complications (e.g., blood clotting in the extracorporeal circuit secondary to inadequate anticoagulation or accidental disconnection of blood lines) [3] and retroperitoneal or intra-renal hemorrhage (spontaneously or as a complication of hereditary or acquired renal cysts) [30]. CT of the abdomen to rule out intra-abdominal bleeding is indicated when there is an unexplained drop in the hemoglobin level in dialysis patients.

Evaluation of the dialysis patient with neurological problems

Presentation of the dialysis patient to the ED with neurological complaints such as headache, symptoms of global encephalopathy (mental status changes and/or depressed level of consciousness), seizures, and/or focal neurological deficits (e.g., hemiplegia) is common [3, 31].

Patients started on HD with severe azotemia (BUN level >150 mg/dL) may experience "dialysis disequilibrium" characterized by headache, global encephalopathy, and (in severe cases) seizures/coma/fatal tentorial herniation, during or after the initial few HD sessions. This syndrome is attributed to rapid decrease in serum osmolality due to removal by HD of osmotically active uremic toxins from the blood with consequent shift of water into relatively hyperosmolar brain tissue. The mildest form of this syndrome (recurrent dialysis-related headache) is still seen, but the more severe manifestations have become rare due to increased awareness of this complication and reduction of delivered dialysis-dose during the initial HD sessions. Dialysis disequilibrium is uncommon in PD patients due to slower removal of uremic waste, which avoids rapid changes in serum osmolality [32].

Another cause of headache, global encephalopathy, and/or seizures in dialysis patients is hypertensive encephalopathy. As already discussed, seizures could also be caused by cerebral ischemia secondary to intra-dialytic hypotension. Global encephalopathy may also result from uremia due to inadequate dialysis, sepsis, hypercalcemia, hypoglycemia, dysna-tremias, hepatic or respiratory failure, meningoencephalitides, and fail-ure to decrease doses of drugs that accumulate in renal failure (e.g., meperidine, penicillins, cephalosporins, acyclovir, amantadine, cimetidine, etc.). Wernicke's encephalopathy secondary to thiamine deficiency has been reported in malnourished dialysis patients. Dialysis dementia at-tributed to aluminum accumulation in the brain has become uncommon with avoidance of chronic aluminum exposure resulting from aluminum-containing phosphate-binders and aluminum-contaminated water for dialysate preparation [3, 31].

Focal neurological deficits (and/or headache) may be the result of a sub-dural hematoma (SDH). The incidence of SDH is increased in dialysis pa-tients due to qualitative platelet dysfunction and heparin administration during dialysis. SDH can occur in ESRD patients without significant head trauma. Chronic dementia secondary to SDH has also been reported [33]. The threshold for neuroimaging to rule out SDH should be low in dialysis patients.

Since cerebral atherosclerosis and hypertension are more prevalent in dialysis patients, cerebrovascular accidents occur commonly with resul-tant focal deficits such as hemiplegia [34]. Even though uremic platelet dysfunction is common in dialysis patients, there is no absolute contraindi-cation to systemic thrombolytic therapy in the ESRD patient presenting with an ischemic stroke [35]. Multi-infarct dementia secondary to cere-bral atherosclerosis is commonly encountered in older dialysis patients [3]. Uremic peripheral neuropathy may cause numbness and (less commonly) motor weakness of distal parts of the extremities or the "restless legs" syndrome [31].

Commonly encountered acid–base and electrolyte disorders in dialysis patients

Uremic, high anion-gap metabolic acidosis

Uremic, high anion-gap metabolic acidosis is corrected during HD by movement of bicarbonate from the dialysate into the blood stream. Af-ter HD there may be transient overcorrection of the acidosis with mild metabolic alkalosis lasting a few hours [3]. Acidosis redevelops over the subsequent 48–72 hours until the next HD. Patients on CAPD have more stable acid–base status due to the continuous correction of acidosis. In HD patients, pre-dialysis acidosis is usually mild with serum bicarbonate levels >15 mmol/L. If a dialysis patient presents with more severe metabolic acidosis (pH <7.15 and/or serum bicarbonate <12 mmol/L), presence of another type of acidosis compounding uremic acidosis will have to be considered (e.g., lactic acidosis, ketoacidosis, volatile alcohol or salicylate poisoning, or respiratory acidosis) [3]. In dialysis patients, intravenous sodium bicarbonate therapy should be used only for severe acidosis and only partial correction acidosis (to pH >7.20) should be attempted because overzealous use of intravenous sodium bicarbonate may cause pulmonary edema, symptomatic hypocalcemia (since rapid increase in pH decreases serum ionized calcium level) and/or hypernatremia [36,37].

Hyperkalemia

Hyperkalemia is more common in HD than in CAPD patients because in the former potassium removal occurs only during dialysis every 48 to 72 hours whereas in PD there is continuous potassium removal. In fact, CAPD patients may require oral potassium supplements to avoid hypokalemia. Fortunately, hyperkalemia is mild (<5.5 to 6.0 mmol/L) in most HD patients. However, dietary potassium excess, use of potassium-rich salt substitutes, severe hyperglycemia and/or acidosis, missing dialysis, prolonged fasting causing suppressed insulin secretion, release of intracellular potassium into the circulation due to severe catabolism (trauma, major surgery, and/or sepsis) or red cell lysis (intravascular hemolysis or breakdown of RBCs in large hematomas), and/or the use of angiotensin-converting enzyme inhibitor or angiotensin-receptor blocker or potassium supplements may cause severe hyperkalemia in dialysis patients [3].

Hyperkalemia >6.5 to 7.0 mmol/L may cause generalized muscle weakness, and the EKG usually shows progressive changes (peaked T waves, prolonged PR interval, disappearance of P waves, widened QRS with a "sine-wave" pattern, and eventual asystole), correlating with increasing serum potassium level. However, even severe hyperkalemia may be totally asymptomatic with a normal EKG, which can evolve directly into asystole. Therefore, therapy for hyperkalemia should be based not just on EKG changes but also on the actual serum potassium level. If serum potassium is >7.0 mmol/L it is advisable to give intravenous calcium even if the EKG is normal to counter the cardiac effects of hyperkalemia. Intravenous hypertonic glucose (50 mL of 50% dextrose), if the patient is not already hyperglycemic, together with 5 to 10 units of intravenous regular insulin is used to shift potassium into the cells and lower the serum potassium to a safer level within 30 minutes. Intravenous or inhaled β-sympathetic agonists (albuterol, terbutaline, or epinephrine) also lower the serum potassium rapidly. Patients who are given β-sympathetic agonists should be monitored for acute coronary syndromes or serious cardiac arrhythmias. Intravenous sodium bicarbonate is not effective in lowering potassium levels except in the very uncommon setting of inorganic metabolic acidosis [38, 39]. Cation-exchange resin (sodium polystyrene sulfonate/Kayexalate®) is used widely to achieve more prolonged (6–12 hours) lowering of serum potassium level. However, both the efficacy and safety (risk of bowel necrosis, perforation, and/or stenosis) of cation-exchange resin therapy have been questioned recently [40]. The above-mentioned treatments are only temporizing measures. To minimize the risk of rebound hyperkalemia, the severely hyperkalemic ESRD patient should generally be hospitalized for dialysis as soon as possible [3]. In the uncommon event of a CAPD patient presenting with severe hyperkalemia, it is better to perform temporary HD because PD does not lower the serum potassium level rapidly.

ESRD-associated hypocalcemia

ESRD-associated hypocalcemia is corrected with supplements of calcium and active vitamin-D analogs, and by the intra-dialytic calcium flux from the dialysate into the patient [41]. The risk of precipitating tetany by the rapid correction of metabolic acidosis with intravenous sodium bicarbonate in dialysis patients has been mentioned earlier. Rapid remineralization of bone following subtotal parathyroidectomy for severe secondary hyperparathyroidism of CKD may cause symptomatic hypocalcemia—"hungry bone syndrome". In a patient with history of recent parathyroidectomy and symptoms of hypocalcemia/tetany, this diagnosis will have to be considered and intravenous calcium infusion and calcitriol administration may be required to correct hypocalcemia rapidly [42].

Hypercalcemia

Hypercalcemia is uncommon in dialysis patients and may be due to blood sampling within a few hours after HD (transient overcorrection of hypocalcemia by calcium influx from the dialysate), severe secondary hyperparathyroidism of CKD, excessive doses of active vitamin D metabolites, and/or causes of hypercalcemia not unique to CKD (e.g., malignancy, and granulomatous disorders) [3].

ESRD-associated hyperphosphatemia

ESRD-associated hyperphosphatemia is only partially corrected by dialysis and the use of oral phosphate binders. Thus, asymptomatic hyperphosphatemia is common in dialysis patients [41]. However, severe hyperphosphatemia (serum phosphorous >10 to 15 mg/dL) may develop if a dialysis patient ingests sodium phosphate as a laxative or in preparation for colonoscopy. Severe hyperphosphatemia can cause life-threatening hypocalcemia and widespread soft tissue calcification. The only effective way to rapidly correct severe hyperphosphatemia is intensive HD [3].

Hypermagnesemia

Hypermagnesemia (magnesium level 2.0 to 3.0 mg/dL) is common in HD patients. This degree of hypermagnesemia is asymptomatic [43]. However, intake of medications with high magnesium content (e.g., magnesium-containing antacids, laxatives, or magnesium sulfate enema) may cause dangerous hypermagnesemia resulting in flaccid, ascending skeletal muscle paralysis, bradycardia, respiratory paralysis, and obtundation. Serum magnesium and potassium levels must be checked in dialysis patients with muscle weakness. Initial therapy for symptomatic hypermagnesemia is intravenous calcium (similar to treatment of hyperkalemia) while awaiting emergent HD for magnesium removal from the body [3].

Hypokalemia, hypophosphatemia and hypomagnesemia

Hypokalemia, hypophosphatemia, and hypomagnesemia are rare in HD patients. Initial replacement doses of potassium, magnesium, and phosphorous are the same in the ESRD patient compared to patients with normal renal function. However, long-term therapy with potassium, magnesium, and/or phosphorous supplements is not safe in ESRD patients unless blood levels are closely monitored [3].

Hyponatremia

Hyponatremia (serum sodium 130 to 135 mEq/L) is common in ESRD patients and is due to excess water intake in the setting of low urine output. This mild, chronic hyponatremia is generally asymptomatic and should not be corrected rapidly. Hyponatremia is partially corrected during HD because of the higher sodium concentration in the dialysate (140 mEq/L) [3].

Special considerations in the management of diabetes-related emergencies in dialysis patients

Diabetic nephropathy is the etiology of ESRD in approximately 40% of dialysis patients [3]. Presentation of the diabetic dialysis patient to the ED with markedly elevated blood glucose (with or without ketoacidosis) or severe hypoglycemia is common.

While insulin therapy of the diabetic patient with hyperglycemia is similar to that in the non-renal population, several special considerations apply [44]:

1. In the oligo-anuric HD patient, urinary losses of sodium, water, potassium, phosphorous, and magnesium (caused by glucosuria) will not occur. Therefore, intravenous saline, bicarbonate, potassium, magnesium, and phosphorous administration have to be cautious with close monitoring of volume status and blood chemistries. In fact, hyperglycemia-induced increase in serum osmolality with attendant shift of water from

the cells into the circulation causing acute pulmonary edema has been reported [45].

2. The high glucose content of peritoneal dialysate may contribute to hyperglycemia in PD patients. However, because salt, water and electrolyte removal is continuous during PD, intravenous fluid and electrolyte replacement can be more liberal in these patients [3].

3. ESRD patients lack the normal renal catabolism and excretion of insulin, and therefore, are more sensitive to the effects of insulin necessitating moderation in insulin dosing (initial dose 50%–75% of that used in the general population).

4. The use of icodextrin-containing peritoneal dialysate may cause spurious hyperglycemia when blood glucose level is checked with glucose dehydrogenase test strips. This is because icodextrin absorbed from the dialysate is metabolized to maltose which cross-reacts with glucose dehydrogenase test strips. Patients should be questioned about the use of icodextrin-containing dialysate and in such patients glucose oxidase or hexokinase test strips should be preferentially used or blood glucose level should be checked by laboratory measurement to avoid inappropriate treatment of spuriously elevated blood glucose level [46].

In ESRD patients, hypoglycemia secondary to insulin or oral hypoglycemic drugs tends to be more prolonged than in the non-renal population because the renal catabolism and/or excretion of these drugs is impaired [44]. Thus, longer observation for recurrence of hypoglycemia after treatment is warranted in dialysis patients and hospitalization for prolonged intravenous 10% dextrose administration may be required. Spontaneous hypoglycemia has been reported in malnourished, non-diabetic ESRD patients [3].

Problems related to the urinary tract in dialysis patients

If a dialysis patient presents with pain over the kidney(s) and/or gross hematuria, in addition to pyelonephritis and nephrolithiasis, the possibility of polycystic kidney disease causing these symptoms will have to be considered. Polycystic disease may be hereditary (ADPKD) or acquired ("degenerative" cysts developing in previously non-polycystic end-stage kidneys). Either type of cysts can be complicated by infection, intra-cystic or retroperitoneal hemorrhage, and development of adenoma or carcinoma within the cysts [30]. CT is the preferred technique for the initial evaluation of these cyst-related complications.

Sterile pyuria may occur in oligo-anuric dialysis patients and does not necessarily indicate urinary infection [47]. Stasis of small volumes of urine in the bladder might be complicated by infection and pyocystis. Since such a patient may not void urine spontaneously, bladder catheterization to obtain urine for culture is indicated in the workup of the febrile, oligo-anuric patient [3].

Special considerations regarding the HD vascular access in the ED

A number of points are worth emphasizing regarding the HD access (external catheter, arteriovenous graft, or fistula) in the patient presenting to the ED:

1. Use of the HD access for drawing blood or administration of parenteral fluids or medication should be avoided, except as a last resort in settings such as cardiopulmonary resuscitation. If a dialysis catheter is used as a venous access, 5 mL of blood should first be drawn out of the catheter and discarded to remove the heparinized saline or sodium citrate with which these catheters are "locked" after dialysis.
2. Blood pressure should not be measured in the extremity with an arteriovenous access to avoid occlusion and thrombosis of the access.
3. If there is no palpable thrill or bruit over the arteriovenous access, thrombosis of the access should be diagnosed, and surgical consultation for prompt declotting is required.
4. Access-related venous thrombosis or stenosis may cause unilateral edema of the extremity, and Doppler venous imaging is indicated. In patients with central venous catheters, right atrial thrombosis, or superior vena cava thrombosis and/or stenosis may develop. These vena caval problems might cause facial and bilateral upper extremity edema.
5. Creation of an arteriovenous access in an extremity may be followed by the "steal syndrome" (diversion of blood flow through the access causing distal ischemia) with numbness and coldness of the fingers.
6. HD patients may return to the ED with bleeding from access needle puncture sites. Initial therapy consists of manual pressure without complete occlusion of the access, and topical thrombin or gelfoam. If bleeding persists, surgical intervention is indicated.
7. Localized aneurysms may develop in long-standing arteriovenous accesses. Aneurysmal rupture can cause life-threatening hemorrhage. Immediate complete occlusion of the access with a tourniquet and surgical intervention are mandatory [3, 6].

Emergencies related to intra-dialytic accidents

The safety systems built into modern HD equipment have made life-threatening complications secondary to intra-dialytic accidents (e.g., air embolism, intravascular hemolysis due to copper or cupramine contamination of dialysate, and severe dysnatremia due to incorrect dialysate sodium level) very rare. Anaphylactoid reaction to either residual disinfectant in the dialyzer or to polyacrylonitrile dialyzer membrane (in ACE-inhibitor-treated patients) occur rarely [48, 49].

Approach to the dialysis patient presenting with joint or musculoskeletal problems

Dialysis patients are prone to a variety of articular and musculoskeletal problems. Acute monoarthritis or polyarthritis in dialysis patients is usually due to pseudogout, gout, or septic arthritis due to hematogenous spread of access infection. Prompt arthrocentesis with analysis of the aspirate for total and differential WBC count, crystals, Gram's stain and culture is indicated. Other causes of joint pains in the ESRD patient include periarticular bone resorption as a result of secondary hyperparathyroidism or periarticular deposition of dialysis-related β-2 microglobulin amyloid. Renal osteodystrophy also increases the susceptibility to fractures and rupture of tendons, particularly the Achilles and patellar tendons [50]. Tendon rupture is best diagnosed by soft tissue ultrasonography or MRI [3].

Calciphylaxis

This is the major dermatological emergency likely to be encountered in dialysis patients and warrants hospitalization. It is most commonly seen in obese, diabetic women. Presentation is with painful, red nodules in the lower abdomen, buttocks, thighs, and/or legs that ulcerate quickly with black eschar formation. Hyperphosphatemia and/or secondary hyperparathyroidism causing cutaneous arteriolar calcification with downstream ischemic necrosis is the suggested pathogenic mechanism [51].

Issues regarding choice of diagnostic tests and medications in dialysis patients

Radiological imaging studies involving the intravascular administration of iodinated contrast (e.g., CT, arteriography) are frequently required in the ED. Iodinated contrast-induced acute kidney injury is not a concern in the oligo-anuric ESRD patient on dialysis. However, in the minority of dialysis patients with daily urine output >1 L, contrast may have to be avoided to preserve residual renal function. Pulmonary edema following administration of hyperosmolar contrast is rare even in oligo-anuric dialysis patients [3].

Gadolinium use for MRI is contraindicated in patients with advanced CKD (GFR <30 mL/min/1.73 m^2) and in dialysis patients because of the known association of gadolinium use with the development of nephrogenic systemic fibrosis [52].

Table 5.3 Dose-adjustment for commonly used medications in dialysis patients

1. **Anticoagulation:** No dose adjustment for *heparin*. *Enoxaparin* accumulates—use is not recommended
2. **Antihypertensives/diuretics:** No dose adjustment except for the following:
   (a) *Angiotensin-converting enzyme inhibitors (except fosinopril):* Initial dose to be reduced by 50%. No dose adjustment for angiotensin-receptor blockers
   (b) *Atenolol:* Initial dose to be decreased by 50%. No dose adjustment for other β-blockers
   (c) *Furosemide:* Not effective unless patient has residual urine output greater than 1 L/day. Maximum single dose: 240 to 320 mg PO or 160–240 mg IV—risk of transient deafness with higher doses
3. **Analgesics:**
   (a) *Nonsteroidal anti-inflammatory drugs and COX-2 inhibitors:* Best avoided—increased risk of gastrointestinal bleeding
   (b) *Meperidine:* Contraindicated—its metabolite, normeperidine, accumulates causing encephalopathy and/or seizure
   (c) *Morphine, hydromorphone, oxymorphone, codein, methadone:* initial dose to be reduced by ∼50%. No accumulation, but possible increased sensitivity to neuro-depressive effect
4. **Anticonvulsants:**
   (a) *Phenytoin:* No dose adjustment. Free (not total) blood level to be checked because of decreased protein-binding of the drug in renal failure
   (b) *Gabapentin:* Dose to be reduced to 300 mg once daily or 300 mg after each hemodialysis—risk of neurological and other adverse effects
5. **Antimicrobials:**
   (a) *Gentamicin/tobramycin:* No modification in loading dose (1.0 to 1.7 mg/kg). Subsequent dosing only after each hemodialysis treatment or based on blood levels in peritoneal dialysis patients, to avoid vestibular toxicity
   (b) *Cephalosporins:* 1 g daily or 2 g after each hemodialysis. Risk of encephalopathy and/or seizures with standard dose
   (c) *Pencilillin, ampicillin, ticarcillin, pipracillin:* Dose reduction by 50% to avoid risk of encephalopathy and/or seizures. No dose adjustment needed for *oxacillin*
   (d) *Nitofurantoin:* Contraindicated—increased risk of neuropathy
   (e) *Quinolones (ciprofloxacin, levofloxacin, ciprofloxacin, ofloxacin):* Reduce dose by 50%. No dose adjustment needed for *moxifloxacin*
   (f) *Vancomycin:* No change in loading dose—15 to 20 mg/kg IV. Subsequent dosing only after each hemodialysis treatment or based on blood levels in peritoneal dialysis patients to avoid ototoxicity
   (g) *Acyclovir: Herpes simplex*—200 mg twice daily oral; *Herpes zoster* 800 mg twice daily oral. Risk of neuropsychiatric adverse effects with standard dose
   (h) *Valacyclovir:* 500 mg oral only after each hemodialysis. Risk of neuropsychiatric adverse effects with standard dose
6. **Miscellaneous:**
   (a) ***Colchicine** for gout is best avoided:* Risk of pancytopenia, peripheral neuropathy, myopathy, and hepatotoxicity. If used, reduce dose to 0.6 mg orally every 8 to 12 h for no more than 2 to 3 days

Nonsteroidal anti-inflammatory drug-induced acute kidney injury is not a concern in the dialysis patient. However, these drugs are best avoided because of the increased risk of gastrointestinal bleeding in dialysis patients [3].

Blood transfusion in the oligo-anuric dialysis patient may precipitate volume overload and hyperkalemia. The patient should be monitored for these complications if blood transfusion undertaken in the ED [3]. Since many dialysis patients are wait-listed for kidney transplantation, the preferred blood product is leukoreduced/irradiated to reduce the risk of exposure to donor HLA antigens [53].

Another major management issue is the appropriate adjustment of the doses of medications whose pharmacokinetics is affected by renal dysfunction [54]. Table 5.3 above lists the dose adjustment recommendations regarding medications commonly prescribed in the ED.

The next five years

The "fistula first" initiative in the United States has been moderately successful in increasing the number of patients receiving HD through an arteriovenous fistula and decreasing long-term catheter use [55]. Also, catheter design is improving and the use of "antimicrobial-locking" of catheters is increasing. These developments may decrease HD access-related emergencies, particularly infections. If the number of home HD patients increases over the next 5 years, the utilization of emergency services by ESRD patients may decrease since home HD patients in general have fewer medical problems. The advent of expanded health insurance coverage in the United States may enable earlier referral to nephrologists and thereby decrease the burden of co-morbid conditions that develop prior to initiation of dialysis.

However, the following factors may militate against these favorable trends [2]:

• The continuing increase in the age of onset of ESRD and age-related co-morbidities.
• The global epidemic of obesity and diabetes that might increase the number of ESRD patients.

Conclusion

Dialysis patients represent a complex and challenging population for emergency physicians. Careful understanding of the pathophysiology of disease in these patients will aid in the emergency management of the variety of ailments that can cause this population to present to the ED. Close consultation with treating nephrologists can also prevent adverse outcomes for these patients when admitted or discharged from the emergency department.

References

1. United States Renal Data System—2009 annual data report. Atlas of chronic kidney disease & end-stage renal disease in the United States, Chapter 4: treatment modalities. *Am J Kidney Dis* 2010; 55(1 Suppl.): S249–S258.
2. Neil N, Walker DR, Sesso R, et al. Gaining efficiencies: resources and demand for dialysis around the globe. *Value Health* 2009; 12(1): 73–79
3. Venkat A, Kaufmann KR, Venkat K. Care of the end-stage renal disease patient on dialysis in the ED. *Am J Emerg Med* 2006; 24(7): 847–858.
4. Pastan S, Bailey J. Dialysis therapy. *N Engl J Med* 1998; 338(20): 1428–1437.
5. Power A, Duncan N, Goodlad C. Advances and innovations in dialysis in the 21st century. *Postgrad Med J* 2009; 85: 102–107.
6. Konner K, Gersch M. Vascular access for hemodialysis. In: Feehally J, Floege J, Johnson RJ (eds.) *Comprehensive Clinical Nephrology*. 3rd ed. Philadelphia, PA: Mosby Elsevier; 2007: pp. 929–940.
7. Rippe B. Peritoneal dialysis: principles, techniques and adequacy. In: Feehally J, Floege J, Johnson RJ (eds.) *Comprehensive Clinical Nephrology*. 3rd ed. Philadelphia, PA: Mosby Elsevier; 2007: pp. 979–990.
8. Nassar GM, Ayus JC. Infectious complications of the hemodialysis access. *Kidney International* 2001; 60: 1–13.
9. Lafrance JP, Rahme E, Lelorier J, Iqbal S. Vascular access-related infections: definitions, incidence rates, and risk factors. *Am J Kidney Dis* 2008; 52(5): 982–993.
10. Allon M. Treatment guidelines for dialysis catheter-related bacteremia: an update. *Am J Kidney Dis* 2009; 54(1): 13–17.
11. Davies SJ, Williams JD. Complications of peritoneal dialysis. In: Feehally J, Floege J, Johnson RJ (eds.) *Comprehensive Clinical Nephrology*. 3rd ed. Philadelphia, PA: Mosby Elsevier; 2007: pp. 991–1000.
12. Suresh KR, Port FK. Air under the diaphragm in patients undergoing continuous ambulatory peritoneal dialysis (CAPD). *Perit Dial Int* 1989; 9(4): 309–311.
13. Piraino B, Bailie GR, Bernardini J, et al. ISPD Ad Hoc Advisory Committee. Peritoneal dialysis-related infections recommendations: 2005 update. *Perit Dial Int* 2005 25(2): 107–131.
14. Riella LV, Keithi-Reddy SR, Charytan DM, Singh AK. Acute coronary syndrome in ESRD patients. *Kidney Int* 2009; 75(5): 558–562.
15. Tsai TT, Maddox TM, Roe MT, et al. National Cardiovascular Data Registry. Contraindicated medication use in dialysis patients undergoing percutaneous coronary intervention. *JAMA* 2009; 302(22): 2458–2464.
16. Alpert MA, Ravenscraft MD. Pericardial involvement in end-stage renal disease. *Am J Med Sci* 2003; 325(4): 228–236.
17. Stegmayr BG. Ultrafiltration and dry weight-what are the cardiovascular effects? *Artif Organs* 2003; 27(3): 227–229.
18. Dhar S, Pressman GS, Subramanian S, et al. Natriuretic peptides and heart failure in the patient with chronic kidney disease: a review of current evidence. *Postgrad Med J* 2009; 85: 299–302.
19. Saha TC, Singh H. Non-infectious complications of peritoneal dialysis. *South Med J* 2007; 100(1): 54–58.

20. Coppolino G, Lucisano G, Bolignano D, Buemi M. Acute cardiovascular complications of hemodialysis. *Minerva Urol Nefrol* 2010; 62(1): 67–80.
21. Voroneanu L, Covic A. Arrhythmias in hemodialysis patients. *J Nephrol* 2009; 22(6): 716–725.
22. Herzog CA, Mangrum JM, Passman R. Sudden cardiac death in dialysis patients. *Semin Dial* 2008; 21(4): 300–307.
23. Hörl MP, Hörl WH. Hemodialysis-associated hypertension: pathophysiology and therapy. *Am J Kidney Dis* 2002; 39(2): 227–244.
24. Varon J. The diagnosis and treatment of hypertensive crises. *Postgrad Med* 2009; 121(1): 5–13.
25. Hedges SJ, Dehoney SB, Hooper JS, Amanzadeh J, Busti AJ. Evidence-based treatment recommendations for uremic bleeding. *Nat Clin Pract Nephrol* 2007; 3(3): 138–153.
26. Pitchumoni CS, Arguello P, Agarwal N, Yoo J. Acute pancreatitis in chronic renal failure. *Am J Gastroenterol.* 1996; 91(12): 2477–2482.
27. Perrone RD. Extrarenal manifestations of ADPKD. *Kidney Int* 1997; 51(6): 2022–2036.
28. Archodovassilis F, Lagoudiannakis EE, Tsekouras DK, et al. Non-occlusive mesenteric ischemia: a lethal complication in peritoneal dialysis patients. *Perit Dial Int* 2007; 27(2): 136–141.
29. Locatelli F, Becker H. Update on anemia management in nephrology, including current guidelines on the use of erythropoiesis-stimulating agents and implications of the introduction of "biosimilars". *Oncologist* 2009; 14(1 Suppl.): 16–21.
30. Floege J, Eitner F. Acquired cystic kidney disease and malignancies in chronic kidney disease. In: Feehally J, Floege J, Johnson RJ (eds.) *Comprehensive Clinical Nephrology*. 3rd ed. Philadelphia, PA: Mosby Elsevier; 2007: pp. 911–916.
31. Brouns R, De Deyn PP. Neurological complications in renal failure: a review. *Clin Neurol Neurosurg* 2004; 107(1): 1–16.
32. Patel N, Dalal P, Panesar M. Dialysis disequilibrium syndrome: a narrative review. *Semin Dial* 2008; 21(5): 493–498.
33. Sood P, Sinson GP, Cohen EP. Subdural hematomas in chronic dialysis patients: significant and increasing. *Clin J Am Soc Nephrol* 2007; 2(5): 956–959.
34. Khella SL. New insights into stroke in chronic kidney disease. *Adv Chronic Kidney Dis* 2008; 15(4): 338–346.
35. Agrawal V, Rai B, Fellows J, McCullough PA. In-hospital outcomes with thrombolytic therapy in patients with renal dysfunction presenting with acute ischaemic stroke. *Nephrol Dial Transplant* 2010; 25(4): 1150–1157.
36. Horacio J, Adrogué HJ, Madias NE. Management of life-threatening acid–base disorders. *N Engl J Med* 1998; 338: 26–34.
37. Kraut JA, Madias NE. Metabolic acidosis: pathophysiology, diagnosis and management. *Nat Rev Nephrol* 2010; 6(5): 274–285.
38. Putcha N, Allon M. Management of hyperkalemia in dialysis patients. *Semin Dial* 2007; 20(5): 431–439.
39. Sood MM, Sood AR, Richardson R. Emergency management and commonly encountered outpatient scenarios in patients with hyperkalemia. *Mayo Clin Proc* 2007; 82(12): 1553–1561.

40. Sterns RH, Rojas M, Bernstein P, Chennupati S. Ion-exchange resins for the treatment of hyperkalemia: are they safe and effective? *J Am Soc Nephrol* 2010; 21: 733–735.

41. Martin KJ, González EA. Metabolic bone disease in chronic kidney disease. *J Am Soc Nephrol* 2007; 18(3): 875–885.

42. Cruz DN, Perazella MA. Biochemical aberrations in a dialysis patient following parathyroidectomy. *Am J Kidney Dis* 1997; 29(5): 759–762.

43. Navarro-González JF, Mora-Fernández C, García-Pérez J. Clinical implications of disordered magnesium homeostasis in chronic renal failure and dialysis. *Semin Dial* 2009; 22(1): 37–44.

44. Rigalleau V, Gin H. Carbohydrate metabolism in uraemia. *Curr Opin Clin Nutr Metab Care* 2005; 8(4): 463–469.

45. Tzamaloukas AH, Ing TS, Siamopoulos KC, et al. Pathophysiology and management of fluid and electrolyte disturbances in patients on chronic dialysis with severe hyperglycemia. *Semin Dial* 2008; 21(5): 431–439.

46. Pavlicek V, Garzoni D, Urech P, Brändle M. Inaccurate self-monitoring of blood glucose readings in patients on chronic ambulatory peritoneal dialysis with icodextrin. *Exp Clin Endocrinol Diabetes* 2006; 114(3): 124–126.

47. Vij R, Nataraj S, Peixoto AJ. Diagnostic utility of urinalysis in detecting urinary tract infection in hemodialysis patients. *Nephron Clin Pract* 2009; 113(4): 281–285.

48. Davenport A. Intra-dialytic complications during hemodialysis. *Hemodial Int* 2006; 10(2): 162–167.

49. Jaber BL, Upadhyay A, Pereira BJ. Acute complications of hemodialysis. In: Feehally J, Floege J, Johnson RJ (eds.) *Comprehensive Clinical Nephrology*. 3rd ed. Philadelphia, PA: Mosby Elsevier; 2007: pp. 967–978.

50. Kay J, Bardin T. Osteoarticular disorders of renal origin: disease-related and iatrogenic. *Baillieres Best Pract Res Clin Rheumatol* 2000; 14(2): 285–305.

51. Cordova KB, Oberg TJ, Malik M, Robinson-Bostom L. Dermatologic conditions seen in end-stage renal disease. *Semin Dial* 2009; 22(1): 45–55.

52. Pieringer H, Biesenbach G. Nephrogenic systemic fibrosis. A debilitating disease causing fibrosis of the skin and inner organs in patients with kidney failure. *Clin Exp Rheumatol* 2010; 28(2): 268–274.

53. Sharma RR, Marwaha N. Leukoreduced blood components: advantages and strategies for its implementation in developing countries. *Asian J Transfus Sci* 2010; 4(1): 3–8.

54. Brier ME, Aronoff GR (eds). *Drug Prescribing in Renal Failure: Dosing Guidelines for Adults*. 5th ed., Philadelphia: American College of Physicians–American Society of Internal Medicine; 2007.

55. Vascular Access Work Group. Clinical practice guidelines for vascular access. *Am J Kidney Dis* 2006; 48(1 Suppl.): S248–S273.

CHAPTER 6
Adults with cystic fibrosis

Arvind Venkat[1,2] and Joseph M. Pilewski[3,4]
[1]Allegheny General Hospital, Pittsburgh, PA, USA
[2]Drexel University College of Medicine, Philadelphia, PA, USA
[3]Children's Hospital of Pittsburgh of UPMC, Pittsburgh, PA, USA
[4]University of Pittsburgh School of Medicine, Pittsburgh, PA, USA

Introduction and epidemiology

Cystic fibrosis is the most common lethal genetic disease among Caucasians, affecting approximately 1 in 3500 newborns in the United States [1]. Improvements in treatment have resulted in a dramatic increase in life expectancy in patients with cystic fibrosis over the last 10 to 20 years. Median survival has risen from the teens in the 1970s to 37 years today in the United States. It is anticipated that a child born today with cystic fibrosis has the potential to have a life expectancy of 50 years based on improvements in understanding of the pathophysiology and management of complications related to this disease [2]. With the improvements in life expectancy of patients with cystic fibrosis, the number of adults with cystic fibrosis has increased by 400% since the 1970s, with the Cystic Fibrosis Foundation National Data Registry indicating that 43% of all individuals with cystic fibrosis are adults (age $\geq$18 years), and that percentage is anticipated to rise to 50% in the next decade. A growing number of adults with cystic fibrosis are older than age 30 [3]. For reasons that are not well understood, survival among males with cystic fibrosis slightly surpasses that of females, but improvements in life expectancy have been shared across both sexes [4]. It is estimated that there are 30,000 individuals with cystic fibrosis in the United States and over 100,000 worldwide [3].

Cystic fibrosis is caused by mutations in the gene for the cystic fibrosis transmembrane conductance regulator (*CFTR*). Over 1500 disease-causing mutations have been identified. However, diagnosis of cystic fibrosis is made by a combination of sweat chloride testing, genetic testing, clinical

---

Challenging and Emerging Conditions in Emergency Medicine, First Edition. Edited by Arvind Venkat.
© 2011 by John Wiley & Sons, Ltd. Published 2011 by Blackwell Publishing Ltd.

presentation of the patient, and the use of adjunctive methods like nasal potential difference testing [1].

Contrary to the perception of cystic fibrosis as a pediatric ailment, registry data shows that approximately 10% of patients with cystic fibrosis are diagnosed as adults. Unexplained bronchiectasis with less severe pulmonary disease than childhood presenting cystic fibrosis, persistent airway pathogens in sputum (*Pseudomonas aeruginosa*, non-tuberculous mycobacteria, and *Staphylococcus aureus* most prominently), chronic sinusitis, idiopathic recurrent pancreatitis, male infertility, and delayed puberty in males can all lead to consideration and diagnosis of cystic fibrosis in adulthood. Further characterization of mutations in the *CFTR* gene may lead to increased diagnosis of cystic fibrosis in adults [2].

Pulmonary disease in adults with cystic fibrosis

Pulmonary complications remain the most common cause of morbidity and mortality in patients with cystic fibrosis. Chronic pulmonary infections and airway inflammation lead to obstructive pathophysiology, hypoxia, hypercapnia, and respiratory failure. For the emergency physician, adults with cystic fibrosis may present with numerous pulmonary issues ranging from exacerbations of the underlying pulmonary pathology of cystic fibrosis to pneumothoraces, episodes of hemoptysis, and frank respiratory failure [5].

Prior to a discussion of these pulmonary complications of cystic fibrosis, it is important to understand the common maintenance medications that most patients with cystic fibrosis will be using to manage their pulmonary disease. Table 6.1 shows a summary of these treatments and their underlying basis [6–12].

Table 6.1 Common maintenance medications for pulmonary disease in adults with cystic fibrosis

Aerosolized tobramycin and aztreonam	Suppression of chronic infection with *Pseudomonas aeruginosa* with resultant reduction in exacerbations and improvement of pulmonary function
Recombinant DNase	Degradation of free DNA within pulmonary mucus to decrease thickened secretions and cellular breakdown products, thereby reducing exacerbation frequency and increasing pulmonary function
Hypertonic saline	Increased hydration of pulmonary passages and improved mucus clearance
Azithromycin	Combination of antimicrobial and anti-inflammatory effect
β_2-adrenergic agonists	Bronchodilation and potentially increased mucus clearance

The sequence and dosage of these chronic therapies can vary greatly from patient to patient, but these treatments form the basis of the chronic management and improvement in life expectancy of adults with cystic fibrosis. In general, the standing medications for pulmonary health in adults with cystic fibrosis are well tolerated. Studies that have examined the adverse effects of these treatments indicated that most are mild—cough (hypertonic saline) [9], nausea (azithromycin) [10], and laryngitis and rash (recombinant DNase) [6, 8]. Concerns regarding ototoxicity and nephrotoxicity related to long-term inhaled tobramycin use have not been borne out in clinical trials and long-term follow-up. In addition, while investigations have revealed a measurable increase in the minimum inhibitory concentration of *Pseudomonas aeruginosa* by tobramycin after long-term inhalational treatment, to date, this has not generally affected the utility of tobramycin as first-line therapy in the treatment of *Pseudomonas aeruginosa* as an inciting organism for pulmonary exacerbations in patients with cystic fibrosis [7].

A key component of the maintenance of long-term pulmonary function in cystic fibrosis patients is the use of airway clearance therapies. These therapies have been shown to increase sputum production, improve lung function, oxygen saturation, exercise tolerance, and quality of life. However, studies have not shown that airway clearance efforts improve longevity or frequency of acute pulmonary exacerbations of cystic fibrosis. Among the more common airway clearance techniques are percussion and postural drainage, positive expiratory pressure exercises, active cycle of breathing technique, autogenic drainage, oscillatory positive expiratory pressure devices, and high frequency chest compression. Aerobic exercise is also recommended as a means to improve physical strength and cardiovascular health [13].

Pulmonary exacerbations in cystic fibrosis

The diagnosis and treatment of pulmonary exacerbations of underlying disease in adults with cystic fibrosis is a challenge for emergency physicians. Given the continuing pulmonary insults that characterize the progression of cystic fibrosis, differentiating the natural progression of disease from acute exacerbations can be difficult. There are no consensus diagnostic criteria for determining when an acute exacerbation is occurring. Among the signs and symptoms that can suggest this diagnosis are increased cough, changing sputum production in amount, consistency, and color, weight loss, decreased appetite, alteration in pulmonary exam from baseline (wheezing/crackles), hemoptysis, rising white blood cell count, fever, and new radiographic findings on chest X-ray [14]. Since many of these findings rely on the availability of previous medical records and laboratory/X-ray reports, it is appropriate to discuss with patients where such information might be obtained and to rely heavily on their impression of how their symptoms have changed and whether these reflect their previous experience with pulmonary exacerbations in determining when to initiate treatment.

Once the diagnosis of acute pulmonary exacerbation has been made, a number of therapies can be initiated in the emergency department (ED) to aid the patient. The mainstay of therapy is the use of combination intravenous antibiotic therapy to treat underlying bacterial organisms that have been documented in respiratory cultures of the patient. *Pseudomonas aeruginosa* is the most commonly cultured organism in adult patients with cystic fibrosis and should be presumptively treated if recent cultures are not available to guide antibiotic selection. First-line therapy for *Pseudomonas* consists of an aminoglycoside, typically tobramycin, dosed on a once-daily basis, and a β-lactam antibiotic, typically a third-generation cephalosporin such as ceftazidime, or an anti-Pseudomonal β-lactam, such as piperacillin/tazobactam. Fluoroquinolones can serve as an alternative antibiotic class for treatment, but should be carefully chosen for anti-Pseudomonal activity (ciprofloxacin or levofloxacin, rather than moxifloxacin). Antibiotics are generally given for a 14-day course, though no optimal dosing regimen has been established [15].

With the increased longevity of patients with cystic fibrosis, there is increased recognition that the microbiologic flora, typically cultured from the respiratory tract, is evolving. Beyond *Pseudomonas aeruginosa*, *Stenotrophomonas maltophilia*, *Achromobacter xylosoxidans*, *Ralstonia* species, and *Pandorea* have been increasingly cultured. Fluoroquinolone-resistant Pseudomonal organisms have become more prevalent as well [16]. *Staphylococcus aureus* has also become more prevalent as has methicillin-resistant strains (MRSA). MRSA respiratory infection has been associated with decreased pulmonary function (FEV_1), and studies are ongoing as to whether chronic suppression therapy should become part of the standard medications among adults with cystic fibrosis [17].

Though relatively low in prevalence, *Burkholderia cepacia* complex, consisting of nine different species, raises the greatest fear among patients with cystic fibrosis and their physicians, and is worthy of special note by emergency physicians. This complex is easily transmitted by contact and likely respiratory means, is multidrug resistant, and has characteristics that impedes host response and can cause a fulminant pneumonia with bacteremia and endotoxin-mediated shock and multiorgan failure (cepacia syndrome). Given the low prevalence of this organism due to improved infection control techniques and procedures, it is not necessary for emergency physicians to presume the presence of this pathogen when initiating antimicrobial therapy. However, confirmation of the presence of this organism, either by the patient or review of respiratory culture, or clinical suspicion based on presenting signs and symptoms, raises multiple challenges in initiating antibiotic therapy. Synergistic testing, used to determine the optimal antibiotic regimen in patients with cystic fibrosis based on underlying respiratory cultures, can aid in this determination. However, when such test results are not available, antibiotics that may be effective in combination include carbapenems, quinolones, piperacillin, ceftazidime, trimethoprim–sulfamethoxazole, and minocycline [16].

In general, close consultation with the patient's pulmonologist is warranted in determining the optimal antibiotic regimen for adults with cystic fibrosis presenting with acute pulmonary exacerbations. It is common that patients will be well aware of what antibiotics their treating pulmonologists currently recommend for acute therapy based on recent respiratory cultures.

Other therapies that can aid in the treatment of acute pulmonary exacerbations are airway clearance therapies and the continued use of chronic therapies such as hypertonic saline, DNase, β-agonists, and oral anti-inflammatory medications. It is recommended that these therapies be maintained upon admission with perhaps more aggressive airway clearance therapies [15].

Given the common presence of wheezing in cystic fibrosis patients with acute exacerbations, emergency physicians may feel that corticosteroids will benefit the patient due to their anti-inflammatory effects. While airway inflammation clearly contributes to the pathophysiology of acute pulmonary exacerbations and studies have shown that corticosteroids can provide short-term improvement in pulmonary function (FEV_1), investigations have revealed that this short-term benefit is outweighed by adverse side effects such as hyperglycemia. In general, corticosteroids are not recommended in the standard therapy of acute pulmonary exacerbations of cystic fibrosis [18].

For adults with cystic fibrosis who present with acute respiratory failure, Bilevel Positive Airway Pressure (BiPAP) represents the next step in respiratory support in the emergency department. Nasal BiPAP has been studied in this population and has been found to be effective in improving respiratory rate, mechanics, pulmonary function, oxygenation, and hypercapnia [19]. The prognosis of cystic fibrosis patients on ventilators is quite grave, and all efforts should be made to avoid this intervention, if possible, in the ED.

In general, adults with acute pulmonary exacerbations of cystic fibrosis should be admitted to the hospital. While intravenous antibiotics might be provided as an outpatient, other therapies, such as airway clearance techniques and chronic inhalational therapies (tobramycin, hypertonic saline, and DNase), especially in a patient with worsening respiratory parameters, may not be possible [15]. For the emergency physician caring for adults with cystic fibrosis with a pulmonary exacerbation, a decision to discharge a patient should only be made in close consultation with the treating pulmonologist and assurance of aggressive therapy and support in the outpatient setting.

Infection control procedures are also a key component of emergency care of adults with cystic fibrosis. Given the association of respiratory infection and chronic colonization and reduced pulmonary function in this population, rigid precautions should be the rule upon ED presentation for the protection of the patient and potentially other cystic fibrosis patients who might present in the future. All patients require standard precautions with hand washing using sanitizers and soap and water by health care providers. Given the increased prevalence of MRSA among adults with cystic fibrosis, gowns and gloves with contact precautions may be appropriate as a general rule, though current recommendations are to enact this precaution only if respiratory cultures reflect this necessity. Disposable mouthpieces for nebulizer treatment and inline bacterial filters should be used, and wall-humidifiers should be cleaned and dried appropriately. Chronic airway infection with pathogens such as multidrug resistant *Pseudomonas*, MRSA, *Burkholderia* species, or other intrinsically resistant bacteria are common in adults with cystic fibrosis, so admission to a single-patient room without common facilities is preferred [14,20].

Hemoptysis

Hemoptysis represents a common pulmonary complication in patients with cystic fibrosis and may be a sign of acute pulmonary exacerbation. Retrospective series have indicated that 9.1% of cystic fibrosis patients had hemoptysis. While usually mild, 4.1% of patients with cystic fibrosis suffer massive hemoptysis (>240 mL) during their lifetime, with increased incidence in older patients [21].

For emergency physicians, an important consideration is the amount of hemoptysis. Scant or mild hemoptysis (<5 mL) may be managed as an outpatient with close follow-up by pulmonology. Antibiotic therapy should be initiated if mild hemoptysis is associated with other pulmonary symptoms and may be warranted if the amount of hemoptysis is submassive [21].

Cystic fibrosis patients with moderate to massive hemoptysis represent an emergent population who require resuscitation and quick intervention in the ED. Large-bore intravenous access, complete blood count, type and screen, and coagulation profile should be obtained. Impaired absorption of fat-soluble vitamins from pancreatic insufficiency may result in hypoprothrombinemia or other coagulopathy requiring correction in this patient population. Chest radiography can help localize the sight of hemorrhage with the appearance of pulmonary infiltrate, but chest computerized tomography and bronchoscopy generally do not aid in localization of bleeding while delaying definitive management [21].

Bronchial artery embolization represents the most effective therapy for moderate to massive hemoptysis in adults with cystic fibrosis. Embolization of dilated and tortuous vessels, either at the site of suspected hemorrhage or throughout the pulmonary circulation, may be appropriate. Complications of this procedure include chest pain, dysphagia, bronchial necrosis, and transient neurological symptoms. Paraplegia from inappropriate embolization of a spinal artery is exceedingly rare with an experienced angiographer [22]. Intubation and placement of a bronchial balloon in the bleeding segmental airway may temporize the situation while angiography is arranged; however, this should only be employed when patients are unable to clear airway blood or there is significant impairment of gas exchange due to massive hemoptysis.

Lung resection is the therapy of last resort in patients with massive hemoptysis, but should only be initiated where embolization has been unsuccessful. The loss of lung parenchyma can further worsen the pulmonary function in already impaired cystic fibrosis patients [21].

Pneumothorax

Approximately 3.4% of patients with cystic fibrosis will experience a pneumothorax in their lifetime, again with increased incidence among older patients. Given the distorted anatomy of adults with cystic fibrosis with long-standing bronchiectasis and inflammation, chest radiography may be unrevealing of pneumothorax and chest computerized tomography may be required to make this diagnosis [21].

For large pneumothoraces (>3 cm), chest tube placement with admission is appropriate management. However, patients with small pneumothoraces should only have a chest tube placed if there is evidence of clinical instability. It may be appropriate to discharge the patient with close observation and follow-up in the absence of other clinical signs or symptoms. For patients with mild pulmonary symptoms and small pneumothorax, initiation of therapies for acute pulmonary exacerbation is appropriate prior to consideration of chest tube placement [21].

For patients discharged from the ED, BiPAP and certain airway clearance therapies (positive expiratory pressure and intra-pulmonary percussive ventilation) should be discontinued until resolution of the pneumothorax. However, aerosol therapies should continue. Given the risk of pneumothorax progression, patients discharged from the ED should be advised to avoid flying, lifting weights >5 pounds, and spirometry for up to 2 weeks after the pneumothorax has resolved [21].

Gastrointestinal disease in adults with cystic fibrosis

With improvements in longevity in the cystic fibrosis patient, management of gastrointestinal complications of the disease has become more important. Beyond the pancreatic insufficiency and need for nutritional supplementation that can characterize patients with cystic fibrosis who are diagnosed in childhood, a range of gastrointestinal, hepatic, and pancreatic disorders can manifest in late adolescence and adulthood.

Gastrointestinal disease

Distal intestinal obstructive syndrome (DIOS), previously called meconium ileus equivalent, is characterized by partial or complete bowel obstruction due to thickened gastrointestinal mucus and fecal material. Presenting more commonly in late adolescence and adulthood than in childhood in patients with cystic fibrosis (affecting up to 18% of adults with cystic fibrosis), patients will present with typical symptoms of bowel obstruction (bilious and feculent emesis, abdominal pain and distention, decreased or hyperactive bowel sounds) with radiographic appearance similar to patients who present with mechanical bowel obstructions due to other etiologies (Figure 6.1). DIOS has shown a clear association with exocrine pancreatic insufficiency and worsening pulmonary status (FEV_1 and forced vital capacity (FVC)) [23].

Given the presence of mechanical bowel obstruction pathophysiology, there may be a temptation among emergency physicians to determine that rapid surgical consultation and intervention is required for management. However, conservative therapy using enemas (Gastrograffin© or polyethylene glycol) and oral laxatives are often effective, without the need for insertion of nasogastric tube. One study cited a 96% success rate with conservative management in the inpatient setting [24]. In addition, surgical management can be difficult in this patient population due to underlying poor respiratory and nutritional status. In general, surgical intervention is required only after medical therapy has failed or with signs of bowel ischemia or peritonitis [25]. Patients with DIOS generally require admission to the hospital for aggressive medical therapy and analgesia with serial examinations to evaluate for efficacy of treatment.

Clostridium difficile has been reported in up to 43% of stool cultures of patients with cystic fibrosis. However, *Clostridium difficile*-associated disease is rare despite the presence of pathogenic toxin-producing strains. Presentation of colitis due to *Clostridium difficile* in this patient population can be varied, ranging from constitutional symptoms such as fever and nausea to abdominal pain and diarrhea. When there is a suspicion for this diagnosis in the ED among adults with cystic fibrosis, laboratory evaluation should include complete blood count, C-reactive protein, electrolyte panels, stool culture, and *Clostridium difficile* stool toxin testing. Unlike DIOS, *Clostridium difficile* can cause marked elevation in C-reactive protein levels to a range greater than 100 mg/L range. CT may be most sensitive in the ED for diagnosis, with findings including pancolitis and toxic megacolon. First-line

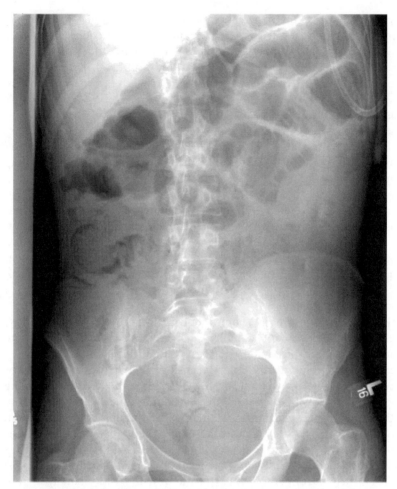

Figure 6.1 Abdominal radiograph of adult cystic fibrosis patient with distal intestinal obstructive syndrome.

therapy continues to be metronidazole, followed by oral vancomycin and, if necessary, surgical intervention [26].

Pancreatic disease

While patients with cystic fibrosis often have pancreatic insufficiency and require enzyme supplementation for exocrine pancreatic function, increased life expectancy in this patient population and diagnosis of patients in adulthood have caused recognition of the prevalence of pancreatitis among adults with cystic fibrosis. Up to 2% of adults with cystic fibrosis will experience acute pancreatitis as a complication of having at least partially preserved exocrine pancreatic function. There is a significant association between acute pancreatitis and the subsequent diagnosis of exocrine pancreatic insufficiency in adults with cystic fibrosis [27]. Small studies have suggested an increased risk of pancreatic cancer in adults with cystic fibrosis who initially have maintained exocrine pancreatic function and develop acute pancreatitis [28].

In general, adults with cystic fibrosis who present with acute pancreatitis will present with typical epigastric pain radiating to the back and associated vomiting. Enzymatic tests using amylase and lipase levels may be unrevealing due to underlying reduced pancreatic function. Imaging studies using CT or magnetic resonance cholangiopancreatography or endoscopic retrograde cholangiopancreatography may be required for definitive diagnosis. Mean age of pancreatitis presentation in this population is in the late twenties, with admission a requirement to maintain hydration and nutritional status, pain control, and evaluation of etiology of acute pancreatitis [29].

Hepatobiliary disease

Up to 20% of adults with cystic fibrosis may show evidence of hepatic disease [30]. Steatosis remains the most common hepatic disorder seen in patients with cystic fibrosis, possibly due to malnutrition and fatty acid deficiency. The likelihood of progression to cirrhosis with this complication is unknown. Focal biliary cirrhosis is the most common clinical hepatic disorder in this patient population. Most commonly presenting with the onset of puberty, focal biliary cirrhosis has been related to worsening pancreatic insufficiency and severe genotype. Patients will present with signs of portal hypertension including hepatosplenomegaly, though variceal bleeding is rare. More than biochemical and laboratory testing, cystic fibrosis liver disease requires imaging and biopsy findings to confirm the diagnosis (echogenicity, nodularity, hepatosplenomegaly with histologic findings of focal biliary, and multinodular cirrhosis). Medical treatment remains the mainstay of therapy with the use of ursodeoxycholic acid as a means of improving cholangiocyte function [31]. A small percentage of patients will progress to end-stage cirrhotic liver disease and require liver transplantation.

Gallstones may be found on imaging in up to 50% of patients with cystic fibrosis. While this can be the etiology of acute pancreatitis, cholecystitis, and ascending cholangitis in this patient population, most adults with cystic fibrosis remain asymptomatic from cholelithiasis. Diagnostic and therapeutic evaluation of complications of cholelithiasis is similar to the non-cystic fibrosis population [31].

Cystic fibrosis related diabetes mellitus (CFRD)

Cystic fibrosis related diabetes mellitus (CFRD) has increased with the life expectancy of patients with cystic fibrosis. As of 2006, 19.2% of cystic fibrosis patients aged >14 and up to 50% of patients aged >30 were insulin-dependent. CFRD is associated with a 6–7-fold increase in mortality in comparison to non-CFRD cystic fibrosis patients, and is related to increased functional decline. CFRD is distinct from both type 1 and type 2 diabetes mellitus in that it has both decreased insulin secretion and relative insulin resistance and requires nutritional support that may include fat and carbohydrate supplementation. Diagnosis is made by either the presence of fasting hyperglycemia (>126 mg/dL) or hyperglycemia after oral glucose tolerance testing (>200 mg/dL) [32]. Insulin therapy is the mainstay of treatment, and emergency physicians may see patients with hypoglycemia due to the combination of poor nutritional intake and use of long-acting insulin agents such as Lantus©. Hypoglycemia may occur in up to 14% of patients with cystic fibrosis, and treatment with supplemental dextrose and glucagon has been shown to be effective [33]. Diabetic ketoacidosis is exceedingly rare in patients with CFRD.

Musculoskeletal and rheumatic disease in adults with cystic fibrosis

It is well recognized that adults with cystic fibrosis commonly have low bone mineral density and associated increased risk for fractures and spinal kyphosis. This decrease in bone mineral density is likely due to a combination of nutritional status, physical activity, and hormonal/vitamin deficiency, specifically vitamin D. Up to 90% of patients with cystic fibrosis may have bone mineral deficiency [34].

As a result of bone mineral deficiency, fractures are more commonly seen in this patient population from low energy mechanisms or spontaneously. Rib fractures, possibly in association with airway clearance techniques, and vertebral fractures, most commonly of the thoracic spine, are most prevalent, though extremity fractures have also been shown to be more prevalent than in the non-cystic fibrosis population. Up to 20% of adults with cystic fibrosis may suffer fractures during their lifetime. Similarly, up to 62% of adults with cystic fibrosis in one study showed evidence of spinal kyphosis that can affect respiratory mechanics and overall functional status. Diagnosis of both fractures and kyphosis is made by plain radiography with management similar to the non-cystic fibrosis population. However, consideration in patient disposition from the ED should take into account how the fracture may affect the underlying functional status and life sustaining airway clearance options of the already impaired patient with cystic fibrosis [35]. Alendronate has been shown in adults with cystic fibrosis to increase bone mineral density, though its effect on preventing fractures is unknown [36].

Patients with cystic fibrosis can present with an arthropathy that is distinct from other polyarthritis conditions. Characterized by recurrent monoarticular and polyarticular inflammation and a rash similar to erythema nodosum, episodes can last up to several weeks and be debilitating with patients complaining of both joint and spine pain. No diagnostic test or imaging study has been found to confirm the diagnosis. Up to 9% of patients with cystic fibrosis may suffer from this condition with increasing likelihood of presentation with age. Treatment largely consists of the use of nonsteroidal anti-inflammatory medications that can also improve pulmonary function. However, episodes of hemoptysis can also be exacerbated with this treatment [37].

Hypertrophic pulmonary osteoarthropathy can occur in up to 5% of patients with cystic fibrosis. Characterized by periosteal inflammation of long bones and clubbing of the digits, this condition is treated by attempting to improve the pulmonary status of patients. By itself, hypertrophic pulmonary osteoarthropathy will not cause patients to present to the ED, but its presence may indicate to the treating physician a higher likelihood of poor underlying pulmonary status in patients with cystic fibrosis [38].

Cardiovascular disease and cor pulmonale in adults with cystic fibrosis

With improvements in survival of patients with cystic fibrosis, it is increasingly recognized that recurrent pulmonary infections and worsening bronchiectasis and pulmonary disease can lead to pulmonary hypertension and cor pulmonale. The finding of pulmonary hypertension and cor pulmonale in patients with cystic fibrosis may be an indicator of likely morbidity and mortality, having been observed in up to 45% of late adolescent and adults with cystic fibrosis in the 2 weeks preceding death. Distinguishing between acute pulmonary exacerbations and the presentation of cor pulmonale in this patient population may be difficult as both may cause dyspnea, tachycardia, hypoxemia, chest pain, and cyanosis. In the ED, making the distinction is less important than recognizing that the mainstay of treatment is both improvement in oxygenation and pulmonary function via treatments for acute pulmonary exacerbation described above. Upon admission to the hospital, ECG may confirm the presence of pulmonary hypertension and cor pulmonale, requiring further management of oxygenation in the outpatient setting [39].

Chronic chest pain has been also found to be prevalent in survey studies of adults with cystic fibrosis, affecting up to 32% of patients who reported chronic pain [40]. No study has shown a clear correlation of this symptom with the presence of underlying atherosclerotic cardiovascular disease, and by itself would not be sensitive for diagnosing acute pulmonary exacerbations. However, pneumothorax and rib fractures may present with chest pain in isolation in this patient population. Lastly, there are reports of a high incidence of deep venous thrombosis, often associated with central venous or peripherally inserted central (PICC) lines, and pulmonary embolism must be considered in the differential diagnosis of chest pain in adults with cystic fibrosis [41, 42].

Psychiatric illness in adults with cystic fibrosis

Registry data suggests that depression may be third highest cause of death in patients with cystic fibrosis and may overall affect up to 46% of this patient population. Studies suggest that depression can be correlated with worsening pulmonary function, though the exact chronological interaction is unknown. Depression is clearly associated with poor adherence to treatment regimens. For emergency physicians, recognition of depression among patients with cystic fibrosis should result in urgent referral for treatment so as to maintain adherence and functional status [43].

Anxiety is also common among adults with cystic fibrosis, affecting up to 31% of this patient population. Treatment involves cognitive behavioral therapy and benzodiazepines. Selective serotonin reuptake inhibitors can be used to treat both anxiety and depression in this patient population. There is also experience with using mirtazapine as an appetite stimulant in depressed cystic fibrosis patients. Benzodiazepines, due to respiratory side effects, are generally prescribed at low doses and only for short periods of time (up to 4–6 weeks) for the acute management of anxiety symptoms [44].

Rhinosinusitis in adults with cystic fibrosis

Nasal obstruction due to changes in mucus characteristics and secretion can often cause chronic rhinosinusitis in patients with cystic fibrosis. Characteristic lesions include panopacification of the sinuses on imaging and nasal polyposis. Treatment involves nasal steroids, saline washes, and surgical removal. For the emergency physician who has a suspicion of acute sinusitis in a patient with cystic fibrosis, treatment should target the possibility of *Pseudomonas aeruginosa* among other organisms as the inciting agent. Ciprofloxacin and trimethoprim–sulfamethoxazole remain the antibiotics of choice in this patient population [45].

Dermatologic disease in adults with cystic fibrosis

Drug hypersensitivity reactions occur in up to 30% of patients with cystic fibrosis. Related to increased antibiotic usage, drug reactions can present with a range of cutaneous signs, including morbilliform rash, urticaria, angioedema, and leukocytoclastic vasculitis. Urticaria and angioedema in these patients may not be related to an acute allergic reaction, nor does the presence of a rash automatically indicate that a particular antibiotic should not be further used in this patient [46]. Given the common use of polypharmacy regimens in the treatment of pulmonary disease in adults with cystic fibrosis, it may be necessary, after careful history and physical examination to determine the inciting agent, for the emergency physician to discuss with the patient's treating physician whether discontinuation of the inciting antibiotic is warranted.

Nutrient deficiency dermatitis of cystic fibrosis represents a primary and secondary disorder of cystic fibrosis, related to both *CFTR* function and nutritional status. This condition can be quite varied in its appearance, including perioral and periorbital dermatitis and erythematous hyperkeratotic desquamating plaques without mucus membrane involvement. This dermatitis may be the presenting symptom for patients who have not been diagnosed with cystic fibrosis to that time [46].

Early aquagenic wrinkling is well recognized in the cystic fibrosis population. While not an emergency diagnosis, it can be recognized and treated with topical aluminum chloride, antihistamines, and iontophoresis as an outpatient [46].

Ocular disease in adults with cystic fibrosis

Ophthalmic disease in patients with cystic fibrosis is often correlated with digestive and nutritional deficiency. Lens transparency is often decreased in patients with cystic fibrosis. Patients with cystic fibrosis can present with cataracts, retinal hemorrhage, papilledema, and functional changes to the optic nerve [47]. Earlier findings include complaints of dry eyes due to changes in the cornea that can create difficulty with contact lenses and resultant presentation to the emergency department [48]. Treatment for these conditions is similar to when present in the non-cystic fibrosis population.

The next five years

While gene therapy remains the ultimate goal for correction of the *CFTR* dysfunction or decreased production that characterizes the underlying genetic disorder in cystic fibrosis patients, this treatment is not likely to be available in the foreseeable future. However, a number of treatments that both attempt to improve *CFTR* function or activate alternative chloride channels on affected cells as well as emerging treatments for the presenting pathology of cystic fibrosis are under active investigation. Table 6.2 classifies the treatments that are discussed below.

Table 6.2 Emerging therapies for cystic fibrosis undergoing active investigation

Ion channel modulating agents	Denufosol
Agents to potentiate or correct *CFTR* function	PTC124, VX-809, and VX-770
Inhaled antibiotics	Fosfomycin/tobramycin combination therapy, liposomal amikacin, ciprofloxacin and levofloxacin
Airway anti-inflammatories	Oral *N*-acetylcysteine

Ion channel modulators such as Denufosol activate alternative chloride channels than *CFTR* with the hopes of improving mucus hydration and clearance. An inhalational therapy, Denufosol has shown in phase II trials improvement in pulmonary function with few adverse effects and would represent a new therapeutic category of treatment for patients with cystic fibrosis [49, 50].

VX-770 is an oral potentiator of normal and a number of mutant *CFTRs* that traffic to the cell membrane, such as *G551D* mutant *CFTR*. PTC124 and VX-809 are recently identified correctors of cystic fibrosis stop mutations, such as *G542X* and *W1282X*, and the most common cystic fibrosis processing mutation, *deltaF508*, respectively. Studies of these agents suggest some restoration of chloride transport via mutant *CFTR* proteins, while further studies are needed to determine clinical efficacy of these potentially disease-modifying or curative drugs [51–53].

Given the constant difficulty with antibiotic selection in patients with cystic fibrosis, particularly adults who have been treated with multiple previous agents, there is a constant need for novel and improved maintenance inhalational antibiotic therapies. Inhaled fosfomycin/tobramycin has shown high levels of activity against common respiratory pathogens in cystic fibrosis patients, including *Pseudomonas aeruginosa* [54]. Liposomal amikacin as an inhalational therapy similarly showed similar improvements in activity against *Pseudomonas aeruginosa* and pulmonary status from baseline in treated patients [55].

Oral *N*-acetylcysteine has been tested as an airway neutrophil anti-inflammatory agent and mucolytic. Trials to date have been inconclusive, but investigation is ongoing as to whether this agent can add to the benefit given by DNase [56].

Conclusion

With improvements in longevity in patients with cystic fibrosis, it is reasonable to expect that emergency physicians will see these patients more commonly and at later stages of disease. As discussed in this chapter, emergency physicians may be required to manage pathology involving a variety of organ systems whose spectrum of disease is changing with the aging of this patient population. Close consultation with treating pulmonologists is invaluable for decisions regarding management and disposition. Novel treatments may over the next 5 years further improve the management and prognosis of adults with cystic fibrosis.

References

1. Farrell P, Rosenstein B, White T, et al. Guidelines for diagnosis of cystic fibrosis in newborns through older adults: cystic fibrosis foundation consensus report. *J Pediatr* 2008; 153(2): S4–S14.
2. O'Sullivan B, Freedman S. Cystic fibrosis. *Lancet* 2009; 373(9678): 1891–1904.
3. Boyle M. Adult cystic fibrosis. *JAMA* 2007; 298(15): 1787–1793.
4. Nick J, Rodman D. Manifestations of cystic fibrosis diagnosed in adulthood. *Curr Opin Pulm Med* 2005; 11(6): 513–518.
5. Flume P. Pulmonary complications of cystic fibrosis. *Respir Care* 2009; 54(5): 618–627.
6. Flume P, O'Sullivan B, Robinson K, et al. Cystic fibrosis pulmonary guidelines: chronic medications for maintenance of lung health. *Amer J Respir Crit Care Med* 2007; 176(10): 957–969.
7. Moss R. Long-term benefits of inhaled tobramycin in adolescent patients with cystic fibrosis. *Chest* 2002; 121(1): 55–63.
8. Fuchs H, Borowitz D, Christiansen D, et al. Effect of aerosolized recombinant human DNase on exacerbations of respiratory symptoms and on pulmonary function in patients with cystic fibrosis. *NEJM* 1994; 331(10): 637–642.
9. Elkins M, Robinson M, Rose B, et al. A controlled trial of long-term inhaled hypertonic saline in patients with cystic fibrosis. *NEJM* 2006; 354(3): 229–240.
10. Saiman L, Marshall B, Mayer-Hamblett N, et al. Azithromycin in patients with cystic fibrosis chronically infected with Pseudomonas aeruginosa: a randomized controlled trial. *JAMA* 2003; 290(13): 1749–1756.
11. Donaldson S, Bennett W, Zeman K, Knowles M, Tarran R, Boucher R. Mucus clearance and lung function in cystic fibrosis with hypertonic saline. *NEJM* 2006; 354(3): 241–250.
12. Ramsey B, Pepe M, Quan J, et al. Intermittent administration of inhaled tobramycin in patients with cystic fibrosis. *NEJM* 1999; 340(1): 23–30.
13. Flume P, Robinson K, O'Sullivan B, et al. Cystic fibrosis pulmonary guidelines: airway clearance therapies. *Respir Care* 2009; 54(4): 522–537.
14. Gibson R, Burns J, Ramsey B. Pathophysiology and management of pulmonary infections in cystic fibrosis. *Amer J Respir Crit Care Med* 2003; 168(8): 918–951.
15. Flume P, Mogayzel Jr. P, Robinson K, et al. Cystic fibrosis pulmonary guidelines: treatment of pulmonary exacerbations. *Amer J Respir Crit Care Med* 2009; 180(9): 802–808.
16. Davies J, Rubin B. Emerging and unusual gram-negative infections in cystic fibrosis. *Semin Respir Crit Care Med* 2007; 28(3): 312–321.

17. Dasenbrook E, Merlo C, Diener-West M, Lechtzin N, Boyle M. Persistent methicillin-resistant Staphylococcus aureus and rate of FEV1 decline in cystic fibrosis. *Amer J Respir Crit Care Med* 2008; 178(8): 814–821.
18. Dovey M, Aitken M, Emerson J, McNamara S, Waltz D, Gibson R. Oral corticosteroid therapy in cystic fibrosis patients hospitalized for pulmonary exacerbation. *Chest* 2007; 132(4): 1212–1218.
19. Granton J, Kesten S. The acute effects of nasal positive pressure ventilation in patients with advanced cystic fibrosis. *Chest* 1998; 113(4): 1013–1018.
20. Saiman L, Garber E. Infection control in cystic fibrosis: barriers to implementation and ideas for improvement. *Curr Opin Pulm Med* 2009 July 30. [Epub ahead of print]
21. Flume P, Mogayzel Jr. P, Robinson K, Rosenblatt R, Quittell L, Marshall B. Cystic fibrosis pulmonary guidelines: pulmonary complications—hemoptysis and pneumothorax. *Amer J Respir Crit Care Med* 2010; 182(3): 298–306.
22. Brinson G, Noone P, Mauro M, et al. Bronchial artery embolization for the treatment of hemoptysis in patients with cystic fibrosis. *Amer J Respir Crit Care Med* 1998; 157(6 Pt 1): 1951–1958.
23. Dray X, Bienvenu T, Desmazes-Duefu N, Dusser D, Marteau P, Hubert D. Distal intestinal obstructive syndrome in adults with cystic fibrosis. *Clin Gastroenterol Hepatol* 2004; 2(6): 498–503.
24. Houwen R, Van Der Doef H, Sermet I, et al. Defining DIOS and constipation in cystic fibrosis with a multicentre study on incidence, characteristics, and treatment of DIOS. *JPGN* 2010; 50(1): 38–42.
25. Speck K, Charles A. Distal intestinal obstructive syndrome in adults with cystic fibrosis: a surgical perspective. *Arch Surg* 2008; 143(6): 601–603.
26. Barker H, Haworth C, Williams D, Roberts P, Bilton D. Clostridium difficile pancolitis in adults with cystic fibrosis. *J Cyst Fibros* 2008; 7(5): 444–447.
27. Modolell I, Alvarez A, Guarner L, De Gracia J, Malagelada J. Gastrointestinal, liver, and pancreatic involvement in adult patients with cystic fibrosis. *Pancreas* 2001; 22(4): 395–399.
28. Krysa J, Steger A. Pancreas and cystic fibrosis: the implications of increased survival in cystic fibrosis. *Pancreatology* 2007; 7(5–6): 447–450.
29. Gooding I, Bradley E, Puleston J, Gyi K, Hodson M, Westaby D. Symptomatic pancreatitis in patients with cystic fibrosis. *Amer J Gastroenterol* 2009; 104(6): 1519–1523.
30. Colombo C, Battezzati P, Strazzabosco M, Podda M. Liver and biliary problems in cystic fibrosis. *Semin Liver Dis* 1998; 18(3): 227–235.
31. Moyer K, Balistreri W. Hepatobiliary disease in patients with cystic fibrosis. *Curr Opin Gastroenterol* 2009; 25(3): 272–278.
32. Fischman D, Nookala V. Cystic fibrosis-related diabetes mellitus: etiology, evaluation, and management. *Endocr Pract* 2008; 14(9): 1169–1179.
33. Battezzati A, Battezzati P, Costantini D, et al. Spontaneous hypoglycemia in patients with cystic fibrosis. *Eur J Endocrinol* 2007; 156(3): 369–376.
34. Stephenson A, Jamal S, Dowdell T, Pearce D, Corey MET. Prevalence of vertebral fractures in adults with cystic fibrosis and their relationship to bone mineral density. *Chest* 2006; 130(2): 539–544.

35. Aris R, Renner J, Winders A, et al. Increased rate of fractures and severe kyphoscoliosis: sequelae of living into adulthood with cystic fibrosis. *Ann Intern Med* 1998; 128(3): 186–193.

36. Papaioannou A, Kennedy C, Freitag A, et al. Alendronate once weekly for the prevention and treatment of bone loss in Canadian adult cystic fibrosis patients (CFOS trial). *Chest* 2008; 134(4): 794–800.

37. Merkel P. Rheumatic disease and cystic fibrosis. *Arthritis Rheum* 1999; 42(8): 1563–1571.

38. Dixey J, Redington A, Butler R, et al. The arthropathy of cystic fibrosis. *Ann Rheum Dis* 1988; 47(3): 218–223.

39. Eckles M, Anderson P. Cor pulmonale in cystic fibrosis. *Semin Respir Crit Care Med* 2003; 24(3): 323–330.

40. Festini F, Ballarin S, Codamo T, Doro R, Loganes C. Prevalence of pain in adults with cystic fibrosis. *J Cyst Fibros* 2004; 3(1): 51–57.

41. Nash E, Helm E, Stephenson A, Tullis E. Incidence of deep vein thrombosis associated with peripherally inserted central catheters in adults with cystic fibrosis. *J Vasc Interv Radiol* 2009; 20(3): 347–351.

42. Barker M, Thoenes D, Dohmen H, Friedrichs F, Pfannenstiel C, Heimann G. Prevalence of thrombophilia and catheter-related thrombosis in cystic fibrosis. *Pediatr Pulmonol* 2005; 39(2): 156–161.

43. Riekert K, Bartlett S, Boyle M, Krishnan J, Rand C. The association between depression, lung function and health-related quality of life among adults with cystic fibrosis. *Chest* 2007; 132(1): 231–237.

44. Cruz I, Marciel K, Quittner A, Schechter M. Anxiety and depression in cystic fibrosis. *Semin Respir Crit Care Med* 2009; 30(5): 569–578.

45. Tandon R, Derkay C. Contemporary management of rhinosinusitis and cystic fibrosis. *Curr Opin Otolaryngol Head Neck Surg* 2003; 11(1): 41–44.

46. Bernstein M, McCusker M, Grant-Kels J. Cutaneous manifestations of cystic fibrosis. *Pediatr Dermatol* 2008; 25(2): 150–157.

47. Fama F, Castagna I, Palamara F, Roszkowska A, Ferreri G. Cystic fibrosis and lens opacity. *Ophthalmologica* 1998; 212(3): 178–179.

48. Castagna I, Roszkowska A, Fama F, Sinicropi S, Ferreri G. The eye in cystic fibrosis. *Eur J Opthalmol* 2001; 11(1): 9–14.

49. Jones A, Helm J. Emerging treatments in cystic fibrosis. *Drugs* 2009; 69(14): 1903–1910.

50. Deterding R, LaVagne L, Engels J, et al. Phase 2 randomized safety and efficacy trial of nebulized denufosol tetrasodium in cystic fibrosis. *Amer J Respir Crit Care Med* 2007; 176(4): 362–369.

51. Van Goor F, Hadida S, Grootenhuis P, et al. Rescue of CF airway epithelial cell function in vitro by a CFTR potentiator, VX-770. *Proc Nat Acad Sci USA* 2009; 106(44): 18825–18830.

52. Accurso F, Rowe S, Clancy J, et al. Effect of VX-770 in persons with cystic fibrosis and the G551D-CFTR mutation. *NEJM* 2010; 363(21): 1991–2003.

53. Kerem E, Hirawat S, Armoni S, et al. Effectiveness of PTC124 treatment of cystic fibrosis caused by nonsense mutations: a prospective phase II trial. *Lancet* 2008; 372(9640): 719–727.

54. MacLeod D, Barker L, Sutherland J, et al. Antibacterial activities of fosfomycin/tobramycin combination: a novel inhaled antibiotic for bronchiectasis. *J Antimicrob Chemother* 2009; 64(4): 829–836.

55. Okusanya O, Bhavnani S, Hammel J, et al. Pharmacokinetic and pharmacodynamic evaluation of liposomal amikacin for inhalation in cystic fibrosis patients with chronic Pseudomonal infection. *Antimicrob Agents Chemother* 2009; 53(9): 3847–3854.

56. Tirouvanziam R, Conrad C, Bottiglieri T, Herzenberg L, Moss R, Herzenberg L. High-dose oral N-acetylcysteine, a glutathione prodrug, modulates inflammation in cystic fibrosis. *Proc Nat Acad Sci USA* 2006; 103(12): 4628–4633.

CHAPTER 7
Adults with sickle-cell disease: implications of increasing longevity

Ward Hagar and Claudia R. Morris
Children's Hospital and Research Center, Oakland, CA, USA

Introduction and epidemiology

Sickle-cell disease (SCD) is an inherited hemolytic anemia that affects nearly 100,000 individuals in the United States, primarily African-Americans, and millions more worldwide. Approximately 8% of African-Americans carry the sickle-cell gene [1]. Sickling conditions occur in individuals of African, Caribbean, Mediterranean, Arab, and other Middle Eastern descent and are appearing in more and more ethnic groups. There are an estimated 60,000 persons with SS-type SCD, 30,000 with SC disease, and 10,000 with S-β-thalassemia conditions in the United States. Although an accurate account of the global burden of SCD is unknown, recent newborn screening analysis for hemoglobinopathies in the State of California revealed an incidence of 1/393 African-American infants born with SCD over an 8.5-year time period [2]. In Sub-Saharan Africa, it is estimated that 1%–4% of the population is born with this disease [3]

Despite the perception that sickle-cell trait and disease are only extant in the African-American community in the United States, there is an increasing realization that this illness exists in other ethics groups as well. In Florida, up to 28% of SCD patients are of Hispanic ethnicity, and in other states, such as New Hampshire, the Hispanic ethnicity prevalence among SCD patients can reach 38% [1]. In California, 12.5% of S-β-thalassemia infants were of Hispanic origin [2]. Despite the high global prevalence, SCD remains a rare and orphan disease in the United States. Continuity of care is a challenge, and transitioning from pediatric to adult care can be difficult, as practitioners familiar with SCD are limited. The small number

Challenging and Emerging Conditions in Emergency Medicine, First Edition. Edited by Arvind Venkat.
© 2011 by John Wiley & Sons, Ltd. Published 2011 by Blackwell Publishing Ltd.

of patients makes it unlikely that any particular health care provider sees any appreciable number of sickle-cell patients. In fact, it is estimated from insurance data that of the sickle-cell patients that see a physician regularly, half see a physician for whom they are the only sickle-cell patient that that provider sees (Cage Johnson, personal communication).

Genetics and pathophysiology

The myriad clinical features of the disease result from a deceptively simple amino acid substitution of valine for glutamic acid in the 6th position of the β-subunits of hemoglobin. The result is intracellular polymerization under hypoxia and dehydration. Sickled RBCs are less deformable than normal cells and fragment in the circulation, resulting in shortened RBC survival of only 10–12 days compared to 120 days for normal erythrocytes. Oxidative stress, chronic endothelial damage, and hemolysis initiate a cascade of events that results in episodic vaso-occlusion and subsequent ischemia-reperfusion injury, which clinically amounts to a cytokine bomb [4, 5]. The clinical phenotype of SCD varies widely and is characterized by anemia, severe pain, and potentially life-threatening complications such as bacterial sepsis, splenic sequestration, acute chest syndrome (pneumonia), stroke, and chronic organ damage. These and other manifestations result from chronic hemolysis and intermittent episodes of vascular occlusion that cause tissue injury and organ dysfunction [4, 6, 7].

The single sickle mutation is not sufficient to explain the heterogeneity of the disease phenotype. Two subphenotypes of SCD have recently emerged: that of "Viscosity–Vaso-Occlusion" that involves erythrocyte sickling complications such as pain crisis, acute chest syndrome, and osteonecrosis; and a second subphenotype of "Hemolysis–Endothelial Dysfunction", a proliferative vasculopathy that involves pulmonary hypertension, priapism, leg ulcers, stroke [8] (Figure 7.1) [7], and possibly asthma [5, 9]. The quantification of hemolytic intensity can be estimated by evaluating tertiles or quartiles of lactate dehydrogenase values [10], or using a recently published hemolytic "index" determined by a principal component analysis of the levels of reticulocyte count, lactate dehydrogenase, aspartate aminotransferase, and bilirubin [11]. The variable disease severity is likely the result of complex genetic modifiers and polymorphisms that affect the individual phenotype. For example, SCD patients with single or double α-hemoglobin gene deletions or genetically influenced elevations of fetal hemoglobin (Hb-F) experience milder disease. Since fetal hemoglobin is protective, the newborn will not have clinical manifestation of SCD until the switch from Hb-F to Hb-S occurs after the first few months of life. The enhanced survival for these RBCs results from the improved erythrocyte survival and deformability from the inhibition of Hb-S

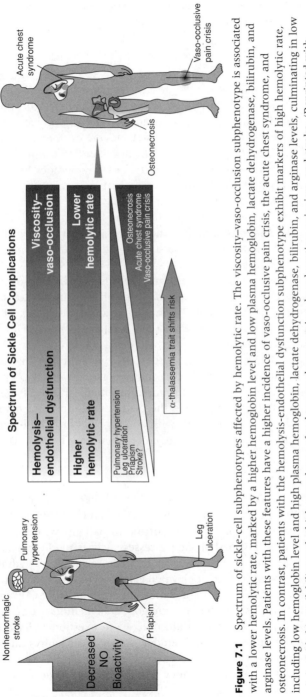

Figure 7.1   Spectrum of sickle-cell subphenotypes affected by hemolytic rate. The viscosity–vaso-occlusion subphenotype is associated with a lower hemolytic rate, marked by a higher hemoglobin level and low plasma hemoglobin, lactate dehydrogenase, bilirubin, and arginase levels. Patients with these features have a higher incidence of vaso-occlusive pain crisis, the acute chest syndrome, and osteonecrosis. In contrast, patients with the hemolysis–endothelial dysfunction subphenotype exhibit markers of high hemolytic rate, including low hemoglobin level and high plasma hemoglobin, lactate dehydrogenase, bilirubin, and arginase levels, culminating in low nitric oxide bioavailability and a high prevalence of pulmonary hypertension, leg ulceration, priapism, and stroke. (Reprinted with permission from Gladwin MT, Vichinsky E. Pulmonary complications of sickle cell disease. *N Engl J Med* 2008; 359(21): 2254–2265. Copyright© [2008] Massachusetts Medical Society. All rights reserved.)

polymerization by Hb-F. The success of hydroxyurea, the only FDA-approved drug intervention for SCD, is mechanistically based on its ability to increase Hb-F.

Life expectancy

Patients with SCD have a shortened life expectancy, and death in infancy and childhood is still a significant risk, with approximately 15% mortality in patients with homozygous Hb-S prior to 20 years of age, peaking between 1 and 3 years of age [12]. These statistics are even more unfavorable in areas where access to care is limited, particularly in countries of the Third World. However, advances during the last few decades in medical management have significantly improved patient survival. Patients with SCD are now expected to survive into at least late middle age, and a large proportion to well over 50 years. With improved longevity comes the development of complications unique to the adult with SCD that are present alongside the usual medical issues that typically develop for the patient's current age and ethnic group [13–15].

In recent decades, several practices emerged that vastly improved patient survival. In particular, the childhood use of transfusions for stroke risk [16], penicillin prophylaxis [17], and better splenic care has led to a marked increase in longevity. However, there is currently no cure for SCD. Even bone marrow transplantation does not consistently prevent ongoing vasculopathy and delayed symptoms. Ironically, with the fact that this is the first time in human history that so many persons with SCD are living into adulthood, new, unique, and important medical issues have also emerged [18]. This chapter discusses the acute evaluation and management of the adult patient with SCD, with an emphasis on both emerging and common complications that require emergency department (ED) care.

Sickle-cell trait

Sickle-cell disease is an autosomal recessive condition. Sickle-cell trait (hemoglobin AS) is not regarded as a disease state, and individuals are typically asymptomatic. Complications occurring in patients with sickle-cell trait are uncommon, but pathologic processes such as methemoglobinemia, high altitude and other causes of hypoxia, acidosis, dehydration, hyperosmolality, hypothermia, or elevated erythrocyte 2,3-DPG can transform silent sickle-cell trait into a syndrome resembling SCD. Established associations with sickle-cell trait include renal medullary carcinoma, hematuria, splenic infarcts at high altitude, acute exertional rhabdomyolysis, urinary tract infection, and sudden death during physical exertion [19]. Hyphema complications, venous thromboembolic events, fetal loss/neonatal deaths, and pregnancy complications have also been reported [20]. Although rare, reports of increased mortality risk in young African-American athletes and military recruits have generated attention to the risks of sickle-cell trait. Athletes with sickle-cell trait and their instructors must be aware of the dangers of the condition during anaerobic exertion, especially in hot and dehydrated conditions [21]. Awareness of these risks and aggressive early intervention may improve survival. Whether collapse with exercise in sickle trait is more common than in hematologically normal athletes is unknown. However, collapse in a sickle-cell trait patient is a medical emergency. Management should include assessment of vital signs, administration of high flow oxygen (15 L/min with a non-rebreather face mask), cooling of the athlete, intravenous hydration, cardiac monitoring for patients with vital sign abnormalities, or, if obtunded, close evaluation for severe rhabdomyolysis and metabolic complications. Early transfusions or red cell exchange may be important if the hemoglobin is low (less than 6.5 g/dL) and biological markers of ongoing hemolysis (high total bilirubin and lactate dehydrogenase levels) are high.

Complications of sickle-cell disease

Vaso-occlusive episodes

Pain is the hallmark of SCD. Pain is also the most vexing problem of sickle-cell care in the ED [22] and accounts for nearly 80% of the approximately 200,000 annual ED visits for SCD [23]. All severe pain should be considered a precursor of a more severe sickle-cell complication. The pain is often excruciating and debilitating and is a true medical emergency. Pain is typically managed at home using acetaminophen with codeine, fluids, rest, and hot packs; the ED visit is often the final resort only after conservative outpatient measures have failed. The challenge for the emergency physician is to understand that severe pain is often the harbinger of life-threatening conditions. The most common medical mistakes for the ED staff revolve around pain. The first is not fully evaluating a patient presenting even with their typical pain episode. The sickle-cell patient may present with pain for several visits and then come in with a life-threatening condition whose main manifestation is pain. The second mistake, and one that has again led to deaths in the ED, is not recognizing the wide variation in pain in different sickle-cell patients. This may result in assuming that a sickle-cell patient is tolerant to medications and using a higher dose than that particular patient is used to. This mistake is then compounded by failing to monitor the patient for respiratory depression after narcotics are given. Furthermore, it is important to remember that pain is damage—damage to some tissue, organ, or neuronal pathway. Most adults have accumulated enough damage that they have chronic mixed pain with or without acute sickle-cell pain flares, as opposed to the more pure sickle-cell pain of children.

Most studies find that emergency physicians misunderstand sickle pain and are not satisfied with ED pain treatment, just as patients are unsatisfied with the knowledge of the ED staff with SCD and their treatment [22]. Successful use of opioids and adjuvants requires expertise and skill in pain assessment and experience in using potent pain medications. Negative attitudes toward patients with painful sickle crises have been compounded by racial stereotypes, the effects of the disease in limiting educational and employment opportunities, suboptimal medical coverage, and the large doses of opioids often required to obtain pain relief [24]. Disparities in pain management practices have also been reported, as adults with SCD experience longer delays in the initiation of analgesics despite higher pain scores and acuity levels compared to other patients with pain [25]. A recent study found that 53% of emergency physicians believe that over 20% of sickle-cell patients are addicted to opioids, with 22% of emergency physicians believing that over 50% are addicted to opioids. Behaviors such as being a clock-watcher, knowing names and doses of specific opioids, requesting and requiring large doses of medications, and multiple ED visits are taken as evidence of addiction. A recent study of 232 sickle-cell patients that kept detailed pain diaries found that 35.5% were high ED utilizers, defined by three or more ED visits a year. However, the same study showed that these patients had lower hemoglobin, lower quality of life, more pain and distress, more pain days, more crises, and more transfusions than those who were not high ED users [26]. Indeed, controlling for the severity of their illness, high ED utilizers did not use more opioids any more often. In short, they were sicker and they hurt more.

It is important to keep in mind that by the time a person with SCD is an adult, they have had over 15 years of opioid exposure. Such exposure leads to an experience of care, ideas of what has worked in the past, and tolerance to low doses of opioids. The usual pain of SCD is classically felt to be vaso-occlusive and ischemic. Recent work has also implicated numerous cytokines that suggest the release of a cytokine bomb involving adhesion factors, endothelial activation, and nitric oxide changes. Because of this, pain can have roving locations over several days as the vascular beds and nerves respond to these signals, but would tend to be located with stability during a single ED visit. Recent studies with sickle mice suggest the profound changes in the nerves and pain pathways that come not only from chronic pains, but also from chronic use of opioids and other medications. In fact, chronic use of medication may cause hypersensitivity to pain and a decrease in the effectiveness of further treatment. Other studies have shown that some patients worsen their pains with the chronic use of specific opioids, an effect called hyperalgesia [27, 28].

One of the most important questions an emergency physician can ask is whether this pain episode is similar to the patient's prior episodes. Sickle-cell pains are as varied as the persons with SCD. Some patients present so seldom for emergency care that any ED visit warrants admission. Asking about prior treatments, or better yet, having an individualized pain plan accessible from the patient's electronic medical record, allows the consistency of treatment necessary to fine-tune an ED care plan for complex pain. An account of the patient's sickle-cell history is important, including past history of stroke, bony sickling and avascular necrosis, asthma, allergies, or priapism. Treatment plans should include information on which opioids and their amounts and routes work best, along with adjuvants, such as lorazepam, ketorolac, and diphenhydramine. Lastly, set criteria for admission (such as admit if three rounds of opioids are not controlling pain, or hemoglobin is less than 7 g/dL) are helpful.

One major factor in the care of sickle-cell pain is the psychology of pain itself. As patients become stressed, their pain increases when they start thinking about how severe their pain can get. Experience with this population has revealed that one of the most important factors in improvement in a patient's pain is the perception that the health care practitioner cares about them. Having a policy of rapid treatment of sickle-cell pain can allay the worsening of anticipatory pain. This can be especially important since by the time a patient comes to the ED, he or she has had hours, often days, of uncontrolled pain.

Another challenge for patients and emergency physicians is that once they start recovering from their last crisis or medical event, their bone marrow increases production of sickle cells, releasing sickle reticulocytes. Unfortunately, these sickle reticulocytes are the most sticky of sickle cells and often cause a rebound crisis. This has led some to question the utility of using readmission after hospitalization as a "quality" indicator as it is part of the natural history of the disease. For the emergency physician, this manifests itself as a patient returning to the ED several times in a short period of time [29].

Approach to the sickle-cell patient with pain

1. Start analgesics as soon as possible.
2. Patients with severe pain or anxiety may benefit from anxiolytics to decrease anticipatory pain, such as lorazepam (1–2 mg IV q4h).
3. Obtain a history of pain, type, location, and quantity. See if any triggers can be identified. Ascertain if this is similar to usual pain crisis. Note any differences between past episodes and this episode.
4. Acknowledge patient's pain, and ask what has worked in the past. Assure patient that you will work to relieve their pain, regularly assess the success of pain treatment, and adjust treatment accordingly.

5. Give opioids with short duration between doses if pain is unrelieved. Morphine IV can be given every 10 minutes, hydromorphone every 40 minutes. Attempt to get ahead of pain by repeated doses. If no IV, use the IM or subcut route.
6. Evaluate for other causes of pain.
7. Start hydration with D5/0.5 normal saline at 100–120 mL/h, using some free water to aid in cellular, and especially red cell, rehydration.
8. If chest pain, fever, or low pulse oximetry measurement (<93%) that isn't reversed by deep breathing is present, check a chest radiograph for early infiltrates. Utilize supplemental oxygen for low pulse oximetry measurements.
9. Compare hemoglobin to prior values. If the current value is lower by more than 1–1.5 g/dL, consider transfusions or admission.
10. If no better after three rounds of analgesics, consider admission.

Fever/infections

Patients with SCD often present with mild fever. The etiology can be the inflammation of sickle cell itself (up to about 100.5°F). Atelectasis from pulmonary splinting, medications' effects, and infections are common causes for fever in this patient population. There are reports of increased incidence of *Salmonella* osteomyelitis in sickle-cell patients presenting with fever, but these seem rare [30]. In an adult, a fever over 101°F should be evaluated as in a non-sickle-cell adult. Fever can be a harbinger of more severe sickle-cell complications such as acute chest syndrome [31], leg ulcerations, large bony infarcts, thrombosis, and infections. Also, sickle-cell patients often have, or have had, indwelling lines or vascular access devices. What little data is available suggests that patients with SCD are somewhat more susceptible to line infections, possible from small clots caused by their hypercoagulable state [32]. In general, the workup is like any other patient with a fever, but admission is warranted for any symptomatic fever without a clear, treatable source. Some studies suggest that sickle-cell patients are also prone to more atypical infections than the general population [33]. In treating a patient without an identified source, a macrolide or quinolone antibiotic, such as levofloxacin, should be included in addition to a parenteral broad-spectrum antibiotic appropriate to local infective organisms.

Approach to the sickle-cell patient with fever

1. Temperature >100.5°F
   (a) Obtain blood, urine, and line cultures (if present).
   (b) Evaluate the skin for ulcers.
   (c) Obtain chest X-ray (CXR) (posteroanterior and lateral views). Evaluate CXR for signs of infiltrates.
   (d) Evaluate bones for infarcts or infections.

2. Is the fever symptomatic?
   (a) Is the patient fatigued, sweating, or weak?
   (b) Is there localized pain or difficulty in breathing?
3. If the source of fever can be identified, such as a urinary tract infection, sexually transmitted disease, or skin infection, and the patient is not symptomatic, then the patient can be treated as an outpatient with appropriate follow-up.
4. If the source of fever cannot be identified, then the patient should be admitted for evaluation and observation and covered with broad-spectrum antibiotics, including an IV second- or third-generation cephalosporin and an oral or IV macrolide or quinolone antibiotic.

Acute anemic complications

The average lifespan of a sickle red cell is 10 days. So, if there is a process that decreases the reticulocyte count, then the patients can lose up to 10% of their hemoglobin daily. Add that baseline drop in hemoglobin to the drop from active hemolysis, and a patient can suddenly have a hemoglobin level of 3 g/dL or less. In addition, the hemoglobin in the ED often is artificially high from dehydration. In sickle-cell patients with active mild disease, the hemoglobin can drop by 1 g/dL each day and is often significantly lower the day after admission. Patients vary greatly in their baseline hemoglobin levels. Some patients with chronically low hemoglobin levels may decline transfusions even when their hemoglobin level is less than 6 g/dL.

Transfusions in the ED are best started for symptomatic anemia—weakness, dizziness, orthostatic hypertension, chest pains, dyspnea, and sweating—or other signs of poor end organ perfusion. Acute transfusions (as opposed to monthly transfusions) may not be helpful for sickle-cell pain and complications, as once a pain episode has started, the numerous cytokine and endothelial processes already have been released and will run their course. If transfusions are indicated, then red cell transfusions that are negative for the antigens Kell, E, and C may help stabilize the patient's hemoglobin level. Although uncommon, delayed hemolytic transfusion reactions can occur; so obtaining a history of transfusions in the last month could point to a transfusion reaction. Most of these occur within 10 days of transfusions, but delays of weeks have been reported [34, 35]. If a delayed transfusion reaction is suspected, then the patient is best managed by admission where the appropriate follow-up tests, and transfusion under observation, can be more safely performed.

In adults, as compared to children, splenic or hepatic sequestration is rare. Most adults with SS hemoglobin have autoinfarcted their spleens. Hemoglobin SC and S-β-thalassemia patients may have some degree of splenic or hepatic red cell sequestration, but the larger body mass of an adult makes the condition far less life threatening than in a child and is usually treated as a simple anemia. If transfusions are indicated, it is important to keep the hemoglobin under about 11 g/dL. In vitro and in vivo studies find that unless the percentage of sickle cells in the circulation is less than 50%, as measured by quantitative hemoglobin electrophoresis (as it would be from a chronic transfusion program), increasing the hemoglobin over 11.5 g/dL increases red cell viscosity and decreases peripheral tissue oxygen delivery [36, 37].The formulas that can be used to keep the amount transfused in a safe range are discussed in the section below entitled "Transfusion therapy". If a patient with a high hemoglobin level otherwise needs transfusion, then consultation for exchange transfusion is needed.

There are two rare, but potentially deadly, hemolytic complications of SCD. The first is the hyperhemolysis syndrome, where both transfused and non-transfused cells lyse. The more the patient is transfused, the more the hemolysis is accentuated [38]. If a patient presents with a lower hemoglobin level in the ED just after their recent transfusions and with no obvious source of blood loss, then urgent hematologic consultation is warranted. The second complication is aplastic crisis [39, 40]. This condition is defined by hypermetabolic bone marrow, due to necrosis or infection, failing to produce the tens of millions of red cells per second needed to balance the ongoing hemolysis of SCD. This can rapidly result in a dangerously low hemoglobin level. The hallmark of this condition is a low or even nonexistent reticulocyte count in the face of dropping hemoglobin levels. Parvovirus infection, with its propensity to infect reticulocytes, is the most commonly identified cause of this condition [41].

Approach to the sickle-cell patient with anemia

1. Routinely obtain a complete blood count, including reticulocyte count. Ascertain the patient's baseline hemoglobin. See if the reticulocyte count is appropriately higher than normal. If not, then anticipate a further drop in hemoglobin of about 1–2 g/dL over the next 24 hours.
2. Has the patient been transfused in the last month?
3. Ascertain if the patient has symptomatic anemia (weakness, dizziness).
4. If the patient is symptomatic and the hemoglobin is more than 1 g/dL below the patient's baseline, consider transfusing with phenotypically matched, sickle hemoglobin negative and leukoreduced red cells.
5. If the patient has signs of increased hemolysis (higher bilirubin, lactate dehydrogenase, or aspartate transaminases) and an inappropriately low or normal reticulocyte count, consider transfusion.
6. If the patient was transfused within the last month and has a significantly lower hemoglobin level on presentation than after transfusions, consider delayed hemolytic transfusion reactions.

7. If the patient seems to have any severe sickle-cell complications and anemia, then consider transfusions to stabilize the acute sickling cycle. This is especially true for acute chest syndrome as early transfusion may interrupt the severity and duration of this condition.
8. Remember that the hemoglobin in the ED is often elevated from dehydration.
9. Any symptomatic anemia with a history or signs that suggest a possible delayed transfusion reaction, hyperhemolysis, or aplastic crisis necessitates admission and hematologic consultation.
10. Keep the post-transfusion hemoglobin less than 11.5 g/dL. If there is concern about exceeding this value, hematologic consultation is needed for possible manual exchange transfusion or automated exchange transfusion (erythrocytopheresis).

Pulmonary complications

Acute chest syndrome is one of the hallmark complications of sickle-cell disease. It is a complex condition of bone marrow emboli, infection, and vascular shunting [42]. Physician recognition of acute chest syndrome is suboptimal, given that few respiratory symptoms may be present early on [31]. About 50% of acute chest syndromes present as a pain crisis with a normal CXR. Interestingly, one risk factor for developing acute chest syndrome is having severe limb pain, likely secondary to marrow infarct leading to marrow emboli [33]. Any new CXR infiltrate with a fever in a person with SCD should be treated as acute chest syndrome. Macrolide antibiotics are recommended to cover the high percentage of atypical bacteria noted in bronchoscopy studies of SCD [33]. Early transfusions anecdotally seem to abort or to lessen the severity of acute chest syndrome [43]. Some studies have used intravenous corticosteroids to good effect, but rebound has been noted [44, 45]. Keeping the oxygenation greater than 93% by nasal cannula is important to decrease the shunting that keeps the sickled cells in the sickle state. Also, patients short of breath or with chest pain severe enough to keep them from inspiring fully are at risk for development of acute chest syndrome or pneumonia.

Separating acute chest syndrome from pulmonary embolism in the ED is challenging. Hypoxia and chest pain, elevated D-dimer levels, abnormal V/Q scan, and even positive CT angiograms can be due to either condition. Patients with SCD are often in a hypercoagulable state [46], with increased markers of activation of the coagulation system and decreased levels of antithrombotic factors such as protein C and protein S [47]. If a pulmonary embolism is suspected, it should be treated as in a person without SCD. If the CT angiogram is negative, despite an elevated D-dimer, treating the patient as with acute chest syndrome is usually appropriate. Little data support anticoagulation for acute chest syndrome, and such treatment is not routinely recommended.

By adulthood, baseline pulmonary function is abnormal in approximately 90% of patients with SCD [48]. Regardless of the cause, severe pulmonary disease requires admission and inpatient follow-up and evaluations. Sickle-cell patients often present with wheezing and have a history of asthma [49]. Asthma is also common in the background populations where SCD is most prevalent. Treatment with aerosolized β-agonists with pre- and post-peak flows often results in substantial clinical improvement. Incentive spirometry alone has also shown marked improvement in outcomes [50]. Improving lung oxygenation by treating the bronchoreactive component of the disease may decrease the sickling process and prevent further progression. Arterial blood gases usually show partial pressures of oxygen lower than the pulse oximetry would indicate, and should be obtained to guide therapy if the patient has severe pulmonary compromise. The use of corticosteroids for acute chest syndrome is controversial [51–53]. Although they may improve the course of illness, concern for rebound symptoms have affected clinical utilization among many practitioners. However, patients with moderate-to-severe acute chest syndrome are more likely to receive corticosteroids, which may, in part, account for the rebound phenomenon. In a more recent study, a short course of prednisone did not significantly increase readmission rate after discharge for acute chest syndrome [53]. If a patient has severe chest symptoms, transfusions and steroids may be initiated in discussion with the inpatient treatment team, to be evaluated and tapered slowly after admission. Sickle-cell patients can be safely intubated. These patients are more sensitive to barotrauma than the general patient, but acutely require adequate oxygenation. Keeping the airway peak filling pressures as low as possible may help prevent barotrauma.

Pulmonary hypertension is an increasingly recognized complication of chronic hemolytic anemias, including SCD. Approximately a third of adults with SCD have an abnormally elevated tricuspid regurgitant jet velocity (>2.5 mg/s) measured by Doppler echocardiography at steady state, suggestive of pulmonary hypertension. This finding alone is associated with a ten-fold risk of early mortality [54]. Advancing age is a clinical risk factor for pulmonary hypertension. In addition, pulmonary pressures rise acutely during vaso-occlusive crisis [55] and even more so during the acute chest syndrome [56]. A recent study examined 84 consecutive hospitalized patients with the acute chest syndrome and found that 13% had clinical manifestations of right heart failure, placing them at the highest risk for mechanical ventilation and death [56]. These data suggest that acute pulmonary hypertension and right heart dysfunction represent major co-morbidities during the acute chest syndrome. In some EDs, bedside echocardiograms are available. If right-sided pressures are high in a patient that has severe dyspnea, chest pains, or hypoxia despite external oxygen, oral arginine [57] and intravenous L-arginine hydrochloride (0.1 g/kg tid up to 10 g tid) (unpublished series) have safely and temporarily lowered the right-sided pressures while pulmonary or cardiology consultation is sought. Sildenafil has been shown to increase pain episodes in SCD and is not currently recommended in the acute setting. Guidelines for the evaluation and treatment of pulmonary hypertension in SCD are currently under development by a committee commissioned by the American Thoracic Society and will be available in the near future.

Approach to the sickle-cell patient with pulmonary complaints

1. Ascertain rapidity of onset and other historical factors such as asthma, severe limb pain, or a past history of thromboembolism.
2. Ascertain temperature and severity of hypoxia, using arterial blood draw if needed. Attempt to correct low pulse oximetry by deep breathing, thereby showing low tidal volumes secondary to splinting from pain. Give enough analgesics to allow deep breathing.
3. Examine lungs for signs of consolidation, air trapping, wheezing, and pleural changes. Egophony and vesicular breath sounds are often present before radiographic changes are seen.
4. CXR is indicated with any severe chest symptoms, hypoxia, or fever. Heart size is often enlarged secondary to anemia, but compare to prior films for acute changes. Any new infiltrate and a fever should be considered acute chest syndrome and warrants admission.
5. Remember that half of the acute chest syndrome patients present with pain and a normal CXR that will become positive with time and hydration, usually within 72 hours. (Figures 7.2a–c).
6. If acute chest syndrome is suspected, keep the patient hydrated and oxygenated. Empiric antibiotics, including a quinolone or a macrolide, in addition to a parenteral broad-spectrum antibiotic appropriate to local infective organisms, should be routinely started. If symptoms are severe, then consider steroids and early transfusion. If the hemoglobin is too high for simple transfusions, hematology consultation for erythrocytopheresis is needed.
7. If the patient is wheezing, then treatments directed at bronchospasm and asthma should be started.
8. If the history and physical examination suggest a pulmonary embolism, then duplex venous evaluation and CT angiogram should be obtained. SCD is not a contraindication to contrast. However, renal dysfunction is common in adults with SCD and poses the same relative risks as in other patients. D-dimer levels in acute sickling are often high and can overlap the range for pulmonary embolism; thus, this is not a sensitive test alone for pulmonary embolism.
9. For severe dyspnea or chest pain without a clear cause, Doppler echocardiography is indicated to screen for pulmonary hypertension.

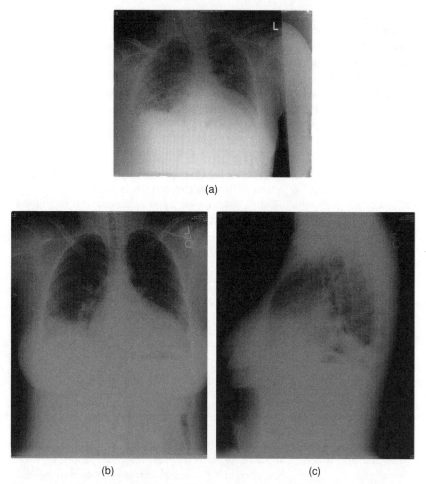

Figure 7.2   Chest radiographs of evolving acute chest syndrome. (a) A CXR taken in the ED of a patient presenting with a vaso-occlusive pain episode that included leg and lower back pain. The official reading by radiology was "mild congestion, no infiltrate." (b, c) CXRs taken 24 hours after admission, with an official reading of right lower lobe infiltrate and atelectasis, consistent with acute chest syndrome.

If increased pulmonary pressure is suspected (over approximately 35 mm Hg), then admission is warranted for further observations and evaluation. Brain natriuretic peptide (BNP) may be helpful diagnostically as most patients with significant pulmonary hypertension have a BNP >500 pg/mL [58].

10. Any acute lung compromise warrants admission for further observation and treatment.

Cardiovascular complications

Chronic inflammation in most patients with SCD was once believed to be protective from classic epicardial heart disease, in part, by keeping the cholesterol levels low [59]. This may have some truth, but as the sickle-cell population ages, more heart abnormalities are becoming increasingly prevalent. These divide into vascular, electrical, and myocardial conditions. There may also be a vasculopathy associated with SCD. This may manifest itself as decreased left ventricular systolic and diastolic function, or pulmonary hypertension. Indeed, chest discomfort may be a sign of increased pulmonary pressures. Electrical cardiac disease may manifest as conduction abnormalities and prolonged QT intervals [60]. Lastly, a decreased left ventricular ejection fraction may be chronic or episodic. Pulmonary hypertension, as shown by echocardiography, may be secondary to volume overload or increased pulmonary vascular resistance. Several publications suggest that if the tricuspid regurgitant jet velocity is greater than 2.5 m/s, sickle-cell patients have a mortality of about 40% at 40 months [54, 61–64]. The pathophysiology of pulmonary hypertension may involve nitric oxide and arginine dysregulation [65], among other abnormalities. Sickle-cell patients may also have a higher incidence of prolonged QTc, likely reflecting many factors including methadone [66] and other opioid use, genetic factors [67], possibly transfusional iron overload [68], hemolysis, and other cardiac abnormalities [69, 70]. Therefore, before giving medications that have a known side effect of prolonging QTc, checking an ECG may be important in the ED. Although less common than in the general population, as patients age, the likelihood of classical atherosclerotic heart disease increases, and patients should be screened for epicardial disease as otherwise age appropriate. For severe chest pains, checking troponin, creatine kinase and its isoenzymes, and BNP levels, along with an ECG, can help delineate the etiology of the chest pain.

Approach to the sickle-cell patient with chest complaints

1. Assess for classic causes of chest pain and discomfort. A high proportion of chest complaints can be reproduced by rib or sternal palpation, showing these as manifestations of soft tissue and bone sickling and pain. Often, these are accompanied by splinting. If age and symptom appropriate, screen for epicardial heart disease by ECG and cardiac markers.
2. If the pain is not musculoskeletal or pleuritic, evaluate the lungs (as above) and the heart. ECGs often show various abnormalities related to acute pain and medications, such as prolonged QTc and nonspecific T-wave abnormalities. Many sickle-cell patients have reduced chest wall muscle mass, and so high voltage in the anterior leads is common. Comparison to prior tracings may be helpful. CXR may show an enlarged

heart and vascular congestion. BNP levels are helpful in assessing for the presence of pulmonary hypertension.

3. Chest pain may be a symptom of acute chest syndrome. Evaluate as per the protocol outlined above.

4. Echocardiograms with estimation of pulmonary artery pressures may identify patients with right and left ventricular abnormalities. Pulmonary artery pressures can rise with acute chest syndrome, pneumonia, pain, and bronchospasm. If increased pulmonary artery pressures (over approximately 35 mm Hg) are present in a symptomatic patient, admission is warranted for further observation and evaluation.

Central nervous system complications

Stroke is a devastating complication of SCD. This is most common in young children not receiving regular transfusions [71]. Adults often have subtle manifestations of clinical and subclinical infarcts [72]. This may manifest from seizures to impulse control to memory issues. A recent neuropsychologic study found profound neurologic and functional deficits even among sickle-cell patients with no overt signs of neurologic problems or any past history of neurologic or psychiatric history [73]. Adults tend to have hemorrhagic strokes [74], possibly related to secondary moyamoya, although occlusive infarcts still occur.

Approach to the sickle-cell patient with suspected stroke

1. In adults, stroke presents with the typical neurologic signs and symptoms. Any unexplained focal neurologic finding, such as tingling or twitching in a cranial nerve distribution, new onset seizures, or loss of sensation or strength, may herald either transient ischemic attacks or a stroke.

2. If a stroke is suspected, emergent erythrocytopheresis is indicated.

3. A CT scan is often needed to look for acute hemorrhagic stroke. Other imaging (contrast CT or MRI) would be indicated in the appropriate clinical setting, such as clinical signs of acute cerebral vascular obstruction.

4. The use of thrombolytics in SCD is understudied, but not contraindicated in the appropriate clinical setting.

Ocular complications

Three acute sickle-cell ocular conditions may present in the ED. One is hyphema, which is blood in the anterior chamber of the eye and, usually, is the result of trauma or surgery [75]. Although this is rare, because of the high risk of complications in patients with sickle trait as well as SCD, a sickledex preparation to rule out sickle trait should be ordered on every hyphema patient, regardless of ethnic background. A second ocular emergency is vitreous hemorrhage. This is a consequence of the neovascularization of the retina, similar to that in diabetic patients. The third complication is arterial occlusion. The treatment for all is similar. The patient needs to reduce the viscosity of blood, increase oxygenation to the tissues, and reduce the amount of sickle cells that cause activation of the endothelium that leads to more occlusion, inflammation, and end organ damage.

Approach to the sickle-cell patient with an ocular emergency

1. The treatment of choice for the acute complications of all the three eye emergencies is erythrocytopheresis, where sickle blood is removed while non-sickle blood is transfused. This reduces the percentage of sickled cells to less than 30% rapidly and is often the best stabilization for the sickling red cell cycle. If pheresis is not available and the patient's hemoglobin is less than 9 g/dL, then straight red cell transfusions may be helpful. However, unless the percentages of sickled cells is less than about 50%, increasing the hemoglobin over 11.5 g/dL will both increase blood viscosity and decrease tissue oxygen delivery.
2. Urgent ophthalmologic consultant is needed for possible surgical interventions.

Pregnancy in SCD—emergency management

Pregnancy in SCD is often uncomplicated. A recent review of pregnancy in SCD shows that although many complications of pregnancy are increased in sickle-cell patients, the management is similar to that of the non-sickle-cell patient [76]. A randomized controlled trial showed that for single, uncomplicated pregnancies, the baby does equally well whether the mother is transfused or not [77]. The mothers, however, often feel better when transfused. The babies are often small for gestational age and delivered slightly earlier than the due date would predict, but otherwise do well. The small size and early delivery is likely from placental infarcts noted in sickle-cell patients. This may also explain the slight increase in preeclampsia and placenta previa in sickle-cell patients. A complicating factor is that sickle-cell patients often have proteinuria, elevated liver transaminases, and hypertension at baseline, making surveillance for many complications of pregnancy challenging. Sickle-cell patients should be followed by high-risk obstetrics.

Approach to the pregnant sickle-cell patient

1. A rule of thumb for the ED is that a distressed mother causes a distressed fetus; so any treatment that relieves the mother's distress helps the baby. Narcotics are not contraindicated. The worry about opioids affecting the fetus, although real, is often outweighed by controlling the distress of the mother.

2. Women with SCD may find that their usual sickle-cell pains worsen, improve, or stay the same during different parts of the pregnancy. Closer to term, separating sickle pain from pain related to the body changes of pregnancy is difficult. The best guide is to ask the patient whether the pain is consistent with their prior sickle episodes.

3. Experienced obstetrics consultation is mandatory in any complex ED presentation.

Priapism

Priapism is one of the more challenging issues for men with SCD [78]. Priapism arises most commonly early in the mornings and persists for several hours. Whether the pathophysiology of priapism in SCD is the same as in other conditions is unclear [79]. One hallmark on physical exam in sickle-cell priapism is that the corpus spongiosum does not become engorged. Urination and a warm shower may help at home. By the time the patient has presented to the ED, usually the priapism has persisted for hours. The pain can be excruciating, and treatment can be challenging. Hydration and alkalization have been used as treatments. Adequate analgesia is essential, and using adjuvants such as lorazepam to address the anticipatory pain helps relax the patient and his muscles. Sometimes the priapism is stuttering, with turgidity increasing and decreasing. In such a case, pseudoephedrine orally, 60 mg to 120 mg up to q6h, may be helpful. Subcutaneous terbutaline can also help. Case reports of intravenous sildenafil, antitestosterone medication, and L-arginine (Claudia Morris, unpublished data) have reportedly been helpful [80, 81]. If the priapism persists with turgidity, then aspiration and injection with epinephrine should be attempted in concert with urologic consultation. Exchange transfusions are often used, but their effectiveness is variable [82].

Approach to the sickle-cell patient with priapism

1. Ascertain history of current and prior episodes, including duration, and exacerbating and relieving factors. Priapism can be stuttering, meaning it can cycle between being present and absent.

2. Hydration, analgesics, and alkalization of the blood may be helpful.

3. Physical examination may vary from a turgid erection to no active priapism (in the case of stuttering priapism).

4. If no relief, penile aspiration and injection of epinephrine should be attempted.

5. If no relief occurs within a few hours, urologic consultation is needed, along with admission for simple or exchange transfusions.

Leg ulcers

Leg ulcers are a recalcitrant symptom of SCD [83]. In the ED, the history can help determine the chronicity. A complex series of factors initiate and maintain sickle-cell ulcers. These ulcers are usually on the lateral and medial malleolus, but can affect any areas of the lower leg. The contribution of increased venous pressure is suspected from the fact that bed rest for several weeks is one of the most effective treatments for these ulcers [84]. For the ED provider, the main issue is whether there is a secondary infection of the ulcer.

Approach to the sickle-cell patient with leg ulcers

1. Determine the chronicity of the ulcers, past history, and any change in size, location, exudates, color, or odor.
2. Assess for signs of local or systemic infection.
3. Occasionally, bone X-rays may be helpful to determine if there is underlying osteomyelitis.
4. Cultures are of variable utility, usually will not come back soon enough to be helpful, and often just show skin colonization. If the ulcers are worsening, then a therapeutic trial of antibiotics that cover common skin bacteria may reduce the ulcers. If unsuccessful, then cultures would be warranted to look for more resistant bacteria such as pseudomonas or methicillin-resistant *Staphylococcus aureus*. Wet to dry dressing, and occasionally an Unna boot, may be needed. If the patient has symptoms of bacteremia, he or she requires admission.
5. Bed rest is an effective treatment for most leg ulcers and may warrant admission. Referral to a plastic surgeon for recalcitrant cases may help.

Transfusion therapy

Sickle-cell patients have variable baseline hemoglobin levels. Whether a patient needs an emergent transfusion depends on the change from baseline hemoglobin, symptoms of anemia, and associated conditions. Hemoglobin should not be raised to over 11.5 g/dL to avoid hyperviscosity [85]. The dangers of transfusion are infection, alloimmunization, and iron overload. In the acute setting, the last fact is not a consideration, but in the long term, hemosiderosis can be of paramount importance. Blood-borne infections are rare enough that this shouldn't be a consideration on whether to acutely transfuse a symptomatic patient. Alloimmunizations can be lessened by using red cells negative for the Kell, E, and C antigens, which are responsible for approximately 80% of alloimmunizations [86]. A common empiric formula for determining how much blood to give is: (desired hemoglobin – current hemoglobin) × 4 × weight in kilograms. Alternatively, 10 mg/kg tends to raise the hemoglobin by 2.5 g/dL. These formulae are commonly used, provide an estimate based on clinical experience and are a reasonable guide. The desired level of hemoglobin depends on the condition and on an estimate of how quickly the hemoglobin may be decreasing. Acutely, keeping the hemoglobin over 8 g/dL, with at least 1 mg/dL reserve, is a reasonable rationale to get the hemoglobin to 9 g/dL. Evaluation of the reticulocyte count can be helpful. If the reticulocyte count is low for the hemoglobin, then the patient will likely continue to drop their hemoglobin levels.

Approach to the sickle-cell patient needing transfusion

1. Ascertain transfusion history, frequency, amounts of blood transfused, and history of transfusion reactions.
2. Calculate the number of mL needed to obtain a post-transfusion hemoglobin of 8–9 mg/dL, without exceeding 11.5 mg/dL. Round to the nearest number of units (approximately 250–300 mL red cells/units).
3. If a patient with high hemoglobin needs transfusion for a non-anemia indication, then exchange transfusion is needed, and hematologic consultation is required.
4. Order leukoreduced, sickledex negative red cells, matched for Kell, C, and E antigens. If these units are not available, hematological consultation is needed to find the most compatible units.
5. Premedication before transfusions is not standardized, but often p.o. acetaminophen 650 mg and diphenhydramine 50 mg are common. Loratidine 10 mg p.o. can also be given as premedication for itching. With adults, 20 mg IV furosemide is often given if the number of units exceeds two, or if vascular congestion, dyspnea or high blood pressure develops during transfusions.

The next five years

There is reason for cautious optimism that the next five years will bring relief from pain, decrease of end organ damage, and better quality of life for patients with SCD. On a biologic level, several large trials of intervention for pain have pointed to gaps in our knowledge of sickle pain and sickle complications that are now active areas of research. On a molecular level, there is promise that selected biomarkers of disease severity and hemolytic rate may identify high-risk patients in need of aggressive intervention. Recent correction of SCD in a humanized mouse model by gene replacement therapy in induced pluripotent stem cells [87] sets the stage for the progress of gene replacement therapies in the future. On a social level, better education of physicians about the protean effects of SCD and the best use of current approaches could relieve much pain and suffering. On a pharmacologic level, studies with simple compounds, such as magnesium [88] and arginine [89] for pain and finasteride for priapism [90], and complex compounds, such as selectin inhibitors, to ameliorate acute vaso-occlusion at its inception [91] are ongoing. Pain management remains the most complex and difficult research priority for patients with

SCD. Maximizing the use of existing agents, while looking for better treatments, is critical.

Conclusion

2010 marked the 100th anniversary since SCD was first described. Advances in medical care since that time have significantly improved longevity for patients with sickle-cell disease, who are now expected to survive into their 4th and 5th decade. Improved survival is associated with unique complications in the adult patient as they present at later stages of their disease. Early recognition of complications and aggressive treatment initiated in the ED can dramatically improve patient survival. Early consultation with a hematologist with sickle-cell experience may provide guidance for management and disposition when patients present to the ED with complex issues. Better insight into the pathogenesis of sickle vasculopathy may guide future therapies, while novel therapeutic strategies that target hemolysis, inflammations, and oxidative stress are currently under investigation for this challenging patient population.

References

1. Hassell KL. Population estimates of sickle cell disease in the U.S. *Am J Prev Med* 2010; 38(4 Suppl.): S512–S521.
2. Michlitsch J, Azimi M, Hoppe C, et al. Newborn screening for hemoglobinopathies in California. *Pediatr Blood Cancer* 2009; 52(4): 486–490.
3. Aliyu ZY, Kato GJ, Taylor JT, et al. Sickle cell disease and pulmonary hypertension in Africa: a global perspective and review of epidemiology, pathophysiology, and management. *Am J Hematol* 2008; 83(1): 63–70.
4. Bunn HF. Pathogenesis and treatment of sickle cell disease. *N Engl J Med* 1997; 337(11): 762–769.
5. Morris CR. Mechanisms of vasculopathy in sickle cell disease and thalassemia. *Hematology Am Soc Hematol Educ Program* 2008: 177–185.
6. Stuart MJ, Nagel RL. Sickle-cell disease. *Lancet* 2004; 364(9442): 1343–1360.
7. Gladwin MT, Vichinsky E. Pulmonary complications of sickle cell disease. *N Engl J Med* 2008; 359(21): 2254–2265.
8. Kato GJ, Gladwin MT, Steinberg MH. Deconstructing sickle cell disease: reappraisal of the role of hemolysis in the development of clinical subphenotypes. *Blood Rev* 2007; 21(1): 37–47.
9. Field JJ, Stocks J, Kirkham FJ, et al. Airway hyper-responsiveness in children with sickle cell anemia. *Chest* 2010. [Epub ahead of print]
10. Kato GJ, McGowan V, Machado RF, et al. Lactate dehydrogenase as a biomarker of hemolysis-associated nitric oxide resistance, priapism, leg ulceration, pulmonary hypertension, and death in patients with sickle cell disease. *Blood* 2006; 107(6): 2279–2285.
11. Minniti CP, Sable C, Campbell A, et al. Elevated tricuspid regurgitant jet velocity in children and adolescents with sickle cell disease: association with

hemolysis and hemoglobin oxygen desaturation. *Haematologica* 2009; 94(3): 340–347.

12. Leikin SL, Gallagher D, Kinney TR, Sloane D, Klug P, Rida W. Mortality in children and adolescents with sickle cell disease. Cooperative Study of Sickle Cell Disease. *Pediatrics* 1989; 84(3): 500–508.

13. Hagar W, Vichinsky E. Advances in clinical research in sickle cell disease. *Br J Haematol* 2008; 141(3): 346–356.

14. Lane PA. Sickle cell disease. *Pediatr Clin North Am* 1996; 43(3): 639–664.

15. Platt OS, Brambilla DJ, Rosse WF, et al. Mortality in sickle cell disease: life expectancy and risk factors for early death. *N Engl J Med* 1994; 330(23): 1639–1644.

16. Adams R, McKie V, Hsu L, et al. Prevention of a first stroke by transfusions in children with sickle cell anemia and abnormal results on transcranial Doppler ultrasonography. *N Engl J Med* 1998; 339: 5–11.

17. Gaston MH, Verter JI, Woods G, et al. Prophylaxis with oral penicillin in children with sickle cell anemia: a randomized trial. *N Engl J Med* 1986; 314(25): 1593–1599.

18. Hagar RW, Vichinsky EP. Major changes in sickle cell disease. *Adv Pediatr* 2000; 47: 249–272.

19. Kerle KK, Nishimura KD. Exertional collapse and sudden death associated with sickle cell trait. *Am Fam Physician* 1996; 54(1): 237–240.

20. Tsaras G, Owusu-Ansah A, Boateng FO, Amoateng-Adjepong Y. Complications associated with sickle cell trait: a brief narrative review. *Am J Med* 2009; 122(6): 507–512.

21. Makaryus JN, Catanzaro JN, Katona KC. Exertional rhabdomyolysis and renal failure in patients with sickle cell trait: is it time to change our approach? *Hematology* 2007; 12(4): 349–352.

22. Tanabe P, Artz N, Mark Courtney D, et al. Adult emergency department patients with sickle cell pain crisis: a learning collaborative model to improve analgesic management. *Acad Emerg Med* 2010; 17(4): 399–407.

23. Lanzkron S, Carroll CP, Haywood C, Jr. The burden of emergency department use for sickle-cell disease: an analysis of the national emergency department sample database. Am J Hematol *2010;* 85(10): 797–799.

24. Ballas SK. New era dawns on sickle cell pain. *Blood* 2010; 116(3): 311–312.

25. Lazio MP, Costello HH, Courtney DM, et al. A comparison of analgesic management for emergency department patients with sickle cell disease and renal colic. *Clin J Pain* 2010; 26(3): 199–205.

26. Aisiku IP, Smith WR, McClish DK, et al. Comparisons of high versus low emergency department utilizers in sickle cell disease. *Ann Emerg Med* 2009; 53(5): 587–593.

27. Davis MP, Shaiova LA, Angst MS. When opioids cause pain. *J Clin Oncol* 2007; 25(28): 4497–4498.

28. Liang D, Shi X, Qiao Y, Angst MS, Yeomans DC, Clark JD. Chronic morphine administration enhances nociceptive sensitivity and local cytokine production after incision. *Mol Pain* 2008; 4: 7.

29. Brousseau DC, Owens PL, Mosso AL, Panepinto JA, Steiner CA. Acute care utilization and rehospitalizations for sickle cell disease. *JAMA* 2010; 303(13): 1288–1294.

30. Anand AJ, Glatt AE. Salmonella osteomyelitis and arthritis in sickle cell disease. *Semin Arthritis Rheum* 1994; 24(3): 211–221.
31. Morris C, Vichinsky E, Styles L. Clinician assessment for acute chest syndrome in febrile patients with sickle cell disease: is it accurate enough? *Ann Emerg Med* 1999; 34(1): 64–69.
32. McCready CE, Doughty HA, Pearson TC. Experience with the Port-A-Cath in sickle cell disease. *Clin Lab Haematol* 1996; 18(2): 79–82.
33. Vichinsky EP, Neumayr LD, Earles AN, et al. Causes and outcomes of the acute chest syndrome in sickle cell disease. National Acute Chest Syndrome Study Group. *N Engl J Med* 2000; 342(25): 1855–1865.
34. Petz LD, Calhoun L, Shulman IA, Johnson C, Herron RM. The sickle cell hemolytic transfusion reaction syndrome. *Transfusion* 1997; 37(4): 382–392.
35. Scheunemann LP, Ataga KI. Delayed hemolytic transfusion reaction in sickle cell disease. *Am J Med Sci* 2010; 339(3): 266–269.
36. Eckman JR. Techniques for blood administration in sickle cell patients. *Semin Hematol* 2001; 38(1 Suppl 1): 23–29.
37. Alexy T, Pais E, Armstrong JK, Meiselman HJ, Johnson CS, Fisher TC. Rheologic behavior of sickle and normal red blood cell mixtures in sickle plasma: implications for transfusion therapy. *Transfusion* 2006; 46(6): 912–918.
38. Win N, New H, Lee E, de la Fuente J. Hyperhemolysis syndrome in sickle cell disease: case report (recurrent episode) and literature review. *Transfusion* 2008; 48(6): 1231–1238.
39. Setubal S, Gabriel AH, Nascimento JP, Oliveira SA. Aplastic crisis caused by parvovirus B19 in an adult patient with sickle-cell disease. *Rev Soc Bras Med Trop* 2000; 33(5): 477–481.
40. Pardoll DM, Rodeheffer RJ, Smith RR, Charache S. Aplastic crisis due to extensive bone marrow necrosis in sickle cell disease. *Arch Intern Med* 1982; 142(12): 2223–2225.
41. Rao SP, Desai N, Miller ST. B19 parvovirus infection and transient aplastic crisis in a child with sickle cell anemia. *J Pediatr Hematol Oncol* 1996; 18(2): 175–177.
42. Vichinsky EP, Styles LA, Colangelo LH, et al. Acute chest syndrome in sickle cell disease: clinical presentation and course. *Blood* 1997; 89(5): 1787–1792.
43. Styles LA, Abboud M, Larkin S, Lo M, Kuypers FA. Transfusion prevents acute chest syndrome predicted by elevated secretory phospholipase A2. *Br J Haematol* 2007; 136(2): 343–344.
44. Sobota A, Graham DA, Heeney MM, Neufeld EJ. Corticosteroids for acute chest syndrome in children with sickle cell disease: variation in use and association with length of stay and readmission. *Am J Hematol* 2010; 85(1): 24–28.
45. Kumar R, Qureshi S, Mohanty P, Rao SP, Miller ST. A short course of prednisone in the management of acute chest syndrome of sickle cell disease. *J Pediatr Hematol Oncol* 2010; 32(3): e91–e94.
46. Singer ST, Ataga KI. Hypercoagulability in sickle cell disease and beta-thalassemia. *Curr Mol Med* 2008; 8(7): 639–645.
47. Schnog JB, Mac Gillavry MR, van Zanten AP, et al. Protein C and S and inflammation in sickle cell disease. *Am J Hematol* 2004; 76(1): 26–32.
48. Klings ES, Wyszynski DF, Nolan VG, Steinberg MH. Abnormal pulmonary function in adults with sickle cell anemia. *Am J Respir Crit Care Med* 2006; 173(11): 1264–1269.

49. Morris CR. Asthma management: reinventing the wheel in sickle cell disease. *Am J Hematol* 2009; 84(4): 234–241.

50. Bellet PS, Kalinyak KA, Shukla R, Gelfand M, Rucknagel DL. Incentive spirometry to prevent acute pulmonary complications in sickle cell diseases. *New England Journal of Medicine* 1995; 333: 699–703.

51. Strouse JJ, Takemoto CM, Keefer JR, Kato GJ, Casella JF. Corticosteroids and increased risk of readmission after acute chest syndrome in children with sickle cell disease. *Pediatr Blood Cancer* 2008; 50(5): 1006–1012.

52. Isakoff MS, Lillo JA, Hagstrom JN. A single-institution experience with treatment of severe acute chest syndrome: lack of rebound pain with dexamethasone plus transfusion therapy. *J Pediatr Hematol Oncol* 2008; 30(4): 322–325.

53. Kumar R, Qureshi S, Mohanty P, Rao SP, Miller ST. A short course of prednisone in the management of acute chest syndrome of sickle cell disease. *J Pediatr Hematol Oncol* 2010; 32(3): e91–e94.

54. Gladwin M, Sachdev V, Jison M, et al. Pulmonary hypertension as a risk factor for death in patients with sickle cell disease. *N Engl J Med* 2004; 350: 22–31.

55. Machado RF, Kyle Mack A, Martyr S, et al. Severity of pulmonary hypertension during vaso-occlusive pain crisis and exercise in patients with sickle cell disease. *Br J Haematol* 2007; 136(2): 319–325.

56. Mekontso Dessap A, Leon R, Habibi A, et al. Pulmonary hypertension and cor pulmonale during severe acute chest syndrome in sickle cell disease. *Am J Respir Crit Care Med* 2008; 177(6): 646–653.

57. Morris CR, Morris SM, Jr., Hagar W, et al. Arginine therapy: a new treatment for pulmonary hypertension in sickle cell disease? *Am J Respir Crit Care Med* 2003; 168(1): 63–69.

58. Machado RF, Anthi A, Steinberg MH, et al. N-terminal pro-brain natriuretic peptide levels and risk of death in sickle cell disease. *JAMA* 2006; 296(3): 310–318.

59. Barrett O, Jr., Saunders DE, Jr., McFarland DE, Humphries JO. Myocardial infarction in sickle cell anemia. *Am J Hematol* 1984; 16(2): 139–147.

60. Liem RI, Young LT, Thompson AA. Prolonged QTc interval in children and young adults with sickle cell disease at steady state. *Pediatr Blood Cancer* 2009; 52(7): 842–846.

61. Castro O, Hoque M, Brown BD. Pulmonary hypertension in sickle cell disease: cardiac catheterization results and survival. *Blood* 2003; 101(4): 1257–1261.

62. De Castro LM, Jonassaint JC, Graham FL, Ashley-Koch A, Telen MJ. Pulmonary hypertension associated with sickle cell disease: clinical and laboratory endpoints and disease outcomes. *Am J Hematol* 2008; 83(1): 19–25.

63. Hagar RW, Michlitsch JG, Gardner J, Vichinsky EP, Morris CR. Clinical differences between children and adults with pulmonary hypertension and sickle cell disease. *Br J Haematol* 2008; 140(1): 104–112.

64. Lee MT, Small T, Khan MA, Rosenzweig EB, Barst RJ, Brittenham GM. Doppler-defined pulmonary hypertension and the risk of death in children with sickle cell disease followed for a mean of three years. *Br J Haematol* 2009; 146(4): 437–441.

65. Morris CR, Kato GJ, Poljakovic M, et al. Dysregulated arginine metabolism, hemolysis-associated pulmonary hypertension, and mortality in sickle cell disease. *JAMA* 2005; 294(1): 81–90.

66. Porter BO, Coyne PJ, Smith WR. Methadone-related Torsades de Pointes in a sickle cell patient treated for chronic pain. *Am J Hematol* 2005; 78(4): 316–317.

67. Fugate T, 2nd, Moss AJ, Jons C, et al. Long QT syndrome in African-Americans. *Ann Noninvasive Electrocardiol* 2010; 15(1): 73–76.

68. Dervisoglu E, Yilmaz A, Sevin E, Kalender B. The relationship between iron stores and corrected QT dispersion in patients undergoing hemodialysis. *Anadolu Kardiyol Derg* 2007; 7(3): 270–274.

69. Boga C, Kozanoglu I, Yeral M, Bakar C. Assessment of corrected QT interval in sickle-cell disease patients who undergo erythroapheresis. *Transfus Med* 2007; 17(6): 466–472.

70. Liem RI, Young LT, Thompson AA. Prolonged QTc interval in children and young adults with sickle cell disease at steady state. *Pediatr Blood Cancer* 2009; 52(7): 842–846.

71. Wang WC, Langston JW, Steen RG, et al. Abnormalities of the central nervous system in very young children with sickle cell anemia. *J Pediatr* 1998; 132(6): 994–998.

72. Marouf R, Gupta R, Haider MZ, Adekile AD. Silent brain infarcts in adult Kuwaiti sickle cell disease patients. *Am J Hematol* 2003; 73(4): 240–243.

73. Vichinsky EP, Neumayr L, Gold J, Wiener M, Rul R. Neuropsychological dysfunction and neuroimaging abnormalities in neurologically intact adults with sickle cell anemia. *JAMA* 2010; 303: 1823–1831.

74. Strouse JJ, Jordan LC, Lanzkron S, Casella JF. The excess burden of stroke in hospitalized adults with sickle cell disease. *Am J Hematol* 2009; 84(9): 548–552.

75. Jackson H, Bentley C, Thompson G. Outpatient management of small traumatic hyphaemas. *Eye (Lond)* 1994; 8(Pt 6): 718–719.

76. Rogers DT, Molokie R. Sickle cell disease in pregnancy. *Obstet Gynecol Clin North Am* 2010; 37(2): 223–237.

77. Koshy M, Burd L, Wallace D, Moawad A, Baron J. Prophylactic red-cell transfusions in pregnant patients with sickle cell disease: a randomized cooperative study. *N Engl J Med* 1988; 319(22): 1447–1452.

78. Adeyoju AB, Olujohungbe AB, Morris J, et al. Priapism in sickle-cell disease: incidence, risk factors and complications—an international multicentre study. *BJU Int* 2002; 90(9): 898–902.

79. Bassett J, Rajfer J. Diagnostic and therapeutic options for the management of ischemic and non-ischemic priapism. *Rev Urol* 2010; 12(1): 56–63.

80. Rogers ZR. Priapism in sickle cell disease. *Hematol Oncol Clin North Am* 2005; 19(5): 917–928, viii.

81. Burnett AL, Bivalacqua TJ, Champion HC, Musicki B. Feasibility of the use of phosphodiesterase type 5 inhibitors in a pharmacologic prevention program for recurrent priapism. *J Sex Med* 2006; 3(6): 1077–1084.

82. McCarthy LJ, Vattuone J, Weidner J, et al. Do automated red cell exchanges relieve priapism in patients with sickle cell anemia? *Ther Apher* 2000; 4(3): 256–258.

83. Eckman JR. Leg ulcers in sickle cell disease. *Hematol Oncol Clin North Am* 1996; 10(6): 1333–1344.

84. Keidan AJ, Stuart J. Rheological effects of bed rest in sickle cell disease. *J Clin Pathol* 1987; 40(10): 1187–1188.

85. Koppensteiner R. Blood rheology in emergency medicine. *Semin Thromb Hemost* 1996; 22(1): 89–91.

86. Wahl S, Quirolo KC. Current issues in blood transfusion for sickle cell disease. *Curr Opin Pediatr* 2009; 21(1): 15–21.

87. Hanna J, Wernig M, Markoulaki S, et al. Treatment of sickle cell anemia mouse model with iPS cells generated from autologous skin. *Science* 2007; 318(5858): 1920–1923.

88. Brousseau DC, Scott JP, Hillery CA, Panepinto JA. The effect of magnesium on length of stay for pediatric sickle cell pain crisis. *Acad Emerg Med* 2004; 11(9): 968–972.

89. Morris C, Ansari M, Lavrisha L, Sweeters N, Kuypers FA, Vichinsky EP. Arginine therapy for vaso-occlusive pain episodes in sickle cell disease. *Blood* 2009; 114: Abstract 573.

90. Rachid-Filho D, Cavalcanti AG, Favorito LA, Costa WS, Sampaio FJ. Treatment of recurrent priapism in sickle cell anemia with finasteride: a new approach. *Urology* 2009; 74(5): 1054–1057.

91. Chang J, Patton JT, Sarkar A, Ernst B, Magnani JL, Frenette PS. GMI-1070, a novel pan-selectin antagonist, reverses acute vascular occlusions in sickle cell mice. *Blood* 2010; 116(10): 1779–1786.

CHAPTER 8

HIV-positive adults on HAART

Arvind Venkat[1,2] and Sukhjit S. Takhar[3,4]
[1] Allegheny General Hospital, Pittsburgh, PA, USA
[2] Drexel University College of Medicine, Philadelphia, PA, USA
[3] Brigham and Women's Hospital, Boston, MA, USA
[4] Harvard Medical School, Boston, MA, USA

Introduction and epidemiology

According to the World Health Organization, 33 million individuals globally are HIV-positive [1] while the Centers for Disease Control estimates that 1.1 million individuals are HIV-positive in the United States [2]. Since the emergence of the HIV pandemic in the early 1980s, physicians and other health care providers have treated HIV-positive adults for a variety of ailments. Prior to the advent of highly active antiretroviral therapy (HAART), the majority of HIV-positive adults experienced a progressive and unrelenting decline in their immune status leading to unusual infections and death. They predominantly presented to the emergency department (ED) for acute care due to opportunistic infections [3].

However, HAART regimens have resulted in a marked increase in life expectancy for HIV-positive adults and reduction in the incidence of opportunistic infections. Combined antiretroviral therapy reduces viral replication, increases CD4 cell counts, and restores and preserves immune function [4]. From 1996 to 2005, the life expectancy for a 20-year-old HIV-positive individual has increased from a mean of 36.1 years to 49.4 years [5]. This increase in life expectancy has been contemporaneous with a decrease in the incidence of opportunistic infections as the cause of morbidity and mortality in this patient population. In comparison to the pre-HAART era, hospitalizations among HIV-positive adults are predominantly in those over age 40 [6]. Similarly, single center studies have suggested that hospitalizations for typical late-stage opportunistic infections, such as

---

Challenging and Emerging Conditions in Emergency Medicine, First Edition. Edited by Arvind Venkat.

Cryptosporidium and *Mycobacterium avium* complex, have decreased while those for conditions such as cardiovascular, renal, oncologic, and HAART-related side effects have increased [7]. From the ED perspective, there is also evidence that both ED and hospital discharge diagnoses due to musculoskeletal, endocrine/metabolic, psychiatric, and circulatory conditions have become more prevalent [8]. Finally, there is increasing evidence that HIV itself may play a prominent role in the development of medical conditions in this patient population which are not classically considered AIDS-defining, such as coronary artery disease, stroke, and malignancies, such as non-Hodgkin's lymphoma, anal, and lung cancers [9].

For emergency physicians and other health care providers, this changing epidemiology requires a paradigm shift in their approach to assessing and treating HIV-positive adults. Rather than focusing exclusively on the diagnosis of opportunistic infections, it is now necessary to recognize that there is a broader spectrum of illnesses that can cause HIV-positive adults to present to the EDs. This chapter presents an overview of the evolving ailments that may cause HIV-positive adults to require emergency care as well as how the changing life expectancy and management of HIV-positive adults in the outpatient setting may affect the future ED evaluation and treatment of this patient population.

HAART regimens

With the advent of HAART, numerous studies have been conducted as to the optimal time to begin therapy in HIV-positive patients. The benefit of antiretrovirals must be balanced against the toxicity, cost, and inconvenience of lifelong treatment. Antiretroviral therapy has continued to improve and the current consensus is in favor of initiating HAART in those patients with CD4 counts <500 cells/mm^3 or those patients who show evidence of an AIDS-defining illness as well those who are pregnant, have HIV nephropathy, or who require treatment for a concurrent infection with Hepatitis B or C [10]. Treatment should be considered in asymptomatic patients with a CD4 cell count of >500 cells/mm^3.

First-line regimens consist of one non-nucleoside analog reverse transcriptase inhibitor (NNRTI) and two nucleoside analog reverse transcriptase inhibitors (nRTI) (efavirenz plus tenofovir and emtricitabine), two nRTI plus a boosted protease inhibitor (tenofovir and emtricitabine plus atazanavir/ritonavir or darunavir/ritonavir), or two nRTI and an integrase strand transfer inhibitor (tenofovir and emtricitabine plus raltegravir) [11]. As a result, emergency physicians will more often be seeing HIV-positive patients who are on newer antiretroviral medications and who may have been on these regimens for longer periods of time and may have never experienced an AIDS-defining illness.

Table 8.1 Class side effects of antiretroviral medications

Antiretroviral medications	Class side effects
Nucleoside analog reverse transcriptase inhibitors	Hepatotoxicity, lactic acidosis, pancreatitis, and lipoatrophy
Protease inhibitors	Lipodystrophy, insulin resistance, and gastrointestinal distress
Non-nucleoside analog reverse transcriptase inhibitors	Hepatotoxicity and drug hypersensitivity

HAART side effects and medication interactions of relevance in the emergency department

The combination nature of HAART predisposes HIV-positive patients who are on this regimen to a number of medication side effects that range from mild to potentially life threatening. Many of these side effects are a class effect of the type of agent in the HAART regimen. Table 8.1 shows the common class side effects for those types of antiretroviral medications used most often in HAART [11, 12].

While hepatic steatosis and hepatotoxicity can be seen with all medications in HAART regimens, the degree and clinical significance can vary greatly. The NNRTI nevirapine is most clearly associated with increased risk of fulminant hepatic failure when started on patients with higher CD4 counts [13]. Similarly, while all HAART medications can cause drug hypersensitivity, the nRTI abacavir is associated with the most severe reaction. This reaction can manifest as a macular or urticarial rash with fever, myalgias, and hypotension, is managed by supportive care, and requires immediate cessation of the medication with recording that it should not be used in this patient in future [14].

In addition to these class side effects, there are unique side effects for certain HAART medications that require recognition by emergency physicians. Table 8.2 elucidates those of the most commonly used HAART medications [12, 13].

Table 8.2 Unique side effects of commonly used HAART medications

Commonly used HAART medications	Unique side effects
Atazanavir	Indirect hyperbilirubinemia
Tenofovir	Renal insufficiency
Efavirenz	Neuropsychological symptoms, depression
Tipranavir	Intracerebral hemorrhage (rare)

Finally, the numerous medications required by HIV-positive patients on HAART can result in medication interactions that can be of importance to emergency physicians. Atazanavir's absorption is decreased when patients are given acid-reducing agents. Both protease inhibitors and NNRTIs are metabolized by hepatic p450 enzymes and drug interactions are common and severe. For example, warfarin use by patients on protease inhibitors can cause hyperanticoagulation. In contrast, anticonvulsants such as phenytoin, carbamazepine, and phenobarbital can increase the metabolism of protease inhibitors. It is well advised for emergency physicians to consult with the patient's treating infectious disease specialist and relevant pharmacologic resources prior to prescribing new medications to this patient population [13].

Cardiovascular diseases in HIV-positive patients on HAART

With improved life expectancy among HIV-positive patients on HAART, there has been a concomitant increase in the incidence of cardiovascular disease in this population and specifically acute coronary syndromes. The pathology of coronary artery disease in HIV-infected patients is multifactorial and complex. Some attribute the lipodystrophy and hyperglycemic side effects of protease inhibitors as major causative factors. Newer evidence suggests that HIV replication has inflammatory and atherogenic properties and the risk of ongoing viral replication outweighs that of the small increase in CAD attributed to antiretroviral therapy [9,15–19]. Regardless of the cause, for emergency physicians, this evidence suggests that HIV-positive adults who present with acute coronary syndrome tend to be younger than the general population. There is no difference in the actual evaluation and interventions for HIV-positive adults with acute coronary syndromes, but the pre-test probability of treating physicians should be higher than that in comparably aged HIV-negative adults.

HIV-positive adults can also show evidence of dilated cardiomyopathy. Associated with a poor prognosis, cardiomyopathy is best diagnosed using echocardiography and cardiac catheterization. ED management is similar to other patients with clinical signs and symptoms of congestive heart failure [20].

Pulmonary diseases in HIV-positive adults on HAART

The cause of pulmonary disease in HIV-patients is dependent on the immune status. Unlike the pre-HAART era, where *Pneumocystis jiroveci* was the primary respiratory pathogen, HIV-positive adults on HAART with a high CD4 count are most likely to be afflicted by bacterial pneumonia due to *Streptococcus pneumoniae*. Presentation in the emergency department will be comparable to the HIV-negative population as will radiographic appearance if the patient has had a good clinical response to HAART (CD4 count >350/mm³) [21]. In contrast, patients with a poor response to HAART can manifest bacterial pneumonia with atypical symptoms, including lack of fever, multifocal pneumonia on chest radiograph, and vague constitutional symptoms which can be hard to differentiate clinically from *P. jiroveci* pneumonia [22]. Patients with a good clinical and immunological response to HAART may be removed from *P. jiroveci* prophylaxis if such a response is maintained for 3 months [23].

Tuberculosis can also show great variability in presentation in HIV-positive adults, dependent largely on CD4 count. While cough may be a predominant presenting symptom, tuberculosis should also be suspected in this patient population when encountering a patient with persistent fever or night sweats of unknown origin [24]. HIV-positive adults are also more likely to manifest extrapulmonary tuberculosis than the HIV-negative population. For HIV-positive adults with a poor response or who have not received HAART and have a CD4 count <200, typical cavitary lesions with consolidation are often absent on chest radiograph. Instead, hilar lymphadenopathy and nonspecific pulmonary infiltrates can be all that is seen on chest radiography [25]. Treatment of tuberculosis in HIV-positive adults on HAART requires close consultation with an infectious disease specialist as there can be significant medication interactions between HAART medications and antituberculosis regimens, especially those using rifampin.

In addition to pneumonia, HIV-positive adults can manifest chronic obstructive pulmonary disease, controlling for smoking history, at a higher incidence than the general population [26]. There is also an increased incidence of pulmonary hypertension, which carries a significant mortality risk (47% survival at 3 years from diagnosis) and can manifest with prosaic symptoms such as fatigue and dyspnea [27]. Treatment is limited to sildenafil, prostaglandins, and anticoagulation.

Renal diseases in HIV-positive adults on HAART

As discussed above, HIV-nephropathy is a well-accepted indication for the initiation of HAART [11, 28]. It is characterized by rapid progression to end-stage renal disease that is best arrested by HAART. For the emergency physician, other reversible causes of renal insufficiency, including pre-renal azotemia and obstructive uropathy from nephrolithiasis, should be ruled out prior to concluding that renal insufficiency in this patient population is due to HIV-nephropathy.

Acute renal failure due to any cause is a poor prognostic sign in HIV-positive adults. Studies have suggested a six-fold increase in mortality among hospitalized HIV-positive patients when acute renal failure is present [29]. For patients requiring intensive care, the mortality rate with acute renal failure may be as high as 43% [30]. As such, HIV-positive adults presenting to the ED who are found to have renal injury should have aggressive evaluation and treatment. The algorithm for assessing for pre- and post-renal causes of renal failure is similar to the non-HIV patient population, but an appreciation of the increased severity of illness in this cohort is required.

Atazanavir, the most commonly used protease inhibitor, can occasionally precipitate and cause kidney stones [31]. Such stones should be radio-opaque on CT as the medication-related stones serve as the core for precipitation with calcium oxalate. Treatment is similar to other patients with renal colic.

Neurological disorders in HIV-positive adults on HAART

With the use of HAART in HIV-positive adults, there has been a corresponding reduction in the incidence of cryptococcal meningitis, toxoplasmosis, CNS lymphoma, progressive multifocal leukoencephalopathy (PML), and AIDS dementia [32]. However, all of these late manifestations of AIDS can still present in patients with poor response to HAART as determined by a CD4 count $<200/mm^3$. In contrast, those patients with CD4 counts $>200/mm^3$ are much less likely to present with these conditions.

As with cardiovascular disease, HIV-positive adults on HAART have seen a concomitant increase in the incidence of ischemic and hemorrhagic cerebrovascular diseases. This has been attributed both to the atherogenic effects of HIV itself and the increased use of protease inhibitors and resultant hyperlipidemia, increasing longevity, and other atherosclerosis risk factors [33, 34]. For emergency physicians, a timely history and physical exam should focus upon whether the patient is presenting with focal or diffuse neurological deficits, the CD4 count of the patient, timeline of when the patient was started on HAART, and previous history of AIDS-defining illnesses of the central nervous system (CNS). Patients with focal neurologic findings should, at minimum, receive a noncontrast CT of the brain and, based on the most recent CD4 count and the clinical presentation, the addition of contrast CT of the brain or MRI to look for space occupying lesions. A lumbar puncture should also be performed if it is not contraindicated.

HIV-positive patients on HAART can also present with manifestations of disease involving the peripheral nervous system. Both HIV itself and certain HAART medications (didanosine and stavudine) can cause sensory neuropathies that cause hypersensitivity of the distal extremities. Generally, this is more prevalent in patients with low CD4 counts, and treatment involves discontinuation of suspect medications and the addition of gabapentin for symptomatic relief [35, 36].

Immune reconstitution inflammatory syndrome

Immune reconstitution inflammatory syndrome (IRIS) represents a unique side effect of HAART. With the initiation of HAART and reinvigoration of the immune system, patients can experience a worsening of their clinical status due to immune reconstitution and resultant inflammatory response to dormant opportunistic pathogens or exacerbation of underlying conditions that are autoimmune in nature. Risk factors for IRIS include high viral load and low CD4 count at the time of HAART initiation, rapid reversal of these two conditions, and widespread manifestation of underlying opportunistic infection [37]. Two opportunistic pathogens that deserve special consideration by emergency physicians when considering the diagnosis of IRIS are *Mycobacterium tuberculosis* and JC virus. If HAART is started concomitantly with treatment for tuberculosis, there is a high risk of the patient experiencing IRIS. Up to 43% of patients in this scenario can experience this complication [38]. Such patients usually will present with exacerbation of pulmonary symptoms, but extrapulmonary manifestations of tuberculosis, particularly in the abdomen or CNS, can also recrudesce. Similarly, patients who are infected with JC virus at the time of initiation of HAART can manifest progressive multifocal leukoencephalopathy, which may present with altered mental status, gait disturbances, or even seizures. Unlike classic PML, IRIS-related PML lesions can be contrast enhancing with space occupying lesions on CT and MRI [39, 40].

The important issue for the emergency physician is to recognize that IRIS is largely a self-limited process that should be treated with supportive measures without discontinuation of HAART. As HAART remains the mainstay for therapy for most opportunistic infections or autoimmune illnesses that can manifest with IRIS, patients should be treated symptomatically for constitutional symptoms using NSAIDs. Corticosteroids may be added in close consultation with the treating infectious disease specialist, but their use is largely confined to when the opportunistic pathogen involved has a specific therapy that can be given to treat worsening clinical symptoms [41].

Gastrointestinal and hepatobiliary diseases in HIV-positive adults on HAART

Ailments of the GI tract remain a common problem in HIV-positive patients on HAART. Most of the medications in the HAART regimen have a side effect of nausea, which can lead to poor oral intake, malnutrition, dehydration, and medication noncompliance. The advent of HAART has resulted in a dramatic decrease in the incidence of Candidal esophagitis, though patients with a poor response to HAART can still present with this condition [42]. In contrast, *Clostridium difficile* diarrhea has emerged as a significant concern among HIV-positive adults on HAART. Up to 36% of HIV-infected adults who are hospitalized for diarrhea are found on stool testing to have *C. difficile* as the inciting agent [43]. For the emergency physician, stool testing for this pathogen is highly recommended in this patient population along with aggressive assessment and treatment of dehydration. In addition, a careful history regarding volume and frequency of stool and CD4 count can help the emergency physician to narrow their differential diagnosis in terms of the inciting pathogen causing the diarrhea. In general, patients with CD4 count >200 are as likely to have self-limited and viral causes of diarrhea as the general patient population. For patients with CD4 count <200, bacterial causes, such as *C. difficile*, *Shigella*, and *Salmonella*, along with opportunistic pathogens, such as *Cryptosporidium*, *Microsporidium*, and *Mycobacterium avium*, are more prevalent and often require hospitalization for treatment of dehydration and the underlying inciting agent [44].

Patients on HAART can also present with acute pancreatitis. A recent study showed that the rate of pancreatitis has not decreased from the pre-HAART era and that the incidence in HIV-positive adults on HAART is five times that of the general patient population. Numerous factors contribute to this finding. HAART medications, especially nRTI, have side effects of causing acute pancreatitis. The hypertriglyceridemia from protease inhibitors can also contribute to pancreatitis. Finally, other more common cause of pancreatitis, such as alcohol use and gallstones, can also be seen in this patient population. Taken together, it behooves emergency physicians to consider acute pancreatitis in the differential diagnosis of HIV-positive adults on HAART who present with abdominal pain. Testing for serum lipase levels and CT imaging are the most accurate diagnostic modalities with treatment largely consisting of supportive care (intravenous hydration, analgesia, and discontinuation of inciting medications) [13].

As discussed above, nearly all HAART medications can cause abnormalities in liver function, ranging from mild elevation in transaminases to fulminant hepatic failure. Up to 49% of patients on atazanavir can manifest an indirect hyperbilirubinemia, which is benign and does not require further evaluation [13]. What has emerged as a critical issue in HIV-positive patients on HAART is concomitant infection with hepatitis B and C. Such coinfection can lead to a 2–3 times elevation in risk of developing chronic liver disease. Additionally, hepatitis C coinfection is associated with a faster presentation of AIDS-defining illnesses in this patient population. Certain antiretroviral medications have activity also against hepatitis B (lamivudine, emtricitabine, and tenofovir), and, in general, both hepatitis B and HIV should be treated concurrently [45–47].

Given the broad differential diagnosis that exists for liver disease in HIV-positive adults on HAART, an approach that focuses on history, physical examination, and the pattern of laboratory liver abnormalities can aid the emergency physician in assessing these patients. Focal elevation of transaminases may be attributable largely to medication side effects or chronic hepatitis viral infection or IRIS. Indirect hyperbilirubinemia is largely confined to conditions causing hemolysis or the use of atazanavir. In contrast, synthetic dysfunction and hepatic failure suggest fulminant hepatitis B or C infection or toxicity from HAART medications such as nevirapine. HIV-cholangiopathy may be attributable to *Cryptosporidium* infection. As with HIV-negative adults, disposition decisions for the emergency physician will largely focus on the presence of liver synthetic dysfunction and clinical status, with patients who have isolated laboratory abnormalities being safe to discharge with close outpatient follow-up [13, 48].

Hematologic and oncologic diseases in HIV-positive adults on HAART

The use of HAART in the treatment of HIV-positive adults has resulted in a number of changes in the epidemiology of hematologic and oncologic conditions that can cause this patient population to present to the emergency department. Zidovudine can classically cause a macrocytic anemia and is treated largely symptomatically. Trimethroprim–sulfamethoxazole is also implicated in patients requiring PCP prophylaxis [49]. Neutropenia and thrombocytopenia, which can manifest with the progression of HIV, are largely treated with HAART though these medications can be associated with suppression of these cell lines as well, most prominently zidovudine [50]. It is now recognized that HIV-positive adults are at higher risk of complications of venous thromboembolism than the general population with a result that emergency physicians should have a low threshold for evaluating these patients for this complication [51]. Later stage HIV also has a clear association with thrombotic thrombocytopenic purpura, and emergency physicians should recognize this diagnosis in the presence of hemolytic anemia and thrombocytopenia and initiate treatment with plasmaphoresis [52].

HAART has resulted in a decreased incidence of certain AIDS-defining cancers such as Kaposi's sarcoma and primary CNS lymphoma. However, there has been a concomitant increase in Hodgkin's lymphoma, anal cancer, and lung cancer, which may be age related. For emergency physicians, prompt referral of patients with anal warts for evaluation for anal cancer is important given the higher incidence of human papilloma virus-related anal cancer among HIV-positive adults [53].

Endocrine disease in HIV-positive adults on HAART

The use of protease inhibitors has resulted in a higher incidence of insulin resistance among HIV-positive adults on HAART than the general population. As a result, there is a rising incidence of diabetes mellitus which should be recognized by emergency physicians both as a primary reason for ED presentation and as a risk factor for cardiovascular, cerebrovascular, and renal disorders [54]. IRIS can also cause an autoimmune thyroid disorder than can manifest as Grave's disease or even thyrotoxicosis. Treatment is similar to the HIV-negative adult with these conditions [55].

Psychiatric diseases in HIV-positive adults on HAART

While not a common cause of acute ailments in the HIV-positive adult population, psychiatric disorders have a profound impact on issues of medication compliance and resultant morbidity from non-psychiatric conditions. 40% of all HIV-positive patient referrals for psychiatric treatment are due to depression, and for emergency physicians, recognition of depression in this patient population should lead to prompt referral and aid to the patient who requires long-term psychiatric management [56].

The commonly used NNRTI efavirenz has well recognized neuropsychological side effects. Generally manifesting within the first 4 weeks of treatment, most patients will manifest mild symptoms of sleep disturbance and irritability and do not need to stop the medication. However, psychosis can also present as a side effect of this medication, and this requires prompt discontinuation of its use. Most neuropsychological symptoms caused by efavirenz will resolve within 4 weeks of treatment, though late depressive symptoms can also manifest, requiring concomitant antidepressant use [57].

Dermatologic diseases in HIV-positive adults on HAART

As with psychiatric conditions in this patient population, dermatologic conditions can lead to noncompliance with prescribed medications and resultant morbidity. There are a number of dermatologic conditions that continue to manifest in this patient population even with the use of HAART. Low CD4 counts can cause the presentation of infectious conditions such as bacterial folliculitis due to *S. aureus*, *Herpes zoster*, and disseminated scabies [58]. HAART itself can lead to photosensitivity reactions and increased risk of *Molluscum contagiosum* [59]. Certain HAART medications (atazanavir, delaviridine, and nevirapine) cause an increased risk of developing Stevens–Johnson syndrome [13]. Finally, as discussed above, emergency physicians should recognize that abacavir can cause a drug hypersensitivity reaction that can be quite severe and requires aggressive supportive care and discontinuation of the medication [14].

Ocular diseases in HIV-positive adults on HAART

With the use of HAART, the incidence of CMV retinitis has decreased up to 80% in the HIV-positive adult population [60]. However, IRIS can cause a CMV uveitis that presents with eye pain, photophobia, and inflammatory cells within the anterior chamber of the eye. Treatment involves the use of topical corticosteroids in careful consultation with an ophthalmologist who can follow the patient's response as an outpatient [61].

HIV can also cause a retinopathy that leads to vision abnormalities involving color and light perception. It is not clear what is the pathophysiology of this process nor whether HAART has resulted in a reduced incidence of this condition [62]. For the emergency physician, recognition of this condition should lead to referral of the patient to outpatient ophthalmologic follow-up.

Musculoskeletal diseases in HIV-positive adults on HAART

HIV-infection and antiretroviral therapy cause a variety of musculoskeletal disorders [63]. HIV-infected patients are susceptible to the same types of fractures, dislocations, and other musculoskeletal disorders as non-HIV infected patients. However, there are a number of musculoskeletal conditions that are specific to this patient population. Patients that are profoundly immunosuppressed (CD4 count <50) are predisposed to disseminated and unusual infections, including disseminated bartonella, tuberculosis, pyomyositis, and atypical mycobacterial infections. Non-infectious spondyloarthropathies are also commonly associated with HIV, as are myopathies. With the alteration in clinical course achieved by HAART in HIV-infected patients, there has been a corresponding change in the types of musculoskeletal complications HIV-infected patients may experience. For example, there has been a decrease in opportunistic infections and an increase in both osteopenia and osteonecrosis [64].

Polymyositis can occur at any stage of HIV infection [65, 66]. Patients present with a subacute, progressive, proximal muscle weakness and an elevated creatine kinase (CK) level. It may be the first sign of HIV infection. Treatment with corticosteroids appears to be beneficial. High dose zidovudine is associated with a polymyositis-like picture in a small percentage of patients, and clinical and laboratory features normalize several months after discontinuing therapy [67].

Multiple studies have suggested that HIV-infected patients have lower bone mineral density (BMD) than age-matched controls [68–70]. Causes of this decrease in BMD include HIV itself as well as secondary effects from medications. Antiretroviral therapy, especially protease inhibitors, has been linked to the development of osteopenia and osteoporosis [69, 70]. Not surprisingly, the reduction in bone strength leads to an increased risk of fractures of the hip and spine [70].

Osteonecrosis, previously known as avascular necrosis, refers to bone infarction at the epiphyseal regions of a bone near a joint. The incidence of osteonecrosis is almost 50 times greater in HIV-infected patients [64]. Other predisposing factors that may contribute to this increased incidence of osteonecrosis in HIV-infected adults include hypertriglyceridemia, corticosteroid use, and ethanol abuse. Antiretroviral medications, especially protease inhibitors, have also been implicated [63, 68]. Osteonecrosis occurs most often in the femoral head, but may occur in other locations also. Routine radiographic screening for osteonecrosis in asymptomatic patients is not recommended [71]. However, MRI of the hip is recommended in patients with persistent pain and in those who have abnormal plain radiographs.

Unexplained myalgias, in association with fatigue and vomiting, may be due to lactic acidosis. Most often associated with the use of didanosine and stavudine, the complication is confirmed by an elevated serum lactic acid level. Treatment is largely supportive, and with the advent of newer antiretroviral regimens, this complication has become less prevalent [13].

The next five years

With the advent of HAART, there has been a profound improvement in the life expectancy of HIV-positive adults. However, the requirement of combination therapy creates barriers to adherence, which may increase the risk of treatment failure [10]. In 2006, the FDA approved Atripla (efavirenz plus tenofovir and emtricitabine)—the first single-pill, once daily fixed-dose regimen (FDR)—for HIV-positive adults who are treatment naïve. A handful of FDRs are in late stage development; these include the addition of an integrase inhibitor and a newer generation NNRTI to an nRTI backbone [72]. There is potential that the next 5 years will see more FDR treatments for HIV-positive adults, which will aid in their adherence to treatment and further improvement in clinical outcome.

The next phase of the HIV-epidemic, certainly in the developed world, will involve the management of older adults with HIV. It is estimated that more than half the HIV-positive population in the United States will be over age 50 by 2015 [73]. For emergency physicians, the challenge of the next 5 years in managing older HIV-positive adults will be in assessing the interaction of HIV-related illnesses and treatment with diseases that are a result of the natural course of aging. Research is needed to determine how the management of this patient population may change with the aging of HIV-positive adults.

Conclusion

The use of HAART among HIV-positive adults has resulted in a profound improvement in the longevity and quality of life in this patient population. However, for emergency physicians, HAART has led to a changed spectrum of illness that requires a broader consideration of conditions that may require emergency evaluation and treatment. A better familiarity with this changing epidemiology and close consultation with treating infectious disease and primary care physicians will aid the emergency physician in managing the HIV-positive adult patient who presents to the ED.

References

1. UNAIDS, World Health Organization. *AIDS Epidemic Update*. December 2009 ed. Geneva: United Nations; 2009.
2. Centers for Disease Control. HIV/AIDS Surveillance Report 2007: US Department of Health and Human Services, CDC; 2007.
3. Talan D, Kennedy C. The management of HIV-related illness in the emergency department. *Ann Emerg Med* 1991 December; 20(12): 1355–1365.
4. Autran B, Carcelain G, Li T, et al. Positive effects of combined antiretroviral therapy on CD4+ T cell homeostasis and function in advanced HIV disease. *Science* 1997 Jul 4; 277(5322): 112–116.
5. Antiretroviral Therapy Cohort Collaboration. Life expectancy of individuals on combination antiretroviral therapy in high-income countries: a collaborative analysis of 14 cohort studies. *Lancet* 2008 Jul 26; 372: 293–299.
6. Kozak L, DeFrances C, Hall M. National hospital discharge survey: 2004 annual summary with detailed diagnosis and procedure data. *Vital Health Stat 13* 2006 October; 162: 1–209.
7. Pulivrenti J, Muppidi U, Glowacki R, Cristofano M, Baker L. Changes in HIV-related hospitalizations during the HAART era in an inner city hospital. *AIDS Read* 2007 Aug; 17(8): 390–394, 397–401.
8. Venkat A, Shippert B, Hanneman D, et al. Emergency department utilization by HIV-positive adults in the HAART era. *Int J Emerg Med* 2008 Dec; 1(4): 287–296.
9. Phillips A, Neaton J, Lundgren J. The role of HIV in serious diseases other than AIDS. *AIDS* 2008 Nov 30; 22(18): 2409–2418.
10. Thompson M, Aberg J, Cahn P, et al. Antiretroviral treatment of adult HIV infection: 2010 recommendations of international AIDS Society-USA Panel. *JAMA* 2010 Jul 21; 304(3): 321–333.
11. Panel on Antiretroviral Guidelines for Adults and Adolescents. Guidelines for the use of antiretroviral agents in HIV-1 infected adults and adolescents. Department of Health and Human Services. 2009 December 1:1–161. http:www.aidsinfo.nih.gov, accessed August 30, 2010.

12. Venkat A, Piontkowsky DM, Cooney RR, Srivastava AK, Suares GA, Heidelberger CP. Care of the HIV-positive patient in the emergency department in the era of highly active anti-retroviral therapy (HAART). *Ann Emerg Med* 2008 Sep; 52(3): 274–285.

13. Bartlett J, Gallant J, Pham P. *Medical Management of HIV Infection* 2009–2010 ed. Baltimore, MD: Johns Hopkins Medicine Health Publishing Business Group; 2009.

14. Hewitt R. Abacavir hypersensitivity reaction. *Clin Infect Dis* 2002 April 15; 34(8): 1137–1142.

15. Stein J, Klein M, Bellehumeur J, McBride P. Use of HIV-1 protease inhibitors is associated with atherogenic lipoprotein changes and endothelial dysfunction. *Circulation* 2001 July 17; 104(3): 257–262.

16. Friis-Moller N, Reiss P, Sabin C, Weber R. Class of antiretroviral drugs and the risk of myocardial infarction. *N Engl J Med* 2007 April 26; 356(17): 1723–1735.

17. Friis-Moller N, Sabin C, Weber R, d'Arminio Monforte A. Combination antiretroviral therapy and the risk of myocardial infarction. *N Engl J Med* 2003 Nov 20; 349(21): 1993–2003.

18. Group SS. CD4 count-guided interruption of antiretroviral treatment. *N Engl J Med* 2006 Nov 30; 355(22): 2283–2296.

19. Oh J, Hegele R. HIV-associated dyslipidaemia: pathogenesis and treatment. *Lancet Infect Dis* 2007 December; 7(12): 787–796.

20. Mishra R. Cardiac emergencies in patients with HIV. *Emerg Med Clin N Am* 2010 May; 28: 273–282.

21. Wolff A, O'Donnell A. Pulmonary Manifestations of HIV infection in the era of highly active antiretroviral therapy. *Chest* 2001 December; 120(6): 1888–1893.

22. Everett C, Fei M, Huang L. Respiratory emergencies in HIV-infected persons. *Emerg Med Clin N Am* 2010 May; 28: 283–298.

23. Lazarous D, O'Donnell A. Pulmonary infections in the HIV-infected patient in the era of highly active antiretroviral therapy: an update. *Curr Infect Dis Rep* 2007 May; 9(3): 228–232.

24. Cain K, McCarthy K, Heilig C, et al. An algorithm for tuberculosis screening and diagnosis in people with HIV. *N Engl J Med* 2010 Feb 25; 362(8): 707–716.

25. Perlman D, El-Sadr W, Nelson E, et al. Variation of chest radiograph patterns in pulmonary tuberculosis by degree of HIV-related immunosuppression. *Clin Infect Dis* 1997 Aug; 25: 242–246.

26. Crothers K, Butt A, Gibert C, Rodriguez-Barradas M. Increased COPD among HIV-positive compared to HIV-negative veterans. *Chest* 2006 November; 130(5): 1326–1333.

27. Limsukon A, Saeed A, Ramaswamy V, Nalamati J, Dhuper S. HIV-related pulmonary hypertension. *Mt Sinai J Med* 2006 November; 73(7): 1037–1044.

28. Wyatt C, Klotman P. HIV-associated nephropathy in the era of antiretroviral therapy. *Am J Med* 2007 Jun; 120(6): 488–492.

29. Wyatt C, Arons R, Klotman P, Klotman M. Acute renal failure in hospitalized patients with HIV: risk factors and impact on in-hospital mortality. *AIDS* 2006 Feb 28; 20(4): 561–565.

30. Lopes J, Fernandes J, Jorge S, Neves J, Antunes F, Prata M. An assessment of the RIFLE criteria for acute renal failure in critically ill HIV-infected patients. *Crit Care* 2007; 11(1): 401–402.

31. Couzigou C, Daudon M, Meynard J, Borsa-Lebas F. Urolithiasis in HIV-positive patients treated with atazanavir. *Clin Infect Dis* 2007 Oct 15; 45(8): e105–e108.

32. Manzardo C, Del Mar Ortega M, Sued O, Garcia F. Central nervous system opportunistic infections in developed countries in the highly active antiretroviral therapy era. *J Neurovirol* 2005; 11(3 Suppl.): 72–82.

33. Rabinstein A. Stroke in HIV-infected patients: a clinical perspective. *Cerebrovasc Dis* 2003; 15(1–2): 37–44.

34. Cole J, Pinto A, Hebel J, Bucholz D. Acquired immunodeficiency syndrome and the risk of stroke. *Stroke* 2004 January; 35(1): 51–56.

35. Ferrari S, Vento S, Monaco S, Cavallaro T. HIV-associated peripheral neuropathies. *Mayo Clin Proc* 2006 February; 81(2): 213–219.

36. Hahn K, Arendt G, Braun J, von Giesen H. A placebo-controlled trial of gabapentin for HIV-associated sensory neuropathies. *J Neurol* 2004 October; 251(10): 1260–1266.

37. Shelburne S, Visnegarwala F, Darcourt J, Graviss E. Incidence and risk factors for IRIS during HAART. *AIDS* 2005 March 4; 19(4): 399–405.

38. Breton G, Duval X, Estellat C, et al. Determinants of IRIS in HIV type-1 infected patients with tuberculosis after initiation of antiretroviral therapy. *Clin Infect Dis* 2004 Dec 1; 39(11): 1709–1712.

39. Eng P, Turnbull B, Cook S, Davidson J. Characteristics and antecedents of progressive multifocal leukoencephalopathy in an insured population. *Neurology* 2006 Sep 12; 67(5): 884–886.

40. Du Pasquier R, Koralnik I. Inflammatory reaction in PML: harmful or beneficial? *J Neurovirol* 2003; 9(1 Suppl.): 25–31.

41. Crum-Cianflone N. Immune reconstitution inflammatory syndromes: what's new? *AIDS Read* 2006 Apr; 16(4): 199–206.

42. Mocroft A, Oancea C, van Lunzen J, Vanhems P. Decline in esophageal candidiasis and use of antimycotics in European patients with HIV. *Am J Gastroenterol* 2005 July; 100(7): 1446–1454.

43. Pulvirenti J, Mehra T, Hafiz I, DeMarais P. Epidemiology and outcome of *Clostridium difficile* infection and diarrhea in HIV infected inpatients. *Diagn Microbiol Infect Dis* 2002 Dec; 44(4): 325–330.

44. Beatty G. Diarrhea in patients infected with HIV presenting to the emergency department. *Emerg Med Clin N Am* 2010 May; 28: 299–310.

45. Nunez M, Puoti M, Camino N, Soriano V. Treatment of chronic hepatitis B in the human immunodeficiency virus infected patient: present and future. *Clin Infect Dis* 2003 Dec 15; 37(12): 1678–1685.

46. Monga H, Rodriguez-Barradas M, Breaux K, Khattak K. Hepatitis C virus infection-related morbidity and mortality among patients with human immunodeficiency virus infection. *Clin Infect Dis* 2001 July 15; 33(2): 240–247.

47. De Luca A, Bugarini R, Lepri A, Puoti M. Coinfection with hepatitis viruses and outcome of initial antiretroviral regimens in previously naive HIV-infected patients. *Arch Intern Med* 2002 October 14; 162(18): 2125–2132.

48. Kottilil S, Polis M, Kovacs J. HIV infection, hepatitis C infection, and HAART: hard clinical choices. *JAMA* 2004 July 14; 292(2): 243–250.

49. Volberding P, Levine A, Dietrich D, Mildvan D. Anemia in HIV infection: clinical impact and evidence-based management strategies. *Clin Infect Dis* 2004 May 15; 38(10): 1454–1463.

50. Huang S, Barbour J, Deeks S. Reversal of HIV type-1 associated hematosuppression by effective antiretroviral therapy. *Clin Infect Dis* 2000 March; 30(3): 504–510.

51. Klein S, Slim E, de Kruif M, Keller T. Is chronic HIV infection associate with venous thrombotic disease? A systematic review. *Neth J Med* 2005 April; 63(4): 129–136.

52. Sutor G, Schmidt R, Albrecht H. Thrombotic microangiopathies and HIV infection: report of two typical cases, features of HUS and TTP, and review of the literature. *Infection* 1999 January–February; 27(1): 12–15.

53. Silverberg M, Abrams D. AIDS-defining and non-AIDS defining malignancies: cancer occurrence in the antiretroviral therapy era. *Curr Opin Oncol* 2007 September; 19(5): 446–451.

54. Brown T, Cole S, Li X, Kingsley L. Antiretroviral therapy and the prevalence and incidence of diabetes mellitus in the multicenter AIDS cohort study. *Arch Intern Med* 2005 May 23; 165(10): 1179–1184.

55. Hoffmann C, Brown T. Thyroid function abnormalities in HIV-infected patients. *Clin Infect Dis* 2007 August 15; 45(4): 488–494.

56. Angelino A, Treisman G. Management of psychiatric disorders in patients infected with HIV. *Clin Infect Dis* 2001 Sep 15; 33(6): 847–856.

57. Arendt G, de Nocker D, von Giesen H, Nolting T. Neuropsychiatric side effects of efavirenz therapy. *Expert Opin Drug Saf* 2007 Mar; 6(2): 147–154.

58. Maurer T, Rodrigues L, Ameli N, Phanuphak N. The effect of HAART on dermatologic disease in a longitudinal study of HIV-type 1 infected women. *Clin Infect Dis* 2004 February 15; 38(4): 579–584.

59. Zancanaro P, McGirt L, Mamelak A, Nguyen R. Cutaneous manifestations of HIV in the era of highly active antiretroviral therapy: an institutional urban clinic experience. *J Am Acad Dermatol* 2006 April; 54(4): 581–588.

60. Jacobson M, Stanley H, Holtzer C, Margolis T. Natural history and outcome of new AIDS-related cytomegalovirus retinitis diagnosed in the era of HAART. *Clin Infect Dis* 2000 January; 30(1): 231–233.

61. Karavellas M, Azen S, MacDonald J, Shufelt C. Immune recovery vitritis and uveitis in AIDS: clinical predictors, sequelae, and treatment outcomes. *Retina* 2001; 21(1): 1–9.

62. Freeman W, Van Natta M, Jabs D, et al. Vision function in HIV-infected individuals without retinitis: report of the studies of ocular complications of AIDS research group. *Am J Opthalmol* 2008 Mar; 145(3): 453–462.

63. Biviji A, Paiement G, Steinbach L. Musculoskeletal manifestations of human immunodeficiency virus infection. *J Am Acad Orthop Surg* 2002 Sep–Oct; 10(5): 312–320.

64. Takhar S, Hendey G. Orthopedic illnesses in patients with HIV. *Emerg Med Clin N Am* 2010 May; 28(2): 335–342.

65. Reveille J, Williams F. Infection and musculoskeletal conditions: rheumatologic complications of HIV infection. *Best Prac Res Clin Rheumatol* 2006 Dec; 20(6): 1159–1179.

66. Dalakas M, Pezezshkpour G, Gravell M, Sever J. Polymyositis associated with AIDS retrovirus. *JAMA* 1986 Nov 7; 256(17): 2381–2383.

67. Tehranzadeh J, Ter-Oganesyan R, Steinbach L. Musculoskeletal disorders associated with HIV infection and AIDS: part II: non-infectious musculoskeletal conditions. *Skeletal Radiol* 2004 Jun; 33(6): 311–320.
68. Glesby M. Bone disorders in human immunodeficiency virus infection. *Clin Infect Dis* 2003; 37(2 Suppl.): S91–S95.
69. Paton N, Macallan D, Griffin G, Pazianas M. Bone mineral density in patients with human immunodeficiency virus infection. *Calcif Tissue Int* 1997 Jul; 61(1): 30–32.
70. Tebas P, Powderly W, Claxton S, et al. Accelerated bone mineral loss in HIV-infected patients receiving potent antiretroviral therapy. *AIDS* 2000 Mar 10; 14(4): F63–F67.
71. Aberg J, Kaplan J, Libman H, et al. Primary care guidelines for the management of persons infected with human immunodeficiency virus: 2009 update by the HIV Medicine Association of the Infectious Disease Society of North America. *Clin Infect Dis* 2009 Sep 1; 49(5): 651–681.
72. Este J, Cihlar T. Current status and challenges of antiretroviral research and therapy. *Antivir Res* 2010 Jan; 85(1): 25–33.
73. Rickabaugh T, Jamieson B. A challenge for the future: aging and HIV infection. *Immunol Res* 2010 Dec; 48(1): 59–71.

CHAPTER 9
Adults receiving chemotherapeutic regimens

Moira Davenport[1,2] and Mary Ann Howland[3,4,5]
[1]Allegheny General Hospital, Pittsburgh, PA, USA
[2]Drexel University College of Medicine, Philadelphia, PA, USA
[3]St. John's University, New York, NY, USA
[4]New York University School of Medicine, Bellevue Hospital Center
and New York University Langone Medical Center, New York, NY, USA
[5]New York City Poison Center, New York, NY, USA

Introduction and epidemiology

Cancer is one of the most feared diagnoses that confronts patients on a regular basis. With the aging of the general population, the incidence of cancer in the United States is increasing. According to American Cancer Society data, 292,540 men and 269,800 women died of cancer in 2009 [1]. This growing trend is not isolated to the United States; World Health Organization data from 2004 indicates that 13% of all deaths worldwide (7.4 million deaths) were attributable to cancer [2]. As the number of cancer patients increases, so does the variety of chemotherapeutic agents available to treat these patients. Monotherapy is rarely seen in modern cancer treatment, resulting in increasing number of agents to which each patient is exposed. Side effects are unfortunately common during chemotherapy. The extent of these manifestations varies based on the agent(s) used, the dose administered, and the frequency of therapy.

For emergency physicians, this creates the double challenge when treating cancer patients of determining whether acute illness is due to the underlying disease or its treatment. Given the complexity of modern oncologic treatment protocols, close contact with the treating cancer specialist of the patient is required to avoid serious adverse outcomes. At the same time, a working knowledge of the common chemotherapeutic regimens and their outcomes will aid emergency physicians in managing cancer patients when presenting to the emergency department. This chapter discusses the emergency department (ED) evaluation and management of cancer patients who present with complications related to chemotherapy.

General principles in the emergency department evaluation of cancer patients receiving chemotherapy

When a cancer patient who is receiving chemotherapy presents to the ED, there are some important historical points that should be obtained. Ideally, the patient or a family member will be able to provide the exact regimen that the patient is receiving. However, when that information is not available, it is possible to make an educated assumption as to what chemotherapeutic agents the patient may be receiving based on the underlying cancer diagnosis. Tables 9.1–9.3 summarize the current first-line regimens for chemotherapy based on diagnosis and the commonly used abbreviations that may be provided by patients [3].

Once the presumed or identified chemotherapeutic regimen has been identified, the emergency physician should note the date of the last chemotherapy session as several clinical complications are related to the time of administration. Neutropenia, for example, is typically seen within 7–10 days of chemotherapy; however, this may develop as much as 2–3 months after treatment with rituximab [4]. At the same time, the mechanism of action of the chemotherapeutic regimen in use can, in some cases, predict associated side effects of therapy. Table 9.4 summarizes the mechanisms of action, uniquely associated side effects, and commonly identified serious side effects of chemotherapeutic agents that may cause presentation to the ED.

Targeted therapies have recently been developed that utilize monoclonal antibody therapy and inhibitors of tyrosine kinase. Monoclonal antibody therapy has been developed to take advantage of tumor biochemistry while limiting systemic side effects (Table 9.5). A specific nomenclature is used to describe new antibodies. The ending "-mab" designates a monoclonal antibody while the suffix "-nib" indicates tyrosine and multikinase inhibitors. For monoclonal antibodies, the letter preceding -mab indicates the source of the antibody: "o" is murine, "u" is human, "xi" is a chimera, and "zu" is a humanized origin. The letter preceding the cell line source indicates the type of tumor the therapy is targeting: tu (m) indicates a general or miscellaneous tumor. It is important to consider the origin of the monoclonal antibody being used in a particular treatment plan as

Table 9.1 Common chemotherapeutic regimens for solid tumors

Cancer	Agents	Common abbreviations for regimen
Lung	Mitomycin, vinblastine, cisplatin	MVP
	Mitomycin, ifosfamide, cisplatin	MIC
	Vinorelbine or gemcitabine + cisplatin	NP
Breast	Cyclophosphamide, methotrexate, 5FU	CMF
	Tamoxifen if estrogen+	
	Vinca alkaloid or anthracycline in metastatic disease	
	Trastuzumab (Herceptin©) (for Her2Neu+ patients)	
Esophageal	Cisplatin, 5FU +/– mitomycin	
Gastric	5FU, cisplatin, mithromycin, docetaxol	
	5FU, adriamycin, methotrexate	FAMTX
Pancreas	5FU, gemcitabine, erlotinib	
Hepatocellular	Anthracyclines, 5FU, etoposide, cisplatin	
	Radiolabeled antibodies	
Colorectal	5FU, lecuovorin, mithromycin	
	5FU, leucovorin, oxaliplatin	
Prostate	Excision + luteinizing hormone releasing hormone antagonist	
Bladder	Surgery only; chemotherapy rare	
Renal cell	Surgery and medroxyprogesterone	
	Some benefit with 5FU or tamoxifen	
	Interferon alpha	
	Aldesleukin (IL-2)	
	5FU, interferon alpha, IL-2	
Germ cell of the testes	Bleomycin, etoposide, cisplatin	BEP
Cervix	Surgery + cisplatin	
Ovarian	Cisplatin or carboplatin + paclitaxel	
Brain	Carmustine	BCNU

Table 9.2 Common chemotherapy regimens for hematological malignancies

Cancer	Agents	Common abbreviations for regimen
AML	Daunorubicin or idarubicin, cytosine +/– etoposide, imatinib	
ALL	Vincristine, prednisolone, anthracycline +/– asparginase	
	Cytosine, etoposide and cyclophosphamide once in remission	
CLL	Alkylating agent, prednisone	
	Nucleoside analogues	
	Immunoglobulin	
CML	Allopurinol, hydroxyurea	
	Interferon alpha, imatinib (Gleevec©)	
Multiple myeloma	Vincristine, doxorubicin, methylprednisolone then melphalan	
	Interferon alpha for maintenance	
Hodgkin's lymphoma	Mustine, vincristine, procarbazine, prednisolone	MOPP
	Doxorubicin or adriamycin, bleomycin, vinblastine, dacarbazine	ABVD
	Vincristine, epirubicin, etoposide, prednisolone	VEEP
	Bleomycin, etoposide, doxorubicin, cyclophosphamide, vincristine, procarbazine, prednisone	BEACOPP
Non-Hodgkin's lymphoma	Cyclophosphamide, doxorubicin, vincristine, prednisolone	CHOP
	Prednisolone, doxorubicin, cyclophosphamide, etoposide, cytarabine, bleomycin, vincristine, methotrexate	ProMACE-CytaBOM

murine-based antibodies cause the highest rate of hypersensitivity during infusion; humanized cells the least amount of hypersensitivity. Patients may present to the ED with a variety of hypersensitivity-related concerns, including fever, chills, sweats, gastrointestinal distress, back pain, and anaphylaxis.

Table 9.3 Common chemotherapeutic regimens for skin and bone cancers

Cancer	Agents	Common abbreviations for regimen
Melanoma	Surgery, then interferon alpha/IL-2 Dacarbazine for metastatic disease	
Sarcoma	Doxorubicin and ifosfamide for metastatic disease	
Rhabdomyosarcoma	Dactinomycin, ifosfamide, doxorubicin +/– etoposide or carboplatin	
Osteosarcoma	Cisplatin, doxorubicin, methotrexate	
Ewing's sarcoma	Doxorubicin, ifosfamide, vincristine, etoposide	
Kaposi's sarcoma	Highly active antiretroviral therapy + daunorubicin	

Clinical side effects of chemotherapeutic agents

Neurologic

A variety of neurologic complications are associated with chemotherapy. As a result, a thorough neurovascular examination should be performed early in the physical exam to identify the presence of a neurological abnormality that may be attributable to the chemotherapeutic regimen. Careful attention should be paid to mental status and focal neurological deficits. Cord compression typically results from metastatic lesions to the spine and results in significant neurovascular deficits; this condition is considered a true oncologic emergency. Patients with suspected cord compression typically present with severe back pain with associated weakness. Sensory deficits are also associated with cord compression, as are changes in urinary and fecal control. Emergent imaging, usually MRI, should be performed to determine the extent of the lesion. Intravenous steroids should be administered in an attempt to limit cord damage and potentially spare neurologic function. Ideal dosing of steroids in cord compression cases is somewhat controversial. Current recommendations now focus on using the neurologic exam to guide steroid dosing; high dose steroids (100 mg dexamethasone loading dose with 96 mg per day in divided doses every 6 h) recommended for patients with rapidly deteriorating neurologic exams and a moderate dosing regimen (10 mg dexamethasone loading dose with 16 mg per day in divided does every 6 h) for patients with known lesions but a stable neurologic exam [5].

Table 9.4 Mechanisms of action, and uniquely associated and serious side effects of common chemotherapeutic agents

Class of agent	Mechanism of action	Example	Characteristic side effects
Anthracyclines	Inhibit DNA uncoiling	Doxorubicin, doxorubicin liposomal	Cardiomyopathy, alopecia, infusion reaction with liposomal formulation
		Daunorubicin, daunorubicin liposomal	
Alkylating agents	Binds DNA strands preventing replication	Cyclophosphamide	Hemorrhagic cystitis
	Binds single DNA strands	Cisplatin	Nausea/vomiting, neuropathy, renal insufficiency
Antimetabolites	Inhibit basic cell metabolism	5-fluorouracil (5FU)	Palmar–Plantar syndrome
		Capecitabine (oral prodrug of 5FU)	Cardiotoxicity, hyperbilirubinemia
		Cytarabine (aka cytosine)	Anaphylaxis, sepsis
		Methotrexate	Thrombosis, AML
		Azathioprine	Pancreatitis, hepatotoxicity
		Mercaptopurine (6MP)	Hepatotoxicity, myelosuppression
Microtubular agents	Block microtubule formation necessary for mitosis	Paclitaxel, paclitaxel protein bound	Alopecia, neuropathy
Vinca alkaloids	Prevent mitosis	Vincristine, vinblastine	Neuropathy, constipation
Antibiotics		Bleomycin	Pulmonary fibrosis
		Mitomycin	Hemolytic–Uremic syndrome
Immune therapy	Increase T cell production and function	Aldesleukin (IL-2)	Capillary leak syndrome
	Activate natural killer cells and macrophages	Interferon	Tachycardia pulmonary edema

Table 9.5 Mechanisms of action and common side effects of targeted therapies used in cancer treatment

Mechanism of action	Example	Side effects
Block surface receptor to inhibit cell growth and mediate antibody directed cellular toxicity	Rituximab (Rituxan©)	All can cause hypersensitivity and infusion reactions
		Neutropenia (late onset), thrombocytopenia, multifocal leukoencephalopathy, tumor lysis syndrome
		Severe mucocutaneous reactions
	Gemtuzumab ozogamicin (Mylotarg©)*	Neutropenia, thrombocytopenia hepatotoxicity, myelosuppression
	Ibritumomab tiuxetan (Zevalin©)	Hepatotoxicity, severe cutaneous or mucocutaneous reactions, delayed and prolonged cytopenias
Epidermal growth factor inhibitors	Cetuximab	Sudden cardiac death, rashes
	Trastuzumab (Herceptin©)	Cardiotoxicity
	Gefitinib (Iressa©)	Disseminated intravascular coagulation, hepatotoxicity, rashes
	Erlotinib (Tarceva©)	Stevens—Johnson syndrome, corneal ulcer

Vascular endothelial growth factor inhibitors	Bevacizumab (Avastin©)	Thromboembolism, hemorrhage
	Sunitinib (Sutent©)	Torsades de Pointes, hyperkalemia, cardiotoxicity
	Sorafenib (Nexavar©)	Anemia, stomatitis, cardiotoxicity
Miscellaneous	Imatinib (Gleevec©)	Cardiac tamponade, cardiogenic shock, hypokalemia, cardiotoxicity
	Dasatinib (Sprycel©)	Pleural effusion, GI bleed, cardiotoxicity
	Bortezomib (Velcade©)	Thrombocytopenia, peripheral neuropathy
	Temsirolimus (Torisel©)	GI perforation, acute renal failure
	Thalidomide (Thalomid©)	Stevens–Johnson syndrome, pulmonary embolism, teratogencity

*Voluntarily recalled from the market.

Altered mental status

Patients undergoing chemotherapy may present to the ED with altered mental status. Several clinical conditions must be considered, including return of primary central nervous system lesions, metastatic lesions, and infectious processes. A glucose level and vital signs should be checked upon patient arrival. A thorough neurologic exam should be performed, with attention to cerebellar function, reflexes, speech, and cognitive function. A CT scan of the head (without and possibly with contrast) should be performed early in the course of the ED visit. Imaging is particularly important before a lumbar puncture to assess the risk for possible herniation. CSF analysis should include at least protein, glucose, cell counts (from tubes 1 and 4), and HSV. Additional studies can be added based on individual patient risk factors. Once standard infectious processes have been ruled out, it is important to consider that certain chemotherapeutic agents are associated with mental status changes. Cisplatin, cytosine, 5FU, ifosfamide, and tamoxifen have all been associated with encephalopathy. The newer agents, particularly the monoclonal antibodies, have an increased risk of altered mental status than more traditional therapies. The risk of chemotherapy associated altered mental status increases significantly with intrathecal administration though changes can still be seen with systemic therapies. Cytosine and methotrexate are known to cause aseptic meningitis. Cerebellar dysfunction is often seen following treatment with cytosine and 5FU; MRI should be considered to further evaluate this anatomic region. Delirium must be considered as well. A multitude of chemotherapy agents have been linked to delirium, including bleomycin, cisplatin, cytosine, 5FU, interferon, interleukin (IL), ifosfamide, methotrexate, prednisone, procarbazine, vinblastine, vincristine, carmustine, and combination therapy with BCNU. As with any case of delirium, the emergency physician should rule out infectious etiologies before assuming delirium is the cause of the patient's altered mental status.

Seizures

Seizures are associated with several commonly used chemotherapeutic agents, including cisplatin, vincristine, and ifosfamide. Chemotherapy associated seizures typically respond to standard therapy, with benzodiazepines such as lorazepam being the first-line agent; the phenytoins, barbiturates, and sedation with propofol can be tried in succession if benzodiazepines do not stop seizure activity.

Sensory changes

Hearing loss and tinnitus can result from cisplatin and carboplatin use as these agents increase NADPH oxidase production leading to increased free radicals and significant ototoxicity [6]. Although the exact mechanism of hearing loss has not yet been elucidated, the investigational use of diphenyleneiodonium chloride or apocynin has limited free radical pro-duction and thus limited cisplatin associated ototoxicity [7]. Symptoms rarely resolve with discontinuation of the medication. Peripheral neu-ropathy is also common after treatment with cisplatin, paclitaxel, and vincristine. It is theorized that the chemotherapeutic agents, particularly paclitaxel, induce change in microtubule organization within nerve cells; thus, these deficits tend to be long standing [8]. Combination therapy with cisplatin and paclitaxel has been shown to have a greater effect on nerve conduction than the agents used separately, potentially accelerating the development of peripheral neuropathy [9]. Cisplatin has also been linked to the development of Lhermitte's Sign, transient paresthesias that radiate from the neck into the upper extremities. Alpha-lipoic acid in an in vitro model has been shown to limit the development of cisplatin–paclitaxel in-duced peripheral neuropathy by serving as a potent mitochondrial antiox-idant [10]. IL-6, in a rodent model, has also shown promise in limiting the development of chemotherapy-related peripheral neuropathy, particularly that associated with cisplatin, vincristine, and paclitaxel [11]. An addi-tional area of potential neurotoxicity involves ABVD therapy for Hodgkin's lymphoma in patients who are HIV positive and on antiretroviral therapy. Many chemotherapeutic agents and antiretroviral agents are metabolized through the cytochrome P450 system, thus slowing degradation of both agents and accelerating neurotoxicity, particularly peripheral neuropathy [12]. Bleomycin has been linked to the development of Raynaud's syn-drome [13]. The incidence of Raynaud's also increases with concurrent use of vinblastine during treatment for germ cell tumors of the male geni-tourinary system [13].

Central nervous system toxicity

Direct neurotoxicity can also occur during intrathecal administration of chemotherapy and by agents that cross the blood–brain barrier. Intrathe-cal errors can occur by pump malfunction, improper concentration of chemotherapeutic agent, or by misidentification of the intrathecal pump versus the standard port or PICC line. Patients will typically note almost instantaneous pain; muscle spasms and alterations of hemodynamic pa-rameters are also common. If medication errors are discovered, CSF ex-change should be performed as quickly as possible; isotonic saline or lactated ringer's can be infused intrathecally to replace fluid and ideally reduce additional headaches/pain associated with rapid changes in CSF volume [14]. This should be done in consultation with both neurosurgery and anesthesia as well as the local poison control center. Admission is warranted to monitor neurologic status. Cyclophosphamide and 5FU eas-ily cross into the CNS while agents like doxorubicin and paclitaxel do not. Insulin-like growth factor 1 (IGF-1), in a rodent model, promotes neurogenesis and thus limits direct neurotoxicity of the drugs that do penetrate the blood–brain barrier [15].

Cerebrovascular accident

Patients undergoing chemotherapy are also at risk for cerebrovascular accidents (CVA); underlying co-morbidities also contribute significantly to the likelihood of CVA. Most CVAs associated with cancer tend to be ischemic in nature; tumor embolism may result in ischemic stroke as well [16]. Hemorrhagic CVAs are typically associated with leukemias, lymphomas, and multiple myeloma [16]. Evaluation of these patients should proceed as would the evaluation of a non-cancer patient presenting with stroke like symptoms. It may be beneficial to obtain an MRI early in the workup to facilitate delineation between CVA and metastatic disease. Also, if t-PA is being considered in the chemotherapy patient, it is important to ensure the patient is not thrombocytopenic as platelet count <100,000 is an exclusion criterion for t-PA administration [17]. Cancer patients may also be hypercoaguable, thus increasing the risk of cerebral venous sinus thrombosis. This risk increases even further following therapy with asparaginase [16].

Cardiac

Cardiac manifestations of chemotherapy are very prevalent. Patients often present with shortness of breath, chest pain, and cardiac dysrhythmias. Evaluation of this chest pain should include standard diagnostic testing including EKG, cardiac enzymes, B-natriuretic peptide, and chest X-ray. Pericardial effusion (occasionally progressing to cardiac tamponade) is associated with cancer, both with metastatic lesions and as a side effect of chemotherapy. Bedside ultrasound (or complete echocardiography) is an integral part of the emergent evaluation of chemotherapy patients with chest pain [18].

Cardiomyopathy is also a common cardiac side effect of chemotherapy, with the anthracyclines being the most common causative agent. The exact mechanism of this side effect is not fully understood, but it is believed that the anthracyclines produce oxidative stress in the mitochondria [19]. Use of several naturally occurring antioxidants, including vitamins A, C and E, coenzyme Q, and carotenoids, has been proposed to limit cardiotoxicity [20]. Inhibition of endothelin-converting enzyme-1, thus decreasing the amount of endothelin-1 produced in mitochondria, has also shown promise in limiting anthracycline-induced cardiomyopathy [21]. High-density lipoprotein (HDL) has also been shown to protect cardiac myocytes against the oxidative stresses induced by doxorubicin [22]. Administration of dexrazoxane, a derivative of the iron chelator EDTA, 30–60 minutes before chemotherapy has also been shown to limit the development of chemotherapy-induced cardiomyopathy, particularly that resulting from anthracycline administration [23]. It is believed that iron chelation decreases the amount of free radicals formed, thus limiting cell toxicity. Both the in vivo and in vitro free radical clearances of dexrazoxane have been shown to be superior to both glutathione and uric acid [24]. While dexrazoxane decreases the incidence of anthracycline-associated cardiomyopathy it does raise the risk of clinically significant leukopenia, more so than therapy with the anthracyclines alone [25].

There is some evidence that survivors of childhood cancers treated with high-dose anthracyclines and cardiac radiation have long-term left ventricular dysfunction [26]. There is also evidence that the development of cardiac abnormalities may be delayed, as cardiac parameters often become increasingly more abnormal as the time from therapy increases [27]. Unfortunately, standard therapy for congestive heart failure (CHF), particularly the second-line combination of digitalis and a diuretic, is not effective at treating anthracycline-induced heart failure; heart transplantation is often required for definitive treatment.

The attribution of development of cardiomyopathy to the administration of trastuzumab, commonly used to treat HER2+ breast cancer, has been somewhat controversial as many patients treated with this agent have also been given an anthracycline. The likelihood of cardiomyopathy increases with cumulative doses of anthracyclines previously administered, and also with combination therapy, particularly radiation therapy. The resultant cardiac changes include decreased left ventricular wall mass leading to dilated cardiomyopathy and potentially CHF (systolic dysfunction) [28]. In contrast to the anthracyclines, this effect of trastuzumab is not dose dependent [29]. Cyclophosphamide, cisplatin, vinca alkaloids, and mitomycin have also been implicated in the development of cardiomyopathy. Resveratrol, a naturally occurring antibiotic, limits cisplatin-induced cardiomyopathy by limiting free radical production in a rodent model [30].

Paclitaxel has been linked to cardiac dysrhythmias while 5FU typically results in nonspecific EKG changes. Coronary artery spasm has also been seen following 5FU administration [31]. Myocardial ischemia has been documented after treatment with 5FU and capecitabine; this effect is even more pronounced in patients with pre-existing coronary artery disease. Doxorubicin has also been found to cause prolonged QTc intervals on EKG; dexrazoxane has been shown to limit this development as well [32]. The newly developed tyrosine kinase inhibitors, including imatinib, dasatinib, nilotinib, sunitinib, sorafenib, and lapatinib, contribute to chemotherapy associated cardiotoxicity, including cardiomyopathy, EKG changes, and left ventricular ejection fraction changes, often resulting in heart failure [33]. Gefitibin and erlotinib have not been found to have cardiotoxic effects [33]. Lastly, the emergency physician should not ignore the patient's underlying coronary artery disease risk factors when evaluating chest pain in chemotherapy patients. The use of chemotherapy may add to the acute coronary syndrome risk and is not a contraindication to aggressive management of myocardial ischemia, including cardiac catheterization and possibly cardiac bypass surgery.

Pulmonary

Cancer in general does increase a patient's risk for pulmonary embolism, but the risk is even higher in patients with brain, lung, renal, gynecologic, or GI tract tumors [34]. Patients with multiple myeloma are also at high risk for deep vein thrombosis (DVT) given the increased viscosity seen with the condition. This risk is increased even further with the use of thalidomide or lenalidomide in combination with dexamethasone, the two agents typically used to treat multiple myeloma [35]. Additionally, patients on mitomycin, bleomycin, cisplatin, bevacizumab, or cyclosporine have a higher risk of DVT than those on other forms of chemotherapy [36]. If a pulmonary embolism is diagnosed, a CT scan of the head should be performed to rule out intracranial lesions prior to initiating anticoagulation therapy. Low molecular weight heparin (LMWH) is preferred over unfractionated heparin (UFH) for treating cancer-related DVT/pulmonary embolism. LMWH has several therapeutic advantages over UFH: less bleeding and less associated treatment resistance with LMWH than with UFH. LMWH is also preferred over warfarin therapy for long-term treatment of DVT/PE in cancer patients due to the difficulty in maintaining a therapeutic INR. Oncologic patients on warfarin therapy require more frequent INR checks than cardiac patients on the drug; many chemotherapeutic agents alter the normal metabolism of warfarin and thus can place the patient at higher risk of bleeding or of developing a DVT/pulmonary embolism [34]. Preventive therapy with LMWH is only currently recommended for patients on combination therapy with thalidomide/lenalidomide and corticosteroids; prophylaxis is not recommended for any other patient subgroups [35].

Respiratory complications are commonly associated with chemotherapy. The reason for this is twofold. Several chemotherapeutic agents have pulmonary side effects while others induce immunosuppression, thus making the patient more susceptible to both typical and atypical lung infections. Common pulmonary infections occurring in chemotherapy patients frequently include pneumonia and pleural effusions. Patients with pneumonia should be treated for health care acquired infections given the regularity with which they receive chemotherapy. Extreme infectious cases can result in bronchiolitis obliterans organizing pneumonia (BOOP). Patients with pleural effusions may require thoracentesis to determine if the fluid collections are infectious or malignant in nature. Pulmonary toxicity (diffuse alveolar hemorrhage or fibrosis) is commonly associated with bleomycin therapy; this, too, is dose dependent. In a prospective study of 95 patients, bleomycin injected directly into hemangiomas and vascular malformations had previously not been associated with pulmonary toxicity [37], but use of this therapy in younger patients raises the possibility that pulmonary toxicity be a consideration in these patients [38]. Cyclophosphamide, busulfan, methotrexate [39], mercaptopurine (6MP), cytosine, BCNU, vinca alkaloids, and paclitaxel have also been associated with clinically significant pulmonary complications [40]. Methotrexate toxicity typically results in pulmonary infiltrates; interstitial infiltrates can be seen, but basilar infiltrates are more common. Pneumonitis is also frequently seen with methotrexate therapy. Treatment of early, minimally invasive cervical cancer with the combination of vincristine, bleomycin, and cisplatin has been found to be particularly pulmonary toxic. BOOP and interstitial pneumonitis are characteristic of this therapy [41]. Pulmonary function testing (peak expiratory flow in the ED setting) can help guide therapy and should be incorporated into the acute diagnostic and treatment plan [39]. Chest CT may also help differentiate the type of infiltrate and thus further guide therapy. Steroid use is critical in limiting the progression of the pneumonitis and should be started as soon as possible.

Hematologic

Significant alterations in hematologic parameters can be seen following chemotherapy. Neutropenia is particularly common following chemotherapy; time from last treatment is particularly important as individual agents affect cell lines at different time intervals. Profound neutropenia places the cancer patient at increased risk of infection. Care should be taken to ensure that reverse isolation precautions are applied to these patients to minimize iatrogenic infection risks. Thrombocytopenia is also associated with a variety of agents, including mitomycin, methotrexate, hydroxyurea, 5FU, anthracyclines, carboplatin, vinblastine, and busulfan [3]. Caution should be taken to avoid trauma in this patient subgroup as apparently minor head trauma can have catastrophic complications. Busulfan and BCNU have been associated with prolonged alterations in cell lines; abnormalities have been found as long as 6 weeks from the time of administration [42]. Attention should be paid to platelet counts prior to performing any invasive procedure on a chemotherapy patient; hemostasis may be difficult to achieve in this situation. Etoposide, a DNA topoisomerase inhibitor, significantly increases the risk of subsequent leukemia [13]. Methotrexate toxicity can result in significant myelosuppression; anemia and thrombocytopenia can be clinically significant in cases of severe toxicity [43].

Tumor lysis syndrome

Tumor lysis syndrome is a combination of metabolic abnormalities resulting from partial breakdown of a tumor. Hematogenous tumors are more frequently associated with tumor lysis syndrome than are solid lesions. The incidence of tumor lysis syndrome increases with the increasing size of the tumor being treated as well as with the rapidity with which the lesion is broken down. Additionally, use of interferon alpha, tamoxifen, methotrexate, and rituximab are associated with higher likelihood of tumor lysis syndrome. Hyperkalemia, hypocalcemia, hyperuricemia, and hyperphosphatemia are the most common electrolyte abnormalities associated with tumor lysis syndrome [44]. An EKG should be performed as soon as the diagnosis of tumor lysis syndrome is considered to ensure timely identification of electrolyte abnormalities. Hyperkalemia and hypocalcemia can have significant morbidity and mortality associated and should be treated as soon as the abnormalities are detected. The combination of electrolyte disturbances can also lead to organ failure, particularly renal failure. Care should be taken to ensure proper hydration and thus appropriate urine output during the treatment period. Administration of allopurinol prior to chemotherapy has been shown to significantly decrease the incidence of tumor lysis syndrome by inhibiting xanthine oxidase, effectively limiting uric acid production [44]. Allopurinol therapy is currently recommended in patients at high risk for tumor lysis syndrome. If hyperuricemia develops, alkalinization of the urine is the preferred method of treatment; hyperphosphatemia may worsen after alkalinization of urine. Rasburicase, a recombinant urate oxidase, is also used to limit the development of hyperuricemia associated with tumor lysis syndrome. This agent converts uric acid to allantoin, a highly soluble complex that is easily excreted in the urine, thus enhancing elimination of uric acid. The measurement of uric acid concentrations in patients on rasburicase will be adversely affected unless blood samples are handled appropriately and collected in pre-chilled heparin containing tubes and kept chilled, with analysis occurring within 4 hours of collection. Urine specimens being evaluated for uric acid must also be chilled prior to analysis. Concomitant alkalinization of the urine is not required when using this agent [44]. Rasburicase is currently preferred over allopurinol in the pediatric population as well as in patients with renal insufficiency as dosage does not need to be altered based on renal function [45,46]. Its use should be avoided in patients with concurrent G6PD deficiency as these patients are not able to metabolize the hydrogen peroxide byproduct of the uric acid conversion and thus are at risk for hemolysis. Methemoglobinemia is another reported side effect of rasburicase. Hypersensitivity reactions, including anaphylaxis are common as well following rasburicase administration; such reactions should be treated with standard therapy [45].

Electrolyte abnormalities

Syndrome of inappropriate antidiuretic hormone (SIADH) can result from chemotherapy [47] or from certain ADH secreting tumors, particularly lung cancers. Hyponatremia is the hallmark of this condition, along with excessive urinary sodium excretion. Signs and symptoms of hyponatremia vary based on the absolute sodium value as well as the rapidity with which the level is reached. Severe hyponatremia may result in seizure and coma. Hypertonic saline may be required to correct severe hyponatremia while more moderate levels may be treated with water restriction. Hyponatremia has been reported following intravenous cyclophosphamide administration [48]. Incidence of cyclophosphamide-induced hyponatremia increases when hypotonic saline is used during therapy; isotonic saline is preferred in this situation. Hypercalcemia is common in cancer patients, particularly those with cervical, esophageal, head/neck, and lung cancers. Symptoms typically include dehydration, altered mental status, and vague abdominal pain. As with other electrolyte abnormalities, an EKG should be performed when hypercalcemia is suspected; arrhythmias and QT abnormalities are common. It is important to check total calcium as well as ionized calcium to determine the level of biologically available calcium. Hydration is the hallmark of therapy. Once patients are euvolemic, furosemide, and calcitonin can be used to enhance renal clearance of excess calcium.

Gastrointestinal

Perhaps the most common side effect of chemotherapy is gastrointestinal distress, resulting in patients being persistently nauseated and often with frequent episodes of vomiting. Almost all agents can cause these symptoms, but varying levels of risk are associated with the different drugs. Cisplatin, carboplatin, ifosfamide, and the anthracyclines have a high incidence of GI distress while intravenous cyclophosphamide, the taxanes, etoposide, and methotrexate have a moderate risk of vomiting [49]. The American Society of Clinical Oncology classifies chemotherapeutic agents on the likelihood to cause emesis. Cisplatin, high-dose cyclophosphamide, carmustine, dacarbazine, and dactinomycin are all considered very high risk for emesis while oxaliplatin, carboplatin, ifosfamide, doxorubicin, danorubicin, moderate dose cyclophosphamide, and epirubicin are considered moderate risk (30%–90%). Low-risk medications include paclitaxel, doxitaxel, topotecan, etoposide, methotrexate, mitomycin, low-dose cytarabine, 5FU, and trastuzumab. The vinca alkaloids, oral cyclophosphamide, bleomycin, busulfan, bevacizumab, and rituximab are the least likely to induce nausea [49].

A variety of antiemetic agents are used to limit the discomfort associated with this gastrointestinal distress. Patients receiving high-risk chemotherapeutic agents, anthracyclines, or cyclophosphamides are typically treated prophylactically with three antiemetic agents, including a serotonin 5HT3 receptor antagonist, corticosteroids, and a neurokinin-1 receptor antagonist [49]. Neurokinin-1 receptor antagonists work by blocking substance P, a potent trigger of emesis. The most commonly used agent is aprepitant. Those undergoing therapy with the other moderate-risk agents typically receive both a serotonin receptor ant agonist and corticosteroids. Low-risk patients are typically given only a corticosteroid. Pre-emptive therapy is not usually prescribed for the very low-risk medications [49]. While serotonin 5HT3 receptor antagonists have few side effects, it is important for the emergency physician to inquire about long-term use of dexamethasone as an antiemetic as the effects of frequent corticosteroid use may affect patient presentation, particularly when relatively minor trauma results in significant fractures. Aprepitant itself may cause significant fatigue and diarrhea. Knowledge of the emetic risk class of a particular chemotherapeutic agent can also help guide therapy in the ED as monotherapy may not be adequate for all patients.

Further disruptions to normal bowel function can also be seen as paclitaxel commonly causes diarrhea while vincristine use frequently results in constipation. The diarrhea associated with paclitaxel is often bloody as this drug is also associated with lower GI bleeds [3,50]; corticosteroid use more typically results in an upper GI bleed. Both upper and lower GI bleeds in cancer patients should be treated in the same manner as bleeds not associated with chemotherapy. Constipation from chemotherapeutic agents can be magnified by the concurrent use of opioid analgesics. Bowel regimens are a key aspect of chemotherapy to limit the development of constipation or even fecal impaction. Mucositis is also associated with chemotherapy. This inflammation of mucosa can affect the oral cavity or the entire gastrointestinal tract. Patients typically notice irritation of the mucosal cells within 3–4 days of chemotherapy; symptoms peak within 2 weeks of treatment. Oral mucositis is commonly seen following therapy with 5FU while gastrointestinal mucositis is associated with irinotecan. Symptomatic and supportive care is the mainstay of treatment, but patients should be closely monitored to prevent superinfection of the lesions [51].

Several chemotherapeutic agents have been found to cause pancreatitis, including azathioprine, bleomycin, cisplatin, cyclophosphamide, cytarabine, 5FU, ifosfamide, interferon, methotrexate, mitomycin, and the vinca alkaloids [52]. Ranson criteria should be applied to chemotherapy patients with pancreatitis. Lastly, hepatotoxicity may be seen following the use of cyclophosphamide, cisplatin, carmustine, cytarabine, mercaptopurine, methotrexate, mithromycin, paclitaxel, etoposide, and tamoxifen [3]. Supportive care is crucial in cases of hepatotoxicity. *N*-acetylcysteine should be considered in these patients and any patient with chemotherapy-associated liver failure.

Renal

Nephrotoxicity also results from a variety of chemotherapeutic agents, including cisplatin, IL-2, ifosfamide, mitomycin, interferon, carboplatin, and methotrexate [3]. It is important to maximize the patient's hydration status while on these agents in an effort to prophylactically limit the development of renal insufficiency or failure. Dialysis is a viable temporizing treatment modality for these patients. However, it is not particularly effective for clearing methotrexate. If methotrexate-induced renal failure is identified early, the use of glucarpidase and leucovorin have been shown to limit renal and direct methotrexate toxicity. However, these agents should be administered as soon as possible following the onset of renal toxicity to have maximum benefit [53]. Glucarpidase is an enzyme that inactivates methotrexate (as well as leucovorin) and limits the development of methotrexate toxicity [43,54]. Combination therapy with cisplatin and paclitaxel has been found to be particularly nephrotoxic. Effects are greater than those seen during monotherapy with cisplatin. Given the relatively low renal injury profile associated with paclitaxel use, this is particularly concerning and thus the mechanism of this reaction is the focus of much research [9]. The antidiabetic medication rosiglitazone has been shown to be nephroprotective during cisplatin therapy as has carvedilol, the β-1 blocker/α-1 blocker [55]. It is theorized that rosiglitazone upregulates IL-10, an anti-inflammatory mediator, thus limiting toxicity [56]. IL-6 deficiency in a rodent model contributes to accelerated cisplatin nephrotoxicity [57]. Drug–drug interactions have also been shown to increase methotrexate toxicity; proton pump inhibitors significantly delay methotrexate elimination, resulting in toxicity. If possible, use of this medication class should be limited during methotrexate therapy [58]. Hemorrhagic cystitis is commonly seen with cyclophosphamide and ifosfamide. MESNA (2-Mercaptoethane sulfonate sodium) can be used to limit the development of hemorrhagic cystitis by binding to the toxic metabolites, thus limiting the cellular damage [59]. Again adequate hydration is paramount to maintain renal function and in this case to maintain patient comfort. Intravascular hemolysis may result from Rho immunoglobulin therapy; the first manifestation of this condition is often hematuria. Use of this agent is now limited to closely monitored, extended care units [60].

Dermatologic

Chemotherapy can have devastating consequences for the skin, particularly in cases of extravasation of the chemotherapeutic agent. It is important to consider the diluent used to administer the actual chemotherapeutic agent as this too may contribute to skin changes associated with extravasation. The site of the extravasation can impact the extent of symptoms. If the extravasation is from a chest wall port, the emergency physician should consider the possibility of mediastinitis; CT scanning of the chest may be required to fully evaluate the extent of tissue damage. Peripheral extravasation should be treated with elevation and ice; compression also helps limit the spread of the agent. Anthracycline extravasation result in ulceration that progresses to skin necrosis [61]. Dexrazoxane in a formulation different from that used for cardioprotection has also shown utility as an antidote to anthracycline extravasation if administered as soon as possible and within 6 hours of the extravasation [62]. Vincristine, vinblastine, and vesicants, such as doxorubicin and mitomycin, typically result in necrosis if extravasation occurs. Several antidotes are available to limit the extent of tissue toxicity following extravasation (Table 9.6 below).

Table 9.6 Common antidotes

Chemotherapy agent	Antidote	Mechanism
Anthracycline (extravasation)	Dexrazoxane	Limits free radical synthesis
Mitomycin (extravasation)	DMSO	Free radical scavenger
Vinca alkaloids (extravasation)	Hyaluronidase	Increases systemic absorption to limit local damage
Methotrexate	Leucovorin	Bypasses methotrexate block to provide active folate
	Glucarpidase	Inactivates methotrexate in plasma
5FU, capecitabine	Uridine triacetate	Competes with active 5FU metabolites for incorporation into RNA

Palmar–plantar syndrome is frequently seen following 5FU, doxorubicin, and IL-2 therapy; the oral agents capecitabine and sorafenib have also produced this syndrome [3].This condition results as chemotherapeutic agents are excreted into the skin cells and concentrate in the palms and soles. Typical features of this condition include erythema, exquisite pain, and in severe cases sloughing of the skin. Exposure to hot water should be limited, as should prolonged walking or activities with the hands. Therapy is initially supportive; however, oral antibiotics and steroids may be required. Extreme cases may require IV antibiotics, IV steroids, and hospital admission. Acne like skin eruptions may be seen following cetuximab or erlotinib use. One study did show that topical therapy with nadifloxacin cream was preferred over tetracycline or isotretinoin due to fewer interactions with the chemotherapeutic agents [63]; larger studies are still needed to fully evaluate topical therapy in this situation.

Reproductive system

The reproductive system is particularly susceptible to the effects of chemotherapy. Sperm production is significantly limited, if present at all, following chemotherapy; such suppression can last up to 5 years after therapy. Administration of testosterone along with chemotherapy may limit the negative impact on sperm production [64], but sperm donation should be considered prior to the onset of chemotherapy in men of child-bearing age. Women are also susceptible to alterations in fertility due to exposure to chemotherapy. The alkylating agents, anthracyclines, bleomycin, etoposide, 5FU, methotrexate, the platinums, thalidomide, and the vinca alkaloids, all directly decrease oocyte counts and follicle formation; they also significantly slow down or halt ovulation completely. Egg donation should be considered prior to initiation of therapy in women of child-bearing age. Paclitaxel is commonly used to treat breast and gynecologic tumors. Transient decreases in the number of corpora lutea were noted, but little decrease in the number of follicles has been found in long-term follow-up. This potential fertility sparing treatment is particularly encouraging for women of child-bearing age undergoing chemotherapy [65].

Antidotes

As chemotherapeutic agents gain widespread use and more side effects are identified, research has begun to focus on the development of antidotes to these drugs (Table 9.6 above).

Methotrexate toxicity can be limited by urine alkalinization and the concurrent use of leucovorin, a biologically active form of folic acid. As folic acid synthesis is limited by methotrexate, leucovorin use provides some substrate for normal DNA and RNA syntheses during chemotherapy. Intravenous doses of leucovorin can be titrated based on serum methotrexate concentration [66]. Glucarpidase can also be used as rescue therapy in methotrexate toxicity. This recombinant enzyme, derived from *Pseudomonas*, accelerates methotrexate degradation [53]. Uridine triacetate, formerly known as vistonuridine, has been shown to limit toxicity from 5FU and presumably from capecitabine, a prodrug of 5FU. Uridine triacetate is a pro-drug for uridine and serves as a competitive inhibitor of the toxic metabolites of 5FU, thus limiting incorporation of 5FU metabolites into RNA and limiting systemic toxicity [67]. Any case of suspected chemotherapy-related toxicity should be called into the local poison control center (1-800-222-1222 in the United States). Specialists are on call 24 hours a day to assist with management of these cases.

The next five years

Research continues to further elucidate the mechanisms through which various tumors develop. As a result, it is reasonable to expect that tailored chemotherapeutic regimens based on individual characteristics will become more common. This will confront emergency physicians with further variability in chemotherapy treatment plans that will have unique and potentially dangerous side effects. Monoclonal antibody therapy has been developed to take advantage of tumor biochemistry while limiting systemic side effects (Table 9.5). Patients may present to the ED with a variety of hypersensitivity related concerns, including fever, chills, sweats, gastrointestinal distress, back pain, and anaphylaxis.

Angiogenesis is a critical part of cancer growth, and several new therapies are targeting this aspect of tumor development. The epidermal growth factor-tyrosine kinase inhibitors (EGFR-TKI) have been found to be particularly potent at limiting angiogenesis in certain cancers. In general, the optimal timing of EGFR administration is still controversial, as is the benefit of monotherapy versus combination with standard chemotherapy. Non-small cell lung cancer, particularly in those with no history of smoking, has been sensitive to treatment with this class of agents. Gefitinib was one of the first EGFR agents used; however, resistance to this drug is fairly common and develops early in the therapy process [68]. Secondary treatment with another EGFR-TKI, eroltinib, has also shown promise in treating these tumors [69]. Similarly, bevacizumab is a vascular endothelial growth factor antibody that is becoming an integral part of therapy for colorectal, non-small cell lung and breast cancer patients. Maximum benefit from bevacizumab is achieved when it is administered concurrently with standard chemotherapy regimens. It is, however, currently recommended as monotherapy during the maintenance phase of treatment.

There are significant neurologic side effects linked to bevacizumab, including blindness and reversible posterior leukoencephalopathy syndrome [70]. Typical features of this syndrome include altered mental status, visual changes, hypertension, seizures, and reversible lesions in the white matter, predominantly in the parietal and occipital lobes. Current therapy centers upon controlling hypertension, limiting seizure activity, and general supportive care. Ofatumumab is currently used as salvage therapy in chronic lymphocytic leukemia patients who have failed standard chemotherapy regimens [71]. Small bowel perforation has also been reported following bevacizumab therapy [72]. Overall, angiogenesis targeting has the potential to develop into first-line therapy for a number of malignancies in the next 5 years with research focusing on which malignancies can be targeted and how to limit side effects.

Temsirolimus is a kinase inhibitor that is now being used to treat solid tumors, particularly renal cell tumors. Side effects seen with this medication include hyperglycemia, abnormal liver function tests (particularly ALT), neutropenia, and stomatitis [73].

Cacalol, a free radical derived from an Asian herbal plant, has shown promise in inducing cell death in breast cancer cells. The cytotoxic effect was even greater when cacalol was administered concurrently with taxol or cyclophosphamide and significantly increased tumor necrosis without significant systemic toxicity [74].

Conclusion

Cancer is becoming increasingly common in the United States and worldwide. Therapies used to treat these conditions are continuously evolving; the combination of medications used for a particular diagnosis is changing as well. These agents have many side effects that can alter the patient's presentation to the ED. The emergency practitioner should be familiar with the common and life-threatening side effects of chemotherapeutic agents as well as the standard methods to treat chemotherapy-related side effects. Close consultation with oncology can aid in the management of this challenging ED patient population. In addition, consultation with the poison control center (1-800-222-1222) can aid with antidotal therapy.

Acknowledgement

The authors would like to thank Tina Kanmaz, Pharm.D, Clinical Associate Professor of Pharmacy, St. John's University College of Pharmacy, and Faculty, Queens Cancer Center, Department of Pharmacy for her review of this paper and her insightful comments.

References

1. American Cancer Society. 2010. Available at: http://www.cancer.org/Healthy/InformationforHealthCareProfessionals/cancer_statistics_2009_slides_rev.ppt, accessed August 30, 2010.
2. World Health Organization. 2010. Available at: http://www.who.int/mediacentre/factsheets/fs297/en/index.html, accessed October 1, 2010.
3. Micromedex. 2010. Available at: http://www.thomsonhc.com/home/dispatch, accessed October 1, 2010.
4. Wolach O, Bairey O, Lahav M. Late-onset neutropenia after rituximab treatment: case series and comprehensive review of the literature. *Medicine* 2010; 89(5): 308–318.
5. Sun H, Nemecek AN. Optimal management of malignant epidural spinal cord compression. *Emerg Med Clin N Amer* 2009; 27: 195–208.
6. Dille MF, Konrad-Martin D, Gallun F, Helt WJ, Gordon JS, Reavis KM. Tinnitus onset rates from chemotherapeutic agents and ototoxic antibiotics: results of a large prospective study. *J Am Acad Audiol* 2010; 21(6): 409–417.
7. Kim HJ, Lee JH, Kim SJ, et al. Roles of NADPH oxidases in cisplatin-induced reactive oxygen species generation and ototoxicity. *J Neurosci* 2010; 30(11): 3933–3946.
8. Shemesh OA, Spira ME. Paclitaxel induces axonal microtubules polar reconfiguration and impaired organelle transport: implications for the pathogenesis of paclitaxel-induced polyneuropathy. *Acta Neuropathol* 2010; 119(2): 235–248.
9. Carozzi V, Chiorazzi A, Canta A, et al. Effect of the chronic combined administration of cisplatin and paclitaxel in a rat model of peripheral neurotoxicity. *Eur J Cancer* 2009; 45(4): 656–665.

10. Melli G, Taiana M, Camozzi F, et al. Alpha-lipoic acid prevents mitochondrial damage and neurotoxicity in experimental chemotherapy neuropathy. *Exp Neurol* 2008; 214(2): 276–284.

11. Callizot N, Andriambeloson E, Glass J, et al. Interleukin-6 protects against paclitaxel, cisplatin, and vincristine-induced neuropathies without impairing chemotherapeutic activity. *Cancer Chemother Pharmacol* 2008; 62(6): 995–1007.

12. Cheung MC, Hicks LK, Leitch HA. Excessive neurotoxicity with ABVD when combined with protease inhibitor-based antiretroviral therapy in the treatment of AIDS-related Hodgkin lymphoma. *Clin Lymphoma Myeloma Leuk* 2010; 10(2): E22–E25.

13. Chaudhary UB, Haldas JR. Long-term complications of chemotherapy for germ cell tumors. *Drugs* 2003; 63(15): 1565–1577.

14. Rao RB. Special Considerations: intrathecal administration of xenobiotics. In: Goldfrank LR, Floenbaum N, Hoffman RS, Nelson LS, Howland MA (eds.) *Goldfrank's Toxicologic Emergencies*. 9th ed. McGraw-Hill; 2010: p. 548.

15. Janelsins MC, Roscoe JA, Berg MJ, et al. IGF-1 partially restores chemotherapy-induced reductions in neural cell proliferation in adult C57BL/6 mice. *Cancer Invest* 2010; 28(5): 544–553.

16. Griswold W, Oberndorfer S, Struhal W. Stroke and cancer: a review. *Acta Neurol Scand* 2009; 119(1): 1–16.

17. Brott T, Bogousslavsky J. Treatment of acute ischemic stroke. *N Engl J Med* 2000; 343(10): 710–722.

18. Monsuez JJ CJ, Vignat N, Artigou JY. Cardiac side-effects of cancer chemotherapy. *Int J Cardiol* 2010 Apr 16. [Epub ahead of print]

19. Thompson KL, Rosenzweig BA, Zhang J, et al. Early alterations in heart gene expression profiles associated with doxorubicin cardiotoxicity in rats. *Cancer Chemother Pharmacol* 2010; 68(2): 303–314.

20. Granados-Principal S, Quiles JL, Ramirez-Tortosa CL, Sanchez-Rovira P, Ramirez-Tortosa MC. New advances in molecular mechanisms and the prevention of adriamycin toxicity by antioxidant nutrients. *Food Chem Toxicol* 2010; 48(6): 1425–1438.

21. Miyagawa K, Emoto N, Widyantoro B, et al. Attenuation of doxorubicin-induced cardiomyopathy by endotherlin-converting enzyme-1 ablation through prevention of mitochondrial biogenesis impairment. *Hypertension* 2010; 55(3): 738–746.

22. Frias MA, Lang U, Gerber-Wicht C, James SW. Native and reconstituted HDL protect cardiomyocytes from doxorubicin-induced apoptosis. *Cardiovasc Res* 2010; 85(1): 118–126.

23. Lipshultz SE. Exposure to anthracyclines during childhood causes cardiac injury. *Semin Oncol* 2006; 33(3 Suppl. 8): S8–S14.

24. Galetta F, Franzoni F, Cervetti G, et al. In vitro and in vivo study on the antioxidant activity of dexrazoxane. *Biomed Pharmacother* 2010; 64(4): 259–263.

25. Chow WA, Synold TW, Tetef ML, et al. Feasibility and pharmacokinetic study of infusional dexrazoxane and dose-intensive doxorubicin administered concurrently over 96 h for the treatment of advanced malignancies. *Cancer Chemother Pharmacol* 2004; 54(3): 241–248.

26. Van Der Pal HJ, van Dalen EC, Hauptmann M, et al. Cardiac function in 5-year survivors of childhood cancer: a long-term follow-up study. *Arch Intern Med* 2010; 170(4): 1247–1255.

27. Hudson MM, Rai SN, Nunez C, et al. Noninvasive evaluation of late anthracycline cardiac toxicity in childhood cancer survivors. *J Clin Oncol* 2007; 20(25): 3635–3643.

28. Procter M, Suter TM, de Azambuja E, et al. Longer-term assessment of trastuzumab-related cardiac adverse events in the Herceptin Adjuvant (HERA) trial. *J Clin Oncol* 2010; 28(21): 3422–3428.

29. Perez EA. Cardiac toxicity of ErbB2-targeted therapies: what do we know ? *Clin Breast Cancer* 2008; 8(3 Suppl.): S114–S120.

30. Wang J, He D, Zhang Q, Han Y, Jin S, Qi F. Resveratrol protects against cisplatin-induced cardiotoxicity by alleviating oxidative damage. *Cancer Biother Radiopharm* 2009; 24(6): 675–680.

31. Alter P, Herzum M, Schaefer JR, Maisch B. Coronary artery spasm induced by 5-fluorouracil. *Z Kardiol* 2005; 94(1): 33–37.

32. Ducroq J, Moha ou Maati H, Guilbot S, et al. Dexrazoxane protects the heart from acute doxorubicin-induced QT prolongation: a key role for I(Ks). *Br J Pharmacol* 2010; 159(1): 93–101.

33. Orphanos GS, Ioannidis GN, Ardavais AG. Cardiotoxicity induced by tyrone kinase inhibitors. *Acta Oncol* 2009; 48(7): 964–970.

34. Lyman GH, Khorana AA, Falanga A, et al. American Society of Clinical Oncology guideline: recommendations for venous thromboembolism prophylaxis and treatment in patients with cancer. *J Clin Oncol* 2007; 25(34): 5490–5505.

35. Palumbo A, Rajkumar SV, Dimopoulos MA, et al. Prevention of thalidomide- and lenalidomide-associated thrombosis in myeloma. *Leukemia* 2008; 22: 414–423.

36. Mano MS, Guimaraes JL, Sutmoller SF, Reiriz AB, Sutomller CS, DiLeo A. Extensive deep vein thrombosis as a complication of testicular cancer treated with the BEP protocol (bleomycin, etoposide, and cisplatin): case report. *Sao Paulo Med J* 2006; 124(6): 343–345.

37. Muir T, Kirsten M, Fourie P, Dippenaar N, Ionescu GO. Intra-lesional bleomycin injection (IBI) treatment for haemangiomas and congenital vascular malformations. *Pediatr Surg Int* 2004; 19(12): 766–773.

38. Atwa K, Abuhasna S, Shihab Z, Hashaykeh N, Hasan R. Acute pulmonary toxicity following intra-lesional administration of bleomycin for a lymphovenous malformaton. *Pediatr Pulmonol* 2010; 45(2): 192–196.

39. Lateef O, Shakoor N, Balk RA. Methotrexate pulmonary toxicity. *Expert Opin Drug Saf* 2005; 4(4): 723–730.

40. Millward MJ, Cohney SJ, Byrne MJ, Ryan GF. Pulmonary toxicity following MOPP chemotherapy. *Aust N Z J Med* 1990; 20(3): 245–248.

41. Ki KD, Lee JM, Lee SK, et al. Pulmonary toxicity after a quick course of combinatorial vincristine, bleomycin, and cisplatin neoadjuvant chemotherapy in cervical cancer. *J Korean Med Sci* 2010; 25(2): 240–244.

42. Molyneux G, Andrews M, Sones W, et al. Haematoxicity of busulphan, doxorubicin, cisplatin and cyclophosphamide in the female BALB/c mouse using

a brief regimen of drug administration. *Cell Biol Toxicol* 2010. [Epub ahead of print]

43. Smith SW, Nelson LS. Case files of the New York City Poison Control Center: antidotal strategies for the management of methotrexate toxicity. *J Med Toxicol* 2008; 4(2): 132–140.

44. Coiffier B, Altman A, Pui C-H, Younes A, Cairo MS. Guidelines for the management of pediatric and adult tumor lysis syndrome: an evidence-based review. *J Clin Oncol* 2008; 26: 2767–2778.

45. Sood AR, Burry LD, Cheng DKF. Clarifying the role of rasburicase in tumor lysis syndrome. *Pharmocotherapy* 2007; 27(1): 111–121.

46. Zonfrillo MR. Management of pediatric tumor lysis syndrome in the emergency department. *Emerg Med Clin N Am* 2009; 27: 497–504.

47. Behl D, Hendrickson AW, Moynihan TJ. Oncologic emergencies. *Crit Care Clin* 2010; 26(1): 181–205.

48. Lee YC, Park JS, Lee CH, et al. Hyponatraemia induced by low-dose intravenous pulse cyclophosphamide. *Nephrol Dial Transplant* 2010; 25(5): 1520–1524.

49. Kris MG, Hesketh PJ, Somerfield, Feyer P, et al. American Society of Clinical Oncology guideline for antiemetics in oncology: Update 2006. *J Clin Oncol* 2006; 24(18): 2932–2947.

50. Daniele B, Rossi GB, Losito S, Gridelli C, deBellis M. Ischemic colitis associated with paclitaxel. *J Clin Gastroenterol* 2001; 33(2): 159–160.

51. Adelberg DE, Bishop MR. Emergencies related to cancer chemotherapy and hematopoietic stem cell research. *Emerg Med Clin N Am* 2009; 27(2): 311–331.

52. Chadha MK, Trump DL. Endocrine complications. In: Abeloff MD, Armitage JO, Niederhuber JE, Kastan MB, McKenna WG (eds.) *Abeloff's Clinical Oncology*. 4th ed. Philadelphia, PA: Churchill Livingstone, an Imprint of Elsevier; 2008.

53. Widemann BC, Bails FM, Kim A, et al. Glucarpidase, leucovorin, and thymidine for high-dose methotrexate-induced renal dysfunction: clinical and pharmacologic factors affecting outcome. *J Clin Oncol* 2010; 28(25): 3979–3986.

54. Widemann BC, Adamson PC. Understanding and managing methotrexate nephrotoxicity. *Oncologist* 2006; 11(6): 694–703.

55. Rodrigues MA, Rodrigues JL, Martins NM, et al. Carvedilol protects against the renal mitochondrial toxicity induced by cisplatin in rats. *Mitochondrion* 2010; 10(1): 46–53.

56. Kim MG, Yang HN, Kim HW, Jo SK, Cho WY, Kim HK. IL-10 mediates rosiglitazone-induced protection in cisplatin nephrotoxicity. *J Korean Med Sci* 2010; 25(4): 557–563.

57. Mitazaki S, Kato N, Suto M, Hiraiwa K, Abe S. Interleukin-6 deficiency accelerates cisplatin-induced acute renal failure but not systemic injury. *Toxicology* 2009; 265(3): 115–121.

58. Santucci R, Leveque D, Kemmel V, et al. Severe intoxication with methotrexate possibly associated with concomitant use of proton pump inhibitors. *Anticancer Res* 2010; 30(3): 963–965.

59. Khaw SL, Downie PA, Waters KD, Ashley DM, Heath JA. Adverse hypersensitivity reactions to mesna as adjunctive therapy for cyclophosphamide. *Pediatr Blood Cancer* 2007; 49(3): 341–343.

60. Schmidmaier R, Baumann P. ANTI-ADHESION evolves to a promising therapeutic concept in oncology. *Curr Med Chem* 2008; 15(10): 978–990.
61. Wang RY. Special considerations: extravasation of xenobiotics. In: Goldfrank LR, Floenbaum N, Hoffman RS, Nelson LS, Hoffman MA (eds.) *Goldfrank's Toxicologic Emergencies*. 9th ed. McGraw Hill; 2010: p. 793.
62. Conde-Estevez D, Saumell S, Salar A, Mateu-de Antonio J. Successful dexrazoxane treatment of a potentially severe extravasation of concentrated doxorubicin. *Anticancer Drugs* 2010; 21(8): 790–794.
63. Katzer K, Tietze J, Klein E, Heinemann V, Ruzicka T, Wollenberg A. Topical therapy with nadifloxacin cream and prednicarbate cream improves acneiform eruptions caused by the EGFR-inhibitor cetuximab—a report of 29 patients. *Eur J Dermatol* 2010; 20(1): 82–84.
64. Aminsharifi A, Shakeri S, Ariafar A, Moeinjahromi B, Kumar PV, Kabalaeedoost S. Preventive role of exogenous testosterone on cisplatin-induced gonadal toxicity: an experimental placebo-controlled prospective trial. *Fertil Steril* 2010; 93(5): 1388–1393.
65. Tarumi W, Suzuki N, Takahashi N, et al. Ovarian toxicity of paclitaxel and effect on fertility in the rat. *J Obstet Gynaecol Res* 2009; 35(3): 414–420.
66. Zelcer S, Kellick M, Wexler LH, Gorlick R, Meyers PA. The Memorial Sloan Kettering Cancer Center experience with outpatient administration of high dose methotrexate with leucovorin rescue. *Pediatr Blood Cancer* 2008; 50(6): 1176–1180.
67. Bamat MK, Tremmel R, O'Neill JD, von Borstel R. Uridine triacetate: an orally administered, life-saving antidote for 5-FU overdose. *J Clin Oncol* 2010; 28(15 Suppl.): S15.
68. Belani CP. The role of irreversible EGFR inhibitors in the treatment of non-small cell lung cancer: overcoming resistance to reversible EGFR inhibitors. *Cancer Invest* 2010; 28(4): 413–423.
69. Wong MK, Lo AI, Lam B, Lam WK, Ip MS, Ho JC. Erlotinib a salvage treatment after failure to first line gefitinib in non-small cell lung cancer. *Cancer Chemother Pharmacol* 2010; 65(6): 1023–1028.
70. Hernandez SH, Wiener SW, Smith SW. Case files of the New York City Poison Control Center: paradichlorobenzene-induced leukoencephalopathy. *J Med Toxicol* 2010; 6(2): 217–229.
71. Osterborg A. Ofatumumab, a human anti-CD20 monoclonal antibody. *Expert Opin Biol Ther* 2010; 10(3): 439–449.
72. Lecarpentier E, Ouaffi L, Mir O, et al. Bevacizumab-induced small bowel perforation in a patient with breast cancer without intra-abdominal metastases. *Invest New Drugs* 2010 Jul 31. [Epub ahead of print]
73. Fujisaka Y, Yamada Y, Yamamoto N, Horiike A, Tamura T. A phase 1 clinical study of temsirolimus (CCI-779) in Japanese patients with advanced solid tumors. *Jpn J Clin Oncol* 2010; 40(8): 732–738.
74. Liu W, Furuta E, Shindo K, et al. Cacalol, a natural sesquiterpene, induces apoptosis in breast cancer cells by modulating Akt-SREBP-FAS signaling pathway. *Breast Cancer Res Treat* 2010 July 28. [Epub ahead of print]

CHAPTER 10

The bariatric surgery patient

Melissa B. Bagloo and Alfons Pomp
Weill Medical College of Cornell University and New York Presbyterian Hospital, New York, NY, USA

Introduction and epidemiology

In the United States, the prevalence of obesity has steadily increased since the 1980s. Between 1980 and 2004, the prevalence of obesity increased from 15% to 33% among adults and 6% to 19% among children [1]. The most recent National Health and Nutrition Examination Survey continues to indicate an alarming percentage of individuals who are morbidly obese. These statistics reveal an age-adjusted prevalence of obesity at 33.8% (95% confidence interval, 31.6%–36.0%) overall, 32.3% (95% CI, 29.5%–35.0%) among men, and 35.5% (95% CI, 33.2%–37.7%) among women [2]. The prevalence of overweight and obesity combined (BMI >–25) is even greater at 68.0% (95% CI, 66.3%–69.8%), 72.3% (95% CI, 70.4%–74.1%), and 64.1% (95% CI, 61.3%–66.9%), respectively [2].

Obesity has been linked to a number of medical co-morbidities: hypertension, cardiovascular disease, hyperlipidemia, diabetes mellitus, sleep apnea, several cancers, increased risk of disability, and elevated risk of all-cause mortality [1]. Surgical treatment of obesity (for patients with a BMI ≥40) has been shown to be more effective than non-surgical treatment for long-term management of weight loss [3]. With an overall mortality and morbidity of 0.3% [4], the number of bariatric procedures rapidly expanded in the late 1990s through the first decade of this century [5]. Since then, the number of bariatric procedures has reached a plateau [6]. Given the large number of bariatric cases performed in the United States annually (200,000 cases per year), the emergency physician must be familiar with the common early and late post-operative complications of these procedures. In this chapter, we review the commonly performed bariatric operations and discuss their potential complications.

Challenging and Emerging Conditions in Emergency Medicine, First Edition. Edited by Arvind Venkat.
© 2011 by John Wiley & Sons, Ltd. Published 2011 by Blackwell Publishing Ltd.

Description of bariatric surgical procedures

Laparoscopic adjustable gastric banding

The laparoscopic adjustable gastric banding (LAGB) (Figure 10.1a) was approved by the US Food and Drug Administration (FDA) in 2001. It is a silicone-based adjustable band that is placed around the proximal portion of the stomach, creating a 15–30 cc pouch just distal to the gastroesophageal junction. This pouch is connected to a port, which is placed on the anterior abdominal wall and is accessed percutaneously (similar to the technique used to access implantable IV ports) to allow for adjustments of the band [7]. The LAGB functions purely as a restrictive procedure, limiting caloric intake by adjusting the silicone band.

Roux-en-Y gastric bypass

The Roux-en-Y gastric bypass (RYGBP) (Figure 10.1b) is both a restrictive and malabsorptive procedure in which a 15–30 cc pouch is created along the lesser curvature of the stomach using surgical staplers. The pouch created in the RYGBP is usually completely separated from the remainder of the stomach. Next, the jejunum is transected to create the biliopancreatic and Roux limb of the bypass. Various limb lengths have been described in the literature. The Roux limb is then either stapled or hand sewn to the gastric pouch. A jejunojejunostomy is created to allow continuity between the biliopancreatic limb and the remainder of the bowel [8]. Mesenteric defects that are created during this process are usually closed to prevent internal herniation of bowel contents. RYGBP represents the most commonly performed bariatric surgical procedure.

Laparoscopic longitudinal (sleeve) gastrectomy (LSG)

Laparoscopic longitudinal (sleeve) gastrectomy (LSG) (Figure 10.1c) is a novel procedure in which a narrow tube-like stomach is created by the resection of the greater curvature of the stomach. This functions as a restrictive procedure that aims to decrease appetite by reducing the ability of the stomach to distend and producing a sensation of fullness with minimal oral intake. The operation itself is performed by detaching the attachments of the greater omentum to the greater curvature of the stomach and continuing proximally to ligate the short gastric vessels. A longitudinal portion of the stomach is then transected starting several (usually 4–6) centimeters proximal to the antrum. The dissection is continued along the lesser curvature and is carried to the angle of His (creating a pylorus-preserving vertical subtotal gastrectomy) and this part of the stomach is removed from the abdominal cavity [9].

Biliopancreatic diversion/duodenal switch

Biliopancreatic diversion/duodenal switch (BPD/DS) (Figure 10.1d) combines the restriction of a pylorus-preserving vertical subtotal gastrectomy

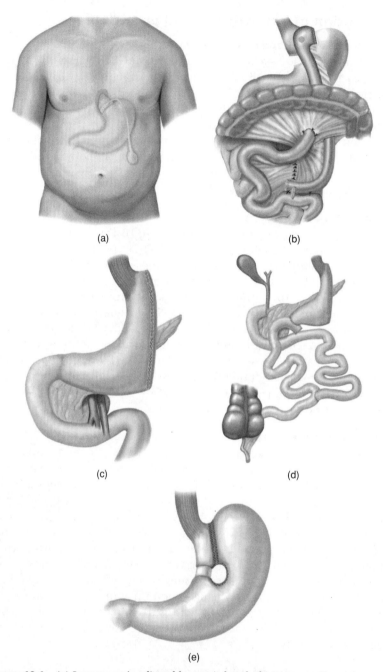

Figure 10.1   (a) Laparascopic adjustable gastric band. (b) Roux-en-Y gastric bypass. (c) Sleeve gastrectomy. (d) Biliopancreatic diversion/duodenal switch. (e) Vertical banded gastroplasty. (Reprinted with permission from Jones DB, et al. *Atlas of Metabolic and Weight Loss Surgery*, Cine-Med, 2010.)

with malabsorption by excluding the majority of the small bowel. Initially, a longitudinal (sleeve) gastrectomy is performed. Then, the duodenum is transected at its first portion a few centimeters distal to the pylorus. Next, a segment of small bowel is measured starting at the ileocecal valve. This segment is anastomosed to the duodenum and serves as the Roux or alimentary limb. The excluded biliopancreatic limb (most of the small bowel) is then anastomosed to the more distal ileum, reestablishing intestinal continuity and flow through a relatively short common channel [10].

Vertical banded gastroplasty

Vertical banded gastroplasty (VBG) (Figure 10.1d) is now primarily only of historical interest and is no longer commonly performed. It is a purely restrictive procedure in which a small vertical pouch is created along the lesser curvature of the stomach using surgical staplers. The pouch is left in continuity with the remainder of the stomach and is not transected; it is simply stapled closed. A non-adjustable Marlex band is then placed around this pouch to create distal constriction and limit passage of food [11]. This can create confusion as patients with the VBG present to the emergency department (ED) stating that they have a "band." The Marlex "band," which is placed during the creation of a VBG should not be confused with the LAGB. It is not adjustable and there is no subcutaneous port. Ultimately, the goal of the VBG was to provide an early sense of satiety in order to limit caloric intake.

Description of emergency diagnosis and treatment of post-bariatric surgery complications

The common risks of any intra-abdominal surgery include bleeding, intra-abdominal or surgical site infection, and even death. Post-operative complications after bariatric surgery are relatively common [12].

Due to the large amount of intra-abdominal and subcutaneous adipose tissue, signs and symptoms of peritonitis are often masked in the bariatric surgery patient. For emergency physicians, the absence of abdominal tenderness should not serve to rule out the possible presence of intra-abdominal pathology in the post-bariatric surgery patient. In fact, many abdominal conditions in the bariatric surgery patient present initially with signs of respiratory distress [13]. Additionally, the lack of physiologic reserve results in rapid decompensation of bariatric surgery patients, making early diagnosis essential in their ED care. Below we describe the commonly encountered complications and outcomes of the most common bariatric operations.

Laparoscopic adjustable gastric band

The laparoscopic adjustable gastric band (LAGB) has only been commonly used in the United States for the last 10 years; however, it has been employed in Europe, Australia, and Israel since the mid-1990s. Studies evaluating the outcomes of the LAGB have shown variable results. Ren et al. showed outcomes of 44.4% excess weight loss (EWL) at 1 year, 51.8% at 2 years, and 52% at 3 years [14]. Long-term European data has also shown promising results with >50% EWL maintained after 7-year follow-up [15]. However, other series in the United States have been less promising showing greater weight loss failure rates with the LAGB [16].

Direct comparisons of the LAGB to the RYGBP have shown greater weight loss, lower BMI, and greater %EWL at each time point across all BMI ranges for RYGBP with a follow-up of approximately 6 years [17, 18]. However, the Longitudinal Assessment of Bariatric Surgery Consortium showed a greater morbidity and mortality associated with the RYGBP when compared to the LAGB [4]. The purported advantages of the lap band system lie in its overall safety profile, maintenance of normal anatomy, and ease of reversibility. Nonetheless, overall, re-operation rates as high as 10% have been reported secondary to the band system [19]. An early complication rate of 3.7% (acute post-operative band obstruction, wound infection, and bleeding) and a late complication rate of 10.1% have been reported for the LAGB [14].

Early post-operative obstruction, often related to surgical technique (leading to an early slip) or gastric edema has been described [20, 21]. The presenting symptoms of patients with a slipped band/obstruction include complaints of inability to tolerate solids and liquids. Diagnosis is easily made by an upper GI series showing malpositioning of the gastric band and herniation of the stomach through the band without passage of contrast into the distal stomach (Figure 10.2). Treatment includes immediate removal of all fluid from the band. The LAGB reservoir resembles the port of intravascular devices used for long-term venous access. In order to access the port, the skin overlying the device is prepped, and the port is stabilized between two fingers of the non-dominant hand. A Huber-type needle (or 16 g bore needle) attached to a 10 cc syringe is inserted through the membrane of the port. Fluid retrieval confirms the needle placement. If this does not immediately resolve the symptoms, early surgical consultation is mandatory. In the acute setting with patients complaining of epigastric pain, the urgency of surgical repair is heightened, as gastric ischemia may be imminent [22].

Gastric prolapse (slip) is the most common delayed complication of LAGB at a rate of 2.9% [14]. However, larger cohort follow-ups have reported higher rates of slippage up to 7.6% [23]. Symptoms of delayed gastric prolapse mimic those of early obstruction, and the workup is identical. Again, surgical consultation is warranted for evaluation.

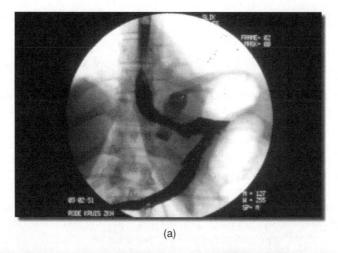

(a)

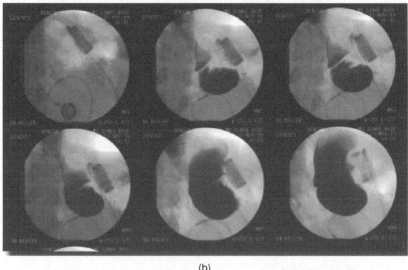

(b)

Figure 10.2   (a) Normal LAGB (Fluoroscopy). (b) Slipped LAGB (Fluoroscopy).

Gastric erosion is also a known complication of the gastric band with an incidence ranging from 0.6%–11% [23–26]. A recent study evaluating 865 bands placed at a single institution noted a band erosion rate of 1.96% over 5 years of follow-up. Fifty-five percent of the erosions presented in the first year after band placement, and only 10% occurred greater than 2 years after surgery [25]. The most common presenting complaint is pain, followed with weight regain, and delayed port-site infection (>60 days). Case studies describing presentation of band erosion with an upper GI bleed have also been reported [24]. Diagnosis with endoscopy is the gold standard. Treatment entails laparoscopic removal of the band with repair of the erosion surgically. There are reports in the literature describing endoscopic removal of the band, though this has not yet become standard [24, 27].

LAGB port/tubing complications (port leak/flip/migration, port abscess, tubing breaks, port protrusion) have been reported to occur at a rate of 2.4%–7.1% [17, 28]. Presentation of these minor complications varies. Port infections present with pain, induration, or overlying cellulitis. Late (>60 days post-operatively) or recurrent port-site infections mandate endoscopic evaluation to exclude an associated band erosion. Treatment may begin with antibiotics; however, the infection may necessitate port removal. Tubing leaks often present with loss of restriction and weight gain. Diagnosis is made by accessing the port and injecting fluid that cannot be retrieved using the procedure described above for removing fluid from the LAGB. The site of the leak can be diagnosed in radiology by injection of contrast. Treatment involves replacement of the damaged portion of the band system [28].

Other more rare complications include erosion of the gastric band tubing into the lumen of the bowel. Tubing breaks often present with abdominal pain and may lead to bowel erosion. Isolated case reports describe erosion into the jejunum and colon [29, 30]. The presenting symptoms are abdominal pain and/or port-site infection. Diagnosis may be difficult and require exploratory laparoscopy, ultimately requiring removal of the band and possible bowel resection. Several case reports of small bowel obstructions secondary to looping of the band tubing have also been described [31, 32]. These patients may not present with the telltale signs of obstruction (nausea/vomiting/abdominal distention) due to creation of a closed loop obstruction by the tubing and may more likely present with unexplained abdominal pain. Diagnosis may be made radiographically with CT scan or necessitate laparoscopic evaluation.

Roux-en-Y gastric bypass

RYGBP has been shown to obtain an EWL of 75% at 5 years follow-up [18]. However, there is a substantial number of patients who are unsuccessful and experience either lack of appropriate weight loss or weight regain post-operatively [33]. The weight loss profile of the gastric bypass has been shown to be better than the LAGB, but not as successful as the BPD/DS. However, the RYGBP has fewer nutritional and metabolic complications than the BPD/DS [33] and requires less post-operative vitamin and mineral supplementation.

Complications associated with the RYGBP are more infrequent, but often more perilous than the band. An early complication associated with gastric bypass is an anastomotic leak (gastrojejunostomy, jejuno-jejunostomy, or bypassed stomach remnant) (Figure 10.3a). If not identified and managed expeditiously, a leak can result in disseminated intra-abdominal sepsis, which can lead to multiorgan system failure and death. Leak rates ranging from 1%–5% in large series have been documented [17, 18,34–36]. A recent study evaluating 3828 RYGBP patients reported an overall leak rate of 3.9%. The overall leak-related mortality after RYGBP was 0.6% [35]. Revision RYGBP has a significantly greater leak rate than both open and laparoscopic RYGBPs, and these patients

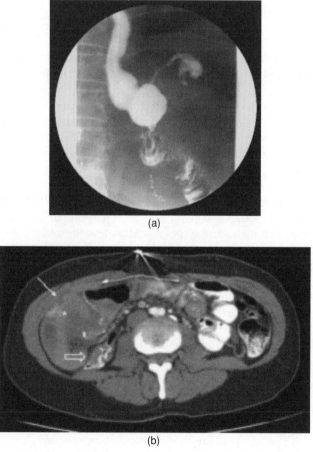

(a)

(b)

Figure 10.3   (a) RYGBP anastomotic leak (Fluoroscopy). (b) RYGBP internal hernia (CT). Open arrow indicates the compressed Roux limb. Thin arrow indicates bypass limb with distention.

deserve particular attention should they present to the ED in the immediate post-operative period.

The most common indicators of a post-operative leak after bariatric surgery are sustained tachycardia (>120), abdominal pain, and fever. Hypotension and shortness of breath may also be present [36]. As mentioned previously, morbidly obese patients with abdominal problems may appear tachypneic with respiratory distress, leading the clinician to believe the most likely diagnosis is a pulmonary embolus. It must be emphasized that presentation with the aforementioned symptoms in the early post-operative period is an anastomotic leak until proven otherwise. Studies to delineate the presence of a leak versus a pulmonary embolus (upper GI series, CT of the chest with intravenous contrast) can be undertaken if done expeditiously. However, if the patient is unstable, further diagnostic testing and attempts at resuscitation should not delay immediate surgical exploration. Treatment in the operating room may entail placement of intra-abdominal drains to create a controlled fistula, antibiotic therapy, and placement of a gastrostomy tube in the gastric remnant for enteral feeds. The patient should be monitored in an ICU setting with supportive care. Contained leaks in a stable patient may be treated non-operatively with broad antibiotic coverage and percutaneous drain placement. Endoscopically placed stents have also been reported for conservative management of leaks [37]; however, patient selection for conservative management is critical.

Post-operative bleeding is another early complication after RYGBP (3.86% incidence in the immediate post-operative period) [38]. Patients can present with abdominal pain, anemia, tachycardia, or hypotension. Hematemesis and melena may be absent as the site of bleeding can be intra-abdominal or along staple lines. The tachycardia that accompanies post-surgical bleeding usually varies from that of the sustained tachycardia of an anastomotic leak and is often progressive, developing over time, and is cyclical, not sustained. Diagnosis can be made with serial hematocrit monitoring. CT scans may also be helpful in identifying an intra-abdominal collection. Management is dependent on the clinical condition of the patient. If stable, anticoagulation medication should be held and the patient typed and crossed for possible transfusions. If unstable, the patient will require a return to the operating room in order to identify and control the source of bleeding. The low physiological reserve in this patient population necessitates aggressive fluid resuscitation in the ED with appropriate large gauge (18 g or better) intravenous access.

The RYGBP patient population is at risk for post-operative development of deep vein thromboses (DVT), and pulmonary embolus is one of the most common causes of post-operative mortality. Prospective studies of patients undergoing gastric bypass have reported DVT rates ranging from

0.16%–3.8% [39,40]. Patients with a history of venous thromboembolism have been observed to have a greater incidence of DVT development, though accurate percentages are difficult to determine due to the low percentage of patients who fit this profile [39]. Other risk factors include venous stasis disease and limited mobility. The PROBE study evaluated the incidence of DVT and pulmonary embolism in the post-surgical bariatric population and found that the greatest risk occurred after cessation of thromboprophylaxis, even if it is stopped weeks after surgery [41]. Thus, patients may present with DVT or pulmonary embolism for several weeks after surgery. Patient presentations may vary from calf pain or swelling to shortness of breath, tachycardia, and right-heart strain. Classic signs of asymmetrical lower extremity edema may not be identified in this population due to their body habitus, which may also preclude adequate evaluation with duplex scans. If respiratory symptoms or tachycardia are present, a spiral chest CT to rule out a pulmonary embolus should be undertaken with extension to the lower extremities to evaluate for DVT. Anticoagulation is the treatment for DVT and pulmonary embolism. In patients where pulmonary embolism is strongly suspected, it is our recommendation to give 60 mg of low molecular weight heparin if their weight is under 250 lbs and 80 mg for those that are heavier.

Gastrojejunostomy anastomotic stricture is also a known complication of RYGBP, whether surgical staplers are used or a hand-sewn anastomosis is constructed. Stricture rates ranging from 3%–27% have been documented [40]. Patients that develop strictures usually present in the first 4–6 weeks after surgery. Presentation includes progressive dysphagia, post-prandial regurgitation, nausea, vomiting, and occasionally pain. Etiology can be secondary to surgical technique, ischemia, or inflammatory processes such as ulcer development in those presenting several months after surgery. Upper GI series contribute very little in the diagnosis of anastomotic strictures due to limitations in determination of the actual anastomotic size. Endoscopy is the diagnostic modality of choice since diagnosis can be made and treatment can often be accomplished with endoscopic dilation of the site. The success rate of endoscopic dilation is high; however, repetitive dilations may be required until clinical resolution of symptoms is achieved [40, 42, 43].

Internal hernias are a known complication for RYGBP with an incidence ranging from 2%–4.5% [44, 45] and can present at any time postoperatively. The incidence of internal hernias is known to be greater after laparoscopic RYGBP than open RYGBP, presumably secondary to a diminished inflammatory response and decreased formation of intra-abdominal adhesions. Potential locations include the transverse mesocolon defect, Petersen's space (the area between the mesentery of the transverse mesocolon and the Roux limb), and the jejunojejunostomy mesenteric defect.

Patients may present with acute or chronic symptoms. Chronic symptoms are typically intermittent in nature with episodes of abdominal pain (97.1%), nausea and emesis (80%) [45]. Acute presentations of internal hernias have symptoms of an acute abdomen and may have tenderness out of proportion to findings at physical exam, the hallmark for intestinal ischemia.

Due to the presence of the bypassed biliopancreatic limb, obstruction symptoms are not always associated with development of internal hernias. In fact, lack of obstructive symptoms should not sway the emergency physician from evaluating the patient for the presence of internal hernias, since a closed loop hernia can present with abdominal pain without signs of obstruction. CT scan is the gold standard for evaluation of internal hernias due to its ability to evaluate the bypassed biliopancreatic limb. Studies evaluating radiologic findings in internal hernias after RYGBP found that 64%–92% of internal hernias were identified with CT scanning [44, 46]. One study noted the presence of four recurring findings: dilated small bowel, distended gastric remnant, excess small bowel loops in the lesser sac, and thick-walled fluid-filled small bowel (Figure 10.3b above). Findings on upper GI series may include dilated fluid-filled small bowel loops, redundant Roux limb in the lesser sac, preponderance of bowel loops in the left upper quadrant, and slow emptying of contrast with prolonged transit times [44]. Once the diagnosis has been made, surgical exploration is mandatory. However, even if imaging modalities are negative, unexplained symptoms of abdominal pain should be referred to a bariatric surgeon to exclude an internal hernia. Intra-operatively, the hernia is reduced and the mesenteric defect is closed. If ischemic, non-viable bowel is present, a bowel resection may also be necessary.

Marginal ulceration in the early post-operative period (30 days) has been reported in 12.3% of patients after laparoscopic gastric bypass. However, when followed out to 1 year, all of these patients healed their ulcers. The incidence of late marginal ulceration (>1 year after surgery) in this population was found to be 0.4%. Twenty-eight percent of these patients with endoscopically diagnosed marginal ulcers were asymptomatic [47]. Patients with marginal ulcers typically present with symptoms of epigastric pain and inability to tolerate oral intake/emesis. Less commonly, patients may present with an upper gastrointestinal bleed or perforation (1%). Risk factors for development of marginal ulcers and perforation include smoking and use of steroids and nonsteroidal anti-inflammatory medications [48]. Diagnosis can be made expeditiously with endoscopy. Medical treatment with proton-pump inhibitors usually suffices. Carafate is often prescribed in addition to proton-pump inhibitors, but may be of minimal efficacy given the lack of an acidic gastric environment when proton-pump inhibitors are used. In cases where ulcers are refractory to treatment, surgical revision of the gastrojejunostomy may be necessary.

Finally, patients undergoing RYGBP are susceptible to mineral and vitamin deficiencies given the bypassed stomach and small bowel. The incidence of deficiencies will increase over time after the surgery. Iron, vitamin B12, folate, calcium, and vitamin D levels should be routinely assessed to evaluate for abnormal values. Parathyroid hormone (PTH) should also be measured to evaluate for secondary hyperparathyroidism due to low calcium levels. Treatment consists of daily supplementation with a multivitamin (MVI), iron, and calcium. Vitamin D deficiency is common and must also be supplemented to maintain physiologic levels. Thiamine is rarely deficient, but must remain part of the assessment of any patient with weight loss surgery who gives a history of recurrent chronic vomiting. Wernicke–Korsakoff encephalopathy has been described in post-RYGBP patients. When thiamine deficiency is identified or suspected in the ED, treatment is initiated with 50–100 mg per day of intravenous thiamine [49].

Longitudinal (sleeve) gastrectomy (LSG)

Laparoscopic sleeve gastrectomy was initially described as the first step in a two-step surgical approach in those morbidly obese patients deemed to be at the highest surgical risk in order to decrease perioperative morbidity and mortality [50]. Early post-operative weight loss profiles were promising, and it has since been accepted as a stand-alone procedure [51]. Long-term results for sleeve gastrectomy are now becoming available. A recent study by Himpens et al. evaluated a small cohort of sleeve gastrectomy patients 3 and 6 years post-procedure with an average EWL of 77.5% and 53.3%, respectively [52]. While data is still limited, these initial findings show promise for sleeve gastrectomy as a primary surgical approach to morbid obesity.

The post-operative complications of sleeve gastrectomy are rare, but their management can be more difficult than those of the gastric bypass. Advantages of this procedure include maintenance of gastrointestinal continuity allowing for future endoscopic intervention. The three main complications of sleeve gastrectomy include: (1) bleeding from the staple line; (2) staple line dehiscence (leak); and (3) stricture formation.

Staple line hemorrhage was reported to occur at a rate of 1.1% at the Second International Consensus Summit for Sleeve Gastrectomy [53]. Patients present in the early post-operative period with typical findings of post-operative blood loss (low hematocrit, tachycardia, melena, and/or hematemesis). Diagnosis is made by following trends of the patient's hematocrit, CT scan, and possibly endoscopy. It should be noted that the site of the bleed is most often not intra-luminal and therefore endoscopy may be of limited value; moreover, the decision to perform endoscopy after recent gastric surgery should not be undertaken without surgical consultation. Based on the clinical condition and hemodynamic stability of the patient, treatment may require correction of coagulation abnormalities, transfusions, endoscopic evaluation, and surgical reexploration.

Staple line dehiscence has been noted to range from 0.7%–5.3% [40, 54] and most commonly occurs in the proximal most portion of the sleeve at the angle of His. Presentation is similar to a leak in an RYGBP patient (tachycardia, fever, abdominal pain, SOB, etc.) and most commonly occurs in the first 10 days post-operatively. Diagnosis can be made with an upper GI series or CT scan with oral water-soluble contrast (Figure 10.4). Management of the leak varies based on the clinical presentation. Early leaks (1–3 days post-operatively) or leaks in unstable patients should be treated with re-operation, repair, and wide drainage. Consideration of a jejunostomy tube placement should also be given for subsequent enteral feeds [54]. Intermediate or late leaks (>3 days post-operatively) can be managed non-surgically in stable patients. Endoscopically placed stents,

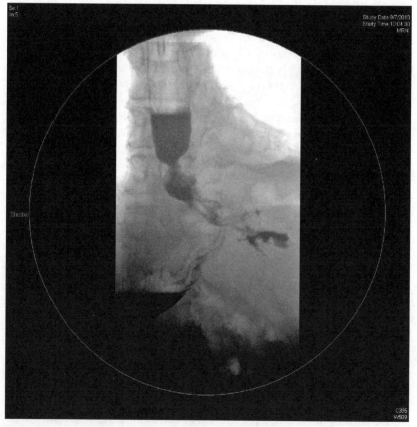

Figure 10.4   Sleeve gastrectomy leak (Fluoroscopy).

application of fibrin glue, and percutaneous drainage have all been used successfully in the management of leaks [55, 56]. It should again be emphasized that a post-operative leak and subsequent peritonitis in a bariatric patient can rapidly lead to multiorgan system failure, and surgical consultation should be sought early in the management of these patients.

Strictures after sleeve gastrectomy usually form at the midpoint (incisura angularis) of the lesser curvature with an incidence of 0.9% [53]. Etiology is related to technical factors, bougie size, and oversewing of staple lines, which lead to stenosis of the gastric sleeve. Patients present weeks to months after surgery with symptoms of dysphagia, post-prandial regurgitation, nausea, and emesis. Diagnosis is made with upper endoscopy or an upper GI series. As previously discussed, strictures that form after gastric bypass are often successfully treated with endoscopic balloon dilation. While this approach is also valid with after-sleeve gastrectomy strictures, the anatomy of the stricture can be a limiting factor. Small, short strictures can be treated with dilation; however, longer strictures may not be amenable to dilation. A recent case series of nine patients with long strictures that were not amenable to endoscopic dilation describes performing a longitudinal seromyotomy, which was successful in all cases [57].

Biliopancreatic diversion/duodenal switch

Biliopancreatic diversion/duodenal switch (BPD/DS) is the most challenging of the bariatric procedures, both in terms of surgical technique and post-operative nutritional management. It is currently the least commonly performed bariatric operation. It does, however, have the best weight loss profile of the bariatric procedures [33] and maintains the pylorus, thereby, in theory, eliminating dumping syndrome. Initial EWL of 73.4% has been reported for patients undergoing BPD/DS. Ten-year follow-up has shown a sustained weight loss of 46.8% [58].

Complications of BPD/DS are similar, but more frequent, to those of gastric bypass, including anastomotic leak, bleeding, marginal ulcers, DVT, and internal hernias [59]. Presenting signs and symptoms are also the same and require the identical workup. BPD/DS, however, appears to have a lower risk of marginal ulceration.

The nutritional complications of the BPD/DS are more frequent than those for any of the other bariatric procedures. Protein deficiency after BPD/DS has been reported in up to 18% of patients and occurs due to bypassing the majority of the small bowel (where protein is absorbed) [49]. Signs of protein deficiency include hypoalbuminemia, peripheral edema, alopecia, and asthenia. Diagnosis is made with routine lab studies, and treatment is initiated with dietary counseling and pancreatic enzyme supplementation. Total parenteral nutrition may be necessary in those patients with severe malnutrition. Care must be taken in the acute period of treatment to monitor for refeeding syndrome. This syndrome is characterized by congestive heart failure, anasarca, respiratory compromise, and, occasionally, neurologic symptoms, such as confusion or even convulsions. Laboratory findings include electrolyte disorders, such as hypokalemia, hypophosphatemia, and hemolysis. Once malnutrition has been corrected, nutritional counseling is necessary to prevent a recurrence. Some patients may need revisional surgery to increase the length of the common channel.

BPD/DS patients are at risk for developing the same vitamin deficiencies as RYGBP patients. Iron, vitamin B12, folate, calcium, and vitamin D are common deficiencies and can be detected by serologic analysis. Again, thiamine levels should also be evaluated. Treatment is the same as for RYGBP patients. Fat-soluble vitamin deficiencies (A, D, E, and K) are more common in BPD/DS patients due to the more limited exposure of ingested foods to biliopancreatic secretions in the relatively short common channel. Magnesium, zinc, and selenium deficiencies have also been identified, though clinical manifestations of deficiency are uncommon [49].

Vertical banded gastroplasty

Vertical banded gastroplasty (VBG) is currently only of historical interest. Despite initially promising results, long-term follow-up studies of the VBG demonstrated poor weight loss outcomes. Initial weight loss over the first year has been shown to be approximately 50%–70% of excess weight; however, weight regain has been shown as early as the second postoperative year [60–62] with 10-year results showing persistent %EWL of >50% in only 26% of patients [63]. The same trend has also been shown with co-morbidity resolution [62].

Due to the lack of malabsorption, the VBG is usually not associated with metabolic complications; however, in patients with a long-standing history of vomiting, thiamine deficiency should also be considered. Late complications are frequent and include staple line disruption (16%), pouch enlargement, gastric outlet stenosis (uncontrollable vomiting), Marlex band erosion/migration, and incisional hernia (41%). Re-operative rates ranging from 17%–21.4% have been documented [63, 64]. Marlex band erosion rates up to 7% have been reported and can occur months to years post-operatively. Patients typically present with symptoms of excessive weight loss and obstruction [65]. Diagnosis is based on endoscopic evaluation. Removal of the band is a complex surgical decision and often conversion to RYGBP or gastrectomy is necessary.

The next five years

As more advanced laparoscopic surgical procedures are developed, there is a constant push to move towards less invasive means of accomplishing the same goals. Newer techniques of single incision laparoscopic approaches and endoscopically performed surgical techniques are currently under investigation.

Endoscopic techniques include a multitude of approaches; however, significant weight loss and co-morbidity data are not yet available for these techniques. Restrictive technique trials are ongoing with transoral gastroplasty (TOGA). TOGA essentially creates an endoluminal sleeve gastrectomy; however, the durability of the device and weight loss data has not been validated. Malabsorptive techniques, mimicking the outcome of a gastric bypass with the *Endobarrier*©, are also under investigation. The *Endobarrier*© is an impermeable polyethylene sleeve that is deployed to essentially exclude the duodenum and jejunum from contact with food. Gastric electrical stimulation is being investigated to determine its effects on food-intake reduction, gastric emptying delay, and appetite suppression via hormonal mechanisms [66].

Single incision and natural orifice surgery (NOTES) have also been applied to the current surgical techniques for bariatric surgery. These approaches may offer a more cosmetically appealing outcome, though safety profiles of the approaches are under evaluation. Single incision surgery, introduced for appendectomy and cholecystectomy, has now been applied to many laparoscopic weight loss procedures, including sleeve gastrectomy and adjustable gastric banding. NOTES for bariatric procedures is currently under investigation in animal and cadaveric models [66].

Finally, the metabolic effects of bariatric procedures are currently under investigation. Specifically, the role of bariatric surgery and its effect on diabetes resolution is an area of intense research. Multiple, case-controlled studies have shown significant improvement in diabetes outcomes with all of the bariatric procedures. RYGBP and BPD/DS have shown improvement and even complete remission of diabetes days to weeks after surgery, before the effects of weight loss would be seen [67]. Thus, it is hypothesized that weight-independent mechanisms for diabetes resolution exist. Animal studies have shown significant improvements in glucose homeostasis in diabetic rat models that underwent duodenojejunal bypass. Additionally, when the operation was reversed in these same rats, glucose tolerance impairment recurred [68]. Such advancements in the field of metabolic and bariatric surgery promise significant advancement in our understanding and treatment of diabetes and provide hope for a possible cure.

Conclusion

Bariatric surgical procedures offer an effective treatment for obesity and the co-morbid conditions associated with obesity. For the emergency physician, the increased prevalence of patients undergoing these procedures requires a knowledge of the post-operative complications that can cause these patients to present to the ED. Close consultation with the bariatric surgical team can aid in the emergency evaluation and management of this patient population.

References

1. Ogden CL, Yanovski, Carroll MD, Flegal KM. The epidemiology of obesity. *Gastroenterology* 2007; 132(6): 2087–2102.
2. Flegal KM, Carroll MD, Ogden CL, Curtin LR. Prevalence and trends in obesity among US adults, 1999–2008. *JAMA* 2010; 303(3): 235–241.
3. Maggard MA, Shugarman LR, Suttorp M, et al. Meta-Analysis: surgical treatment of obesity. *Ann Intern Med* 2005; 142(7): 547–559.
4. Longitudinal Assessment of Bariatric Surgery (LABS) Consortium, Flum DR, Belle SH, King WC, et al. Perioperative safety in the longitudinal assessment of bariatric surgery. *N Engl J Med* 2009; 361(5): 445–454.
5. Davis MM, Slish K, Chao C, Cabana MD. National trends in bariatric surgery, 1996–2002. *Arch Surg* 2006; 141(1): 71–74.
6. Kohn GP, Galanko JA, Overby EW, Farrell TM. Recent trends in bariatric surgery case volume in the United States. *Surgery* 2009; 146: 375–380.
7. Ren CJ, Fielding GA. Laparoscopic adjustable gastric banding: surgical technique. *J Laparoendosc Adv Surg Tech A* 2003; 13(4): 257–263.
8. Schauer PR, Ikramuddin S, Gourash WF. Laparoscopic Roux-en-Y gastric bypass: a case report at one-year follow-up. *J Laparoendosc Adv Surg Tech A* 1999; 9(1): 101–106.
9. Moy J, Pomp A, Dakin G, Parikh M, Gagner M. Laparoscopic sleeve gastrectomy for morbid obesity. *Am J Surg* 2008; 196(5): e56–e59.
10. Gagner M, Matteotti R. Laparoscopic biliopancreatic diversion with duodenal switch. *Surg Clin N Am* 2005; 85(1): 141–149, x–xi.
11. Mason EE, Doherty C, Cullen JJ, Scott D, Rodriguez EM, Maher JW. Vertical gastroplasty: evolution of vertical banded gastroplasty. *World J Surg* 1998; 22(9): 919–924.
12. DeMaria EJ. Bariatric surgery for morbid obesity. *N Engl J Med* 2007; 356: 2176–2183.
13. Pieracci FM, Barie PS, Pomp A. Critical care of the bariatric surgery patient. *Crit Care Med* 2006; 34(6): 1796–1804
14. Parikh MS, Fielding GA, Ren CJ. US experience with 749 laparoscopic adjustable gastric bands: intermediate outcomes. *Surg Endosc* 2005; 19(12): 1631–1635.
15. Miller K, Pump A, Hell E. Vertical banded gastroplasty versus adjustable gastric banding: prospective long-term follow-up study. *Surg Obes Relat Dis* 2007; 3(1): 84–90.
16. DeMaria EJ, Sugerman HJ, Meador JG, et al. High failure rate after laparoscopic adjustable silicone gastric banding for treatment of morbid obesity. *Ann Surg* 2001; 233(6): 809–818.
17. Biertho L, Steffen R, Ricklin T, et al. Laparoscopic gastric bypass versus laparoscopic adjustable gastric banding: a comparative study of 1,200 Cases. *J Am Coll Surg* 2003; 197: 536–544.

18. Christou N, Efthimiou E. Five-year outcomes of laparoscopic adjustable gastric banding and laparoscopic Roux-en-Y gastric bypass in a comprehensive bariatric surgery program in Canada. *Can J Surg* 2009; 52(6): E249–E258.

19. Lyass S, Cunneen SA, Haglike M, et al. Device-related reoperations after laparoscopic adjustable gastric banding. *Am Surg* 2005; 71(9): 738–743.

20. Patel SM, Shapiro K, Abdo Z, Ferzli GS. Obstructive symptoms associated with the lap-band in the first 24 hours. *Surg Endosc* 2004; 18: 51–55.

21. Shen R, Ren CJ. Removal of peri-gastric fat prevents acute obstruction after lap-band surgery. *Obes Surg* 2004; 14: 224–229.

22. Fischer G, Myers JA, Huang W, Shayani V. Gastric migration and strangulation after adjustable gastric banding. *Obes Surg* 2008; 18: 753–755.

23. Kirshtein B, Lantsberg L, Mizrahi S, Avinoach E. Bariatric emergencies for non-bariatric surgeons: complications of laparoscopic gastric banding. *Obes Surg* 2010; Epub. DOI 10.1007/s11695-009-0059-5.

24. Campos J, Ramos A, Neto MG, et al. Hypovolemic shock due to intra-gastric migration of an adjustable gastric band. *Obes Surg* 2007; 17: 562–564.

25. Cherian PT, Goussous G, Ashori F, Sigurdsson A. Band erosion after laparoscopic gastric banding: a retrospective analysis of 865 patients over 5 years. *Surg Endosc* 2010; 24(8): 2031–2038.

26. Suter M, Giusti V, Heraief E, Calmes JM. Band erosion after laparoscopic gastric banding: occurrence and results after conversion to Roux-en-Y gastric bypass. *Obes Surg* 2004; 14: 381–386.

27. Lattuada E, Zappa MA, Mozzi E, et al. Band erosion following gastric banding: how to treat it. *Obes Surg* 2007; 17(3): 329–333.

28. Keidar A, Carmon E, Szold A, Abu-Abeid S. Port complications following laparoscopic adjustable gastric banding for morbid obesity. *Obes Surg* 2005; 15(3): 361–365.

29. Egbeare DM, Myers AF, Lawrance RJ. Small bowel obstruction secondary to intra-gastric erosion and migration of a gastric band. *J Gastrointest Surg* 2008; 12: 983–984.

30. Tekin A. Migration of the connecting tube into small bowel after adjustable gastric banding. *Obes Surg* 2010; 20: 526–529.

31. Van De Water W, Vogelaar FJ, Willems JM. An unusual complication 4 years after laparoscopic adjustable banding: jejunal obstruction due to the connecting tube. *Obes Surg* 2009; Epub. DOI 10.1007/s11695-009-0057-7.

32. Zappa MA, Lattuada E, Mozzi E, et al. An unusual complication of gastric banding: recurrent small bowel obstruction caused by the connecting tube. *Obes Surg* 2006; 16(7): 939–941.

33. Gracia JA, Martinez M, Elia M, et al. Obesity surgery results depending on technique performed: long-term outcome. *Obes Surg* 2009; 19: 432–438.

34. ASMBS Clinical Issues Committee. ASMBS guideline on the prevention and detection of gastrointestinal leak after gastric bypass including the role of imaging and surgical exploration. *Surg Obes Relat Dis* 2009; 5(3): 293–296.

35. Lee S, Carmody B, Wolfe L, et al. Effect of location and speed of diagnosis on anastomotic leak outcomes in 3828 gastric bypass cases. *J Gastrointest Surg* 2007; 11(6): 708–713.

36. Durak E, Inabnet WB, Schrope B, et al. Incidence and management of enteric leaks after gastric bypass for morbid obesity during a 10-year period. *Surg Obes Relat Dis* 2008; 4(3): 389–393.

37. Salinas A, Baptista A, Santiago E, Antor M, Salinas H. Self-expandable metal stents to treat gastric leaks. *Surg Obes Relat Dis* 2006; 2(5): 570–572.
38. Bellorin O, Abdemur A, Sucandy I, Szomstein S, Rosenthal RJ. Understanding the significance, reasons and patterns of abnormal vital signs after gastric bypass for morbid obesity. *Obes Surg* 2010; Epub. DOI 10.1007/s11695-010-0221-0
39. Prystowsky JB, Morasch MD, Eskandari MK, Hungness ES, Nagle AP. Prospective analysis of the incidence of deep venous thrombosis in bariatric surgery patients. *Surgery* 2005; 138(4): 759–765.
40. Escalante-Tattersfield T, Tucker O, Fajnwaks P, Szomstein S, Rosenthal R. Incidence of deep vein thrombosis in morbidly obese patients undergoing laparoscopic Roux-en-Y gastric bypass. *Surg Obes Relat Dis* 2008; 4: 126–130.
41. Hamad GG, Choban PS. Enoxaparin for thromboprophylaxis in morbidly obese patients undergoing bariatric surgery: findings of the prophylaxis against VTE outcomes in bariatric surgery patients receiving enoxaparin (PROBE) study. *Obes Surg* 2005; 15: 1368–1374.
42. Frutos MD, Lujan J, Garcia A, et al. Gastrojejunal anastomotic stenosis in laparoscopic gastric bypass with a circular stapler (21 mm): incidence, treatment and long-term follow-up. *Obes Surg* 2009; 19(12): 1631–1635.
43. Alasfar F, Sabnis AA, Liu RC, Chand B. Stricture rate after laparoscopic Roux-en-Y gastric bypass with a 21 mm circular stapler: the Cleveland clinic experience. *Med Princ Pract* 2009; 18(5): 364–367.
44. Ahmed AR, Rickards G, Johnson J, Boss T, O'Malley W. Radiological findings in symptomatic internal hernias after laparoscopic gastric bypass. *Obes Surg* 2009; 19(11): 1530–1535.
45. Comeau E, Gagner M, Inabnet WB, Herron DM, Quinn TM, Pomp A. Symptomatic internal hernias after laparoscopic bariatric surgery. *Surg Endsoc* 2005; 19: 34–39.
46. Garza E Jr, Kuhn J, Arnold D, Nicholson W, Reddy S, McCarty T. Internal hernias after laparoscopic Roux-en-Y gastric bypass. *Am J Surg* 2004; 188(6): 796–800.
47. Csendes A, Burgos AM, Altuve J, Bonacic S. Incidence of marginal ulcer 1 month and 1 to 2 years after gastric bypass: a prospective consecutive endoscopic evaluation of 442 patients with morbid obesity. *Obes Surg* 2009; 19(2): 135–138.
48. Felix EL, Kettelle J, Mobley E, Swartz D. Perforated marginal ulcers after laparoscopic gastric bypass. *Surg Endosc* 2008; 22(10): 2128–2132.
49. Bloomberg RD, Fleishman A, Nalle JE, Herron DM, Kini S. Nutritional deficiencies following bariatric surgery: what have we learned? *Obes Surg* 2005; 15: 145–154.
50. Regan JP, Inabnet WB, Gagner M, Pomp A. Early experience with two-stage laparoscopic Roux-en-Y gastric bypass as an alternative in the super-super obese patient. *Obes Surg* 2003; 13: 861–864.
51. Brethauer SA, Hammel JP, Schauer PR. Systematic review of sleeve gastrectomy as staging and primary bariatric procedure. *Surg Obes Relat Dis* 2009; 5(4): 469–475.
52. Himpens J, Dobbeleir J, Peeters G. Long-term results of laparoscopic sleeve gastrectomy for obesity. *Ann Surg* 2010; 252(2): 319–324.

53. Gagner M, Deitel M, Kalberer TL, Erickson AL, Crosby RD. The second international consensus summit for sleeve gastrectomy, March 19–21, 2009. *Surg Obes Relat Dis* 2009; 5(4): 476–485.
54. Burgos AM, Braghetto I, Csendes A, et al. Gastric leak after laparoscopic sleeve gastrectomy for obesity. *Obes Surg* 2009; 19(12): 1672–1677.
55. Tan JT, Kariyawasam S, Wijeratne T, Chandraratna HS. Diagnosis and management of gastric leaks after laparoscopic sleeve gastrectomy for morbid obesity. *Obes Surg* 2010; 20(4): 403–409.
56. Casella G, Soricelli E, Rizzello M, et al. Non-surgical treatment of staple line leaks after laparoscopic sleeve gastrectomy. *Obes Surg* 2009; 19(7): 821–826.
57. Dapri G, Cadiere GB, Himpens J. Laparoscopic seromyotomy for long stenosis after sleeve gastrectomy with or without duodenal switch. *Obes Surg* 2009; 19: 495–499.
58. Marceau P, Biron S, Hould FS, et al. Duodenal switch improved standard biliopancreatic diversion: a retrospective study. *Surg Obes Relat Dis* 2009; 5(1): 43–47.
59. Cossu ML, Meloni GB, Alagna S, et al. Emergency surgical conditions after biliopancreatic diversion. *Obes Surg* 2007; 17: 637–641.
60. Del Amo DA, Diez MM, Guedea ME, Diago VA. Vertical banded gastroplasty: is it a durable operation for morbid obesity? *Obes Surg* 2004; 14(4): 536–538.
61. Olbers T, Lonroth H, Dalenback J, Haglind E, Lundell L. Laparoscopic vertical banded gastroplasty: an effective long-term therapy for morbidly obese patients? *Obes Surg* 2001; 11: 726–730.
62. Wang W, Yu PJ, Lee YC, Wei PL, Lee WJ. Laparoscopic vertical banded gastroplasty: 5-year results. *Obes Surg* 2005; 15(9): 1299–1303.
63. Balsiger BM, Poggio JL, Mai J, Kelly KA, Sarr MG. Ten and more years after vertical banded gastroplasty as primary operation for morbid obesity. *J Gastrointest Surg* 2000; 4: 598–605.
64. Marsk R, Jonas E, Gartzios H, Stockeld D, Granstrom L, Freedman J. High revision rates after laparoscopic vertical banded gastroplasty. *Surg Obes Relat Dis* 2009; 5(1): 94–98.
65. Moreno P, Alastrue A, Rull M, et al. Band erosion in patients who have undergone vertical banded gastroplasty: incidence and technical solutions. *Arch Surg* 1998; 133(2): 189–193.
66. Tsesmeli N, Coumaros D. The future of bariatrics: endoscopy, endoluminal surgery, and natural orifice transluminal endoscopic surgery. *Endoscopy* 2010; 42(2): 155–162.
67. Rubino F, Schauer PR, Kaplan LM, Cummings DE. Metabolic surgery to treat type 2 diabetes: clinical outcomes and mechanisms of action. *Annu Rev Med* 2010; 61: 393–411.
68. Rubino F, Forgione A, Cummings DE, et al. The mechanism of diabetes control after gastrointestinal bypass surgery reveals a role of the proximal small intestine in the pathophysiology of type 2 diabetes. *Ann Surg* 2006; 244(5): 741–749.

CHAPTER 11

The obese patient

Andra L. Blomkalns and David W. Silver
University of Cincinnati College of Medicine, Cincinnati, OH, USA

Introduction and epidemiology

Obesity is a growing epidemic in the developed world, and emergency departments (EDs) are frequently the sites for acute care of obese patients [1]. Presently, over 60% of the US population is overweight, and 30% are obese [2]. In addition, health care costs for obese patients are higher than for non-obese patients [3]. It is predicted that by the year 2030, the vast majority—roughly 86%—of Americans age 18 and older could be overweight or obese, and obesity-related costs could climb to over $950 billion per year, or 16%–18% of total US health care costs [4].

Previously obesity was regarded in a more subjective fashion with varied definitions. Research studies on the diagnosis and treatment of acute illnesses have often excluded obese patients. Over time, there has been an agreement on the definitions of the spectrum of obesity: overweight as a body mass index (BMI) of 25–29 kg/m^2, obesity as a BMI$\geq$30, morbid obesity as a BMI$\geq$40, and super obesity as a BMI$\geq$50. Thus, obesity is a clinical diagnosis with specific criteria, not a subjective determination or insult. Obesity is a risk factor for a number of conditions, such as heart disease, diabetes, hypertension, and stroke [5,6]. Just as hospitals will be required to provide care for a growing number of obese patients, EDs will need to adapt to this growing population. Understanding obesity's unique biology, physiology, acute pathological manifestations, and medico–sociological issues are critical for the emergency physician.

On a cellular level, obese patients reside in a chronic inflammatory state, which is associated with features such as endothelial dysfunction, immune system activation, prothrombotic state and insulin resistance. Adipose tissue is not a metabolically inactive storage medium for excess calories, but rather is an active endocrine and immunomodulatory organ. In the event of acute illness or trauma, obese patients manifest an exaggerated

Challenging and Emerging Conditions in Emergency Medicine, First Edition. Edited by Arvind Venkat.
© 2011 by John Wiley & Sons, Ltd. Published 2011 by Blackwell Publishing Ltd.

inflammatory response. Various fat depots, such as subcutaneous, visceral, and perivascular adipose, have a unique phenotype, with both visceral and perivascular adipose being the most inflamed and potentially pathologic [7, 8]. As a result, obese patients manifest a unique physiology that emergency physicians must recognize and, as a result, appropriately modify their diagnostic and treatment decisions. For example, following trauma, obese patients sustain different injuries and have worse outcomes related to co-morbidities. Obese patients with sepsis may require altered doses of antibiotics and ventilator management. Procedures such as endotracheal intubation, venous access, lumbar puncture, and needle thoracostomy require modifications of technique and equipment. A growing scientific interest surrounds the study of adipose tissue and its contribution to a variety of disease processes.

This chapter summarizes the unique pathophysiology of obesity and provides practical suggestions for the diagnosis and treatment of obese patients presenting to the ED.

Acute clinical conditions affected by obesity

Cardiovascular disease

Acute coronary syndrome

Obesity is a traditional and well-known risk factor for the development of acute coronary syndrome (ACS). This condition is often associated with other ACS risk factors, such as metabolic syndrome, diabetes, sedentary lifestyle, and dyslipidemia. Patients with insulin resistance and associated diabetes, in particular, may present with atypical symptoms [9, 10]. Some studies have identified obesity to be a disproportionately more significant risk factor for ACS in the young (<40 years) [11, 12]. Only recently has the attention to obesity brought measures of BMI as part of the demographic parameters collected during clinical trials; therefore, the degree to which classifications of overweight, obese, and morbid obesity should factor into the ED risk assessment of patients presenting with chest discomfort is not yet clear. As such, the obese patient should be viewed by emergency physicians as one at heightened risk of developing ACS deserving careful risk stratification and a lower threshold for further testing and observation unit or hospital admission.

The process of evaluating and risk stratifying obese patients at risk of ACS is problematic in the ED. Obesity and its associated physiologic limitations decrease the utility of exercise treadmill testing [13]. The prognostic value of a normal myocardial perfusion imaging study in this population appears to be less significant than in non-morbidly obese patients as the diagnostic quality of nuclear imaging may be compromised. Duvall et al.

determined that single photon emission CT (SPECT) imaging can be optimized in the obese with the use of a dual-head camera, attenuation correction, and high-stress Tc-99m tracer doses; however, this is not presently available in most institutions [14]. Despite the inherent limitations listed above, perfusion imaging studies continue to be one of the most valuable tools in predicting cardiovascular mortality in the obese and should be utilized in the ED assessment of low- to moderate-risk patients [15]. Patients with nondiagnostic studies should be considered for referral or admission for conventional coronary angiography. The use of dual-source CT coronary angiography (CTCA) possesses similar limitations as myocardial perfusion imaging in the obese patient [16]. Impaired diagnostic accuracy can be explained by scattering and absorption of radiation resulting in poorer image quality due to increase in image noise and decrease in signal-to-noise ratio in obese patients. Moreover, insufficient opacification of the coronary vessels may occur in obese patients due to differences in distribution of blood volume in peripheral venous and central pulmonary circulation when injecting contrast agents [16, 17].

Medications for the initial treatment in ACS may include aspirin, nitroglycerin, anticoagulants, antithrombotics, antiplatelet agents, and fibrinolytics. Aspirin, clopidogrel, and nitroglycerin require no adjustment in dosing for obesity, yet accepted standards for weight-based dosing with other commonly used medications, such as heparin, fondaparinux, bivalirudin, glycoprotein IIb/IIIa inhibitors and fibrinolytics, are not clear. The effects of obesity on drug behavior, clinical efficacy, and safety are unknown for many drugs. Guidelines for the concomitant dosing of these medications is often institutionally based, tends to be more conservative than what the package inserts might recommend and to a large degree depend on the specific combination of medications and regional practice differences. Table 11.1 outlines dosing modifications for commonly used medications in the ED, including those in ACS.

Obesity remains a significant risk factor for the development of cardiovascular disease and ACS and may require increased vigilance in medication dosing. Obese patients with ACS treated with percutaneous coronary intervention paradoxically have a trend for lower mortality and fewer subsequent cardiovascular events [18, 19]. From this we can hypothesize that obesity is a substantial risk factor for ACS, and rapid referral for percutaneous coronary intervention may prove to be more beneficial in this patient population.

Congestive heart failure

Obesity is an important risk factor for acute decompensated heart failure in both women and men, and approximately 11% of cases of congestive heart failure are attributable to obesity alone [20]. For the evaluation and treatment of congestive heart failure, obesity can be particularly

Table 11.1 Medication adjustments in the obese patient population [113, 115–120]

Medication class	Recommendation for dose adjustment for obese patients
Aminoglycosides	Dose by actual body weight; dosing interval dependent on estimated renal function; use therapeutic drug monitoring for peak and trough levels due to the narrow therapeutic window
Beta lactams	Consider doubling dose
Fluoroquinolones	No consistent data; consider using approved dosing range
Linezolid	No empiric change recommended
Carbapenems	No empiric change recommended
Antifungals	No empiric change recommended; use lean body weight as guide for dosing weight-based agents
Enoxaparin	Actual body weight for acute thrombosis at dose of 1 mg/kg; venous thromboembolism prophylaxis at dose of 0.5 mg/kg subcut once daily; venous thromboembolism prophylaxis in morbidly obese trauma patients at dose of 60 mg subcut BID; use antiXa level monitoring
Succinylcholine	Recommended dose is 1 mg/kg of actual body weight
Opioids	Recommended dosing is by lean body weight; increased time for clearance
Muscles relaxants	Dose by lean body weight
Vecuronium	Dose by ideal body weight
Propofol	Dose by lean body weight

problematic. Symptoms of heart failure, such as dyspnea, orthopnea, and lower extremity swelling, can be difficult to interpret in these patients as venous stasis and physical deconditioning are associated with very similar symptoms and presentations. The diagnosis of acute decompensated heart failure is further complicated by laboratory and imaging difficulties. Plain chest radiography in the obese patients is often obscured by the increased amount of soft tissue and can be falsely positive or negative necessitating the risk and expense of further studies [21]. Natriuretic peptide levels tend to be significantly lower in obese patients [22, 23]. For instance, B-natriuretic peptide thresholds to maintain 90% sensitivity for acute heart failure are 170 pg/mL for non-obese patients in contrast to 110 pg/mL for obese patients [24]. Transthoracic echocardiography may be of limited utility due to an inability to obtain an adequate acoustic window necessitating a transesophageal approach. Treatment considerations for obese patients with congestive heart failure are less medication dependent and largely focus upon airway management. Noninvasive positive pressure ventilation (NPPV) should be considered earlier in the course of patient management in obese patients with acute decompensated heart failure due to the potential difficulties associated with emergent endotracheal intubation. Obese patients may also need to be maintained on higher expiratory positive airway pressures.

Similar to ACS, obese patients, while at increased risk for congestive heart failure, tend to have fewer adverse events long term, and this has now been dubbed the "obesity paradox" [25]. Despite the evidence that long-term outcomes for conditions such as ACS and congestive heart failure may be more favorable in the obese patient population, this should not affect the necessary risk stratification performed by emergency physicians in the acute setting. In that obesity can be an independent risk factor for ACS and can complicate the management of congestive heart failure, it is prudent for emergency physicians to have a low threshold for admission of these patients for aggressive inpatient management.

Venous thromboembolism

Obesity is also an independent risk factor for venous thromboembolism, and overall risk appears to be proportional with the degree of obesity [26–28]. Conventional sonography may be limited in obese patients and is largely operator dependent [29, 30]. A lower frequency probe may be required for adequate tissue penetration. No definitive evidence suggests that d-dimer levels might be falsely elevated in obese patients, and, therefore, this test can be used in screening for appropriate patients. The choice between ventilation perfusion scanning and CT pulmonary angiography may depend on the instrument capacities and the practice and experience of the radiologist within the institution. CT pulmonary angiography tends to be favored for the most quality images [31].

Trauma

Trauma in the obese population presents a number of distinct challenges to the emergency physician. Obese patients who experience trauma tend to have higher morbidity than their lean counterparts and have ICU and hospital stays that are double those of the non-obese population [32]. Obese patients also have a significantly higher incidence of multisystem organ failure following trauma [33]. Poor healing, higher incidences of venous thromboembolism, acute renal failure, urinary tract infections, and pulmonary morbidities complicate their hospital course [32, 34, 35]. Obese patients manifest different injury patterns and have inherent obstacles in performing the physical exam, obtaining appropriate images, and performing necessary procedures. Much like identifying the unique features of trauma resuscitation in pediatric or pregnant trauma patients, emergency physicians' strategies for obese patients should be tailored in the context of these unique characteristics.

Traumatic injury patterns

Numerous studies have explored the physical forces and mechanics applied to the human body in the development of vehicle safety restraint systems and designing passenger compartments of vehicles. Results from these studies indicate that obese passengers have very different patterns of body excursion, or movement outside of the neutral position maintained by the restraint, resulting in different injury patterns [36–38]. Standard crash testing for American vehicles currently uses a dummy with a weight of 76.2 kg (167 lbs) and a height of 173 cm (5 feet 8 inches) [36]. A BMI of 24.3 has been artificially set as the standard for the development of safety features in vehicles and is clearly not a fair representation of the American population with nearly 30% having a BMI of greater than 30 [39]. Overall, due to suboptimal positioning or lack of use of safety restraints on the pelvis, as well as greater inertia, obese patients have higher injury-severity scores and abbreviated injury scale extremity scores than their lean counterparts [40, 41].

Obesity appears to be somewhat protective in some trauma situations and in particular from intra-abdominal injuries. One explanation is the "cushion effect" [37, 42]. Other studies, such as that by Wang et al., have demonstrated a protective effect of subcutaneous fat [43]. Biomechanical studies have shown that obese patients have greater forward excursion, but that their increased abdominal fat content serves to lessen the forces to the internal organs [37].

Normal weight or underweight patients tend to sustain more head injuries and abdominal injuries in accidents due to seatbelt restraint as well as the body bending forward during maximal excursion leading to striking the steering column [36, 37]. Obese patients are also less likely to sustain skull fractures as well as traumatic brain injuries, yet, when they do occur, tend to be more severe than in the non-obese patient [35, 44, 45].

Most studies support that obese patients experience more lower extremity and pelvis injuries due to the excursions of the body that results from increased weight, forward momentum, and inefficiencies in lap belt protection in a collision [36, 44, 46–48]. One study, however, demonstrated that in near side collisions, obese patients have a lower incidence of pelvic fractures. This was hypothesized to result from increased subcutaneous fat surrounding the hips or an extrapolation of the abdominal "cushion effect" [49]. Maheshwari demonstrated that obese patients sustain more severe fractures of the distal femur as well as tibia, which is consistent with the fact that obese patients tend to suffer more significant extremity injuries even with minor falls [40, 50, 51].

Obese patients in motor vehicle collisions sustain more thoracic injuries with higher abbreviated injury scale thorax scores [44, 52]. Specifically, broken ribs, pulmonary contusions, and diaphragm injuries are more common and more severe with abbreviated injury scale thorax scores greater than 3 [46, 52]. A study by Reiff et al. demonstrated a strong association between diaphragm injuries in near side collisions in the obese patient population [52]. With these findings the emergency physician should have a lower threshold to order CT imaging of the chest in an obese patient involved in a motor vehicle collision with thoracic complaints or for a high-energy mechanism of injury.

Initial evaluation and imaging

The obese patient presents obstacles to the primary and secondary surveys performed on the trauma patient in the ED. Airway assessment should involve inspection of the soft tissue on and around the neck as well as consideration to appropriate positioning and immobilization. Up to 40% of obese patients have some form of obstructive sleep apnea, and hypertrophied soft tissue within the pharyngeal region may obstruct the airway when lying flat [53]. Specific airway management strategies for obese patients are outlined below in the "Airway Management" section of this chapter. If available cervical collars cannot accommodate the obese patient, inline cervical immobilization may require the use of towel rolls and tape across the patient's forehead and chin.

Obesity affects diagnostic imaging in the trauma setting and should be considered in the diagnostic plan after appropriate injury survey. Cassette size and soft tissue penetration limit the use of plain radiography in the imaging of obese patients [54]. In these cases, CT imaging might be considered, particularly when the lung parenchyma needs to be evaluated. Emergency physicians should consider whether the CT scanner can support the weight or has sufficient gantry size to accommodate the patient. Diagnostic peritoneal lavage may be an option in selected cases [54].

In that physical examination and plain radiography of the lower body may be limited for obese patients, it seems reasonable to have a lower threshold for more advanced imaging if a suspicion for injury of the pelvis exists.

The specific impact of obesity on mortality in trauma patients is less clear. In hospitalized trauma patients, a number of studies have shown a higher mortality for obese patients, while others have only shown increased morbidity with no effect on mortality [32, 33, 44, 55]. It appears that obese patients manifest their higher morbidity and mortality in the long term due to the increased number of complications during hospitalization following trauma [33, 55].

Pulmonary disease

One of the principal organ systems to be affected by obesity is the lungs. In the presence of obesity, the mechanical properties of the respiratory system are profoundly compromised. Conditions such as obstructive sleep apnea (OSA) and obesity hypoventilation syndrome (OHS) are likely caused by obesity, while other conditions, such as asthma, chronic obstructive pulmonary disease (COPD) and pneumonia, can be made worse. Reduced lung expansion reduces the patency of the airways and may lead to greater contractile responses of the airway smooth muscle [56]. Evaluation with auscultation within the din of an ED is more difficult in the obese patient, and imaging with plain radiography can be impaired. There are presently no specific recommendations for the modification of therapeutic approaches to COPD or asthma (e.g., inhalation therapy) in obesity. However, based on the very recent literature, some adjuncts may prove useful in the ED setting.

Asthma

On a population basis, there is a higher prevalence of obesity among adults with asthma, and its severity seems to be proportional to BMI [57]. Ma et al. demonstrated that obesity was independently associated with atopic and non-atopic forms of asthma, even after controlling for insulin resistance and sociodemographic factors. Twelve percent of the obese individuals in this population-based study had asthma, compared to 5% of the normal weight study participants. The risk of asthma was more than tripled for the most obese individuals compared to normal weight people. There is also an association between obesity and poor asthma control. Obese patients experience more exacerbations and emergency visits, a lesser response to therapy, and have higher morbidity compared to non-obese asthma patients [57–60].

The reason why asthma and obesity might be related is still not clear. One hypothesis is that the systemic low-grade inflammation that occurs with obesity may be a factor [61]. Emerging evidence suggests that obese patients have a distinct asthma phenotype and need specialized treatment to control symptoms [62]. Furthermore, obesity-related co-morbidities, such as obstructive sleep apnea, gastroesophageal reflux disease, and vocal cord dysfunction, further complicate asthma control.

Some obese patients with asthma have a non-atopic form and appear to be steroid resistant. One study has found that obese asthma patients respond better to leukotriene inhibitors [62]. The emergency physician does not usually have the benefit of access to spirometry data and what specific asthma phenotype an individual patient expresses. While there are no current recommendations for the routine use of leukotriene inhibitors in the ED, they should be considered in an obese asthmatic patient otherwise not responding to typical therapy. NPPV has gained increased prevalence in ED practice. In asthma, NPPV may have a direct bronchodilating effect, recruit collapsed alveoli, improve ventilation/perfusion mismatch, and reduce the work of breathing. This beneficial effect may be augmented with the use of bronchodilator nebulization together with NPPV [63]. While there are no defined recommendations for the use of NPPV in acute severe asthma exacerbations, it seems reasonable to consider this adjunct in obese patients with acute asthma.

Chronic obstructive pulmonary disease

COPD is caused by the chronic inflammatory response to particles or gases in the lungs, usually from smoking. Obesity is usually associated with chronic bronchitis rather than with emphysema [64]. The prototypical emphysema patient or the "pink puffer" is more likely to be underweight and even cachectic in the final stages. On the other hand, the "blue-bloater" more often fits the description of the obese patients with COPD. This may be due to the fact that patients with COPD lead a more sedentary lifestyle, which would contribute to the development of obesity. Alternatively, obesity may modify the clinical presentation of COPD, although there is little research or clinical evidence on this complex issue. Just as in asthma, it is hypothesized that an increase in circulating pro-inflammatory adipokines may be responsible for COPD pathology [56]. At the present time, there are no alternative pharmacologic recommendations for the obese patient with COPD; however, the efficacy of NPPV in acute COPD exacerbations is well known [65, 66] and should be considered earlier in the care of the obese COPD patient in order to prepare for or even forgo potentially difficult airway management.

Obstructive sleep apnea and obesity hypoventilation syndrome

Obesity is a well-recognized risk factor for OSA. Increased fat tissue deposition in the pharyngeal region and reduced operating lung volumes in obesity act together to reduce upper airway caliber, modify airway configuration and increase their collapsibility; airways are thus predisposed to repetitive closures during sleep [67]. About 70% of people with OSA are obese, and, conversely, the prevalence of the disorder among obese individuals is approximately 40% [68].

A condition related to OSA is OHS characterized by respiratory failure, severe hypoxemia, hypercapnia (daytime $CO_2 > 45$ mm Hg) and pulmonary hypertension. Most patients with OHS also have OSA [69–71]. It has been well established for decades that continuous positive airway pressure is the treatment of choice for obese patients with OSA at home [72]. Due to impaired oxygenation and ventilation physiology at baseline, implementation of NPPV for OSA and OHS patients in the ED with concomitant acute respiratory pathologies is recommended.

Infection and sepsis

Obese critically ill patients represent a challenge in the ED setting. In particular, sepsis is a leading cause of death worldwide, and a growing body of literature is devoted to the increases of morbidity and mortality associated with critically ill obese patients with sepsis. Obese patients also present additional metabolic challenges in resuscitation as they have significantly slower rates of resolving their metabolic acidosis and base deficits [69, 73]. These factors contribute to progression of the patient into multiorgan failure, and continued and recurrent reassessment of these parameters is encouraged. However, there are studies on the association of increased BMI and ICU mortality that yield conflicting results [74–76]. Obesity manifests in a constellation of metabolic disturbances and inflammatory stress. It is difficult to attribute size alone to morbidity and mortality risk, and further assessments and definitions are needed to adequately assess and risk stratify obese patients. As with other medical conditions where obesity by itself does not cause increased mortality, the emergency physician must focus on the acute presentation of the obese septic patient and potential co-morbidities that affect their immediate treatment.

Why obesity may predispose septic patients to increase morbidity is unclear, but it is clear that obese patients are at risk for a number of pre-existing co-morbidities and procedural complications. One possibility is that obesity in itself is not an independent risk factor for infection, but rather associated co-morbidities predispose obese patients to increased risk of suffering community-acquired and nosocomial infections. Extremely obese patients have a higher prevalence of co-morbid conditions that confer higher risk complications with sepsis, including chronic heart, lung, liver, and metabolic diseases [77]. Obesity is a risk factor for ICU-acquired line and blood infections, possibly due to the inherent difficulty of obtaining venous access in this patient population and the reluctance of removing lines once they are established [78]. Obese patients are also predisposed to nosocomial infections after elective surgeries, such as arthroplasty, in comparison to the non-obese [79, 80]. Ironically, many of these patients may require surgery because of complications from or treatment of conditions related to obesity, such as multivessel coronary artery disease and joint degeneration.

Impediments to emergency department management inherent to obesity

Estimating patient weight

The obese patient in need of resuscitation provides a number of challenges for emergency physicians. One of the initial obstacles is estimating the patient's weight. Often, conscious obese patients do not know or grossly understate their weight. Scales in the ED may not have the capacity to weigh patients over 150 kg. While some mechanized beds weigh patients, these are not common in most ED settings. In addition, accurate assessment of patient's weight is critical for safe aeromedical transport. Thus, estimating a patient's weight based on easily obtained information can be a useful clinical skill. A variety of formulas using anthropometric measurements, such as height, waist circumference, hip circumference, and arm circumference, have been derived. Nearly all of these appear to provide more accurate estimations than visual analysis alone. Many of these employ charts or tables and have been derived to accurately allow the use of weight-based medications. Lorenz et al. developed a three input nomogram using height, weight, and hip circumference to assist in the weight estimation of compromised stroke patients receiving weight-based tissue plasminogen activator (tPA) [81]. In another study, height and arm circumference were used to accurately estimate the patient's weight within a 15% error margin [82]. These formulas for weight estimation can be easily used in the ED setting. The authors of this chapter prefer the Crandall et al. formulas as they require the least amount of time and patient manipulation. For non-pregnant females, the formula is:

Weight $= 64.6 + 2.15$ (arm circumference in cm) $+ 0.54$ (height in cm).

For males, the formula is:

Weight $= 93.2 + 3.29$ (arm circumference in cm) $+ 0.43$ (height in cm).

Airway management

Managing the airway is always of concern in obese patients, especially considering the anatomical challenges presented in this patient population. One of the first things to note is that while there may be some mild infiltrations of adipose tissue into the soft tissues of the airway, such as the tonsils and aryepiglottic folds, the airway of the obese patients is approximately the same size as a lean male or female of the same height. The challenge for the emergency physician is aligning of the oral, pharyngeal, and laryngeal axes in the face of anatomical features of obese patients. Obese and lean individuals have the same number and size of cervical vertebrae, but have increased neck mass, volume, and percent adipose tissue. This results in the appearance and functionality of having a short neck [83]. This may be so severe at times that the head and thorax appear to be contiguous. Excess breast or chest wall tissue may fall towards the head and neck when the patient is placed in a recumbent position, acting as a barrier to the laryngoscope handle. Specific short-handled laryngoscope blades may be of use in this circumstance. As mentioned above, OHS is a common baseline condition causing chronic hypercapnia in these patients. Gas exchange and lung function may be improved through the use of a pre-intubation period of NPPV and may assist in the treatment of acute respiratory failure from a variety of causes [84, 85].

Advanced preparation is critical when planning to intubate the obese patient. There is conflicting evidence whether increased BMI can predict a difficult airway [86]. However, if the airway is not successfully intubated in the obese patient, alternative measures such as bag valve mask ventilation or cricothyrotomy are exponentially more difficult. Perhaps the easiest maneuver for the anticipated intubation of the obese patients includes placing them in a "ramp" position. This can be achieved by stacking blankets behind the patient's back, resulting in elevation of the head, upper body, and shoulders significantly above the chest. As a result, the external auditory meatus aligns horizontally with the sternal notch. Similar positioning can be achieved using a commercially available elevation pillow [87–89]. There are several steps that the emergency physician should consider when planning to intubate obese patients:

1. Recruit enough assistance to perform extra maneuvers such as displacing chest tissue caudad, positioning the patient, and acquiring necessary or additional supplies.
2. Advance preparation and acquisition of additional airway adjuncts such as video laryngoscopy (several available devices) and extraglottic devices.

A formula suggested by the authors for the optimal number of people needed to perform a successful intubation is: ((actual body weight in kg)/70 kg) + 2 (round to the highest whole number). Consider a prolonged pre-oxygenation period if time permits and the use of adjustable angle laryngoscopes.

Device considerations may include a number of adjuncts designed for use in managing the difficult airway. Ndoko et al. found that use of the Airtraq™ laryngoscope shortened mean intubation time (56 vs. 24 seconds) and episodes of decreased oxygen saturation in comparison to a Macintosh laryngoscope in the obese patient [90]. Other video-assisted intubation devices (i.e., LMA Ctrach™, Airway Scope™, GlideScope™) may also provide additional aid in managing the airway of obese patients [91, 92]. Sifri et al. demonstrated that emergency physicians can often successfully intubate sick obese trauma patients in the ED setting [93]. In the event that the patient cannot be intubated, ventilation through the use of extraglottic devices, such as the Combitube™ or King Airway™, may be beneficial.

Once intubation has taken place, the emergency physician must be aware that ventilator strategies and settings need to be carefully tailored. Increased BMI has been associated with a higher rate of developing acute respiratory distress syndrome [94]. Ventilation may be improved through slight reverse Trendelenburg angulation of the patient's bed.

Vascular access

Vascular access in obese patients is problematic and often takes additional preparation and time and, despite these efforts, may be unsuccessful. Ideally, whatever technique is decided upon would be safe, efficient, and well tolerated by patients. The advent of bedside ultrasonography has significantly improved the ability to achieve intravenous access in obese patients. Ultrasound-guided peripheral intravenous access has been shown to be more successful than traditional "blind" techniques, requires less time, and decreases the number of percutaneous punctures in patients who were defined to have difficult intravenous access, including obese patients [95]. An alternative to central venous access in the obese patient may be ultrasound-guided brachial vein cannulation. Mills et al. demonstrated the feasibility of using an ultrasound-guided 15-cm catheter to cannulate the brachial or basilic vein in patients with varied reasons for difficult venous access [96]. Regardless, care providers should be prepared with intravenous catheters of sufficient length to avoid dislodgement and potential infiltration.

Central venous access can also be problematic in the obese patient, and there is no clear consensus about which site and approach is most preferable. Femoral access has largely fallen out of favor due to the increased incidence of infection and deep venous thrombosis [97]. Remaining options include standard approaches for the subclavian and internal jugular veins, and both of these approaches can be more difficult in the obese patient due to obscured landmarks. One recent study found that the internal jugular could be accessed with equal success to the subclavian approach in obese patients [98]. These authors recommended that procedural success might be increased by maintaining the head in neutral position where the internal jugular vein would have the least overlap over the carotid artery. Overall, it appears that in any approach and in many special patient populations, including obesity, ultrasound guidance may be the best adjunct in successfully and safely accomplishing central venous access [99–102].

Lumbar puncture

Obese patients have an increased distance from the skin surface to the subarachnoid space. This distance often exceeds that of a routine 9 cm spinal needle. Abe et al. devised a formula for predicting the required lumbar puncture depth, which can aid in the selection of an appropriate-sized spinal needle [103]:

Lumbar puncture depth (cm) = $1 + 17$ (weight (kg))/height (cm)

Awareness of the predicted depth of needle insertion can increase the success rate [104]. Ultrasound may improve the identification of landmarks for lumbar puncture as well [105, 106]. Fluoroscopy may be considered in extreme, technically difficult, or unsuccessful cases.

Needle and tube thoracostomy

Obese patients can have significant adipose tissue on their chest and thorax. This may preclude urgent and emergency procedures such as needle and tube thoracostomy from being rapidly and effectively accomplished [107, 108]. In a study of the effectiveness of needle thoracostomy for tension pneumothorax in the pre-hospital environment, the authors found that nearly 25% of included patients had retained some amount of pneumothorax, with most having subclinical tension, indicating incomplete or total failure of penetration into the pleural space [109]. Procedure failure in this study was attributed to the use of routine 5-cm catheters that were simply too short to adequately decompress the chest. In a similar fashion, Givens et al. retrospectively measured chest wall thickness by chest CT scans in medical and trauma patients and found that 5-cm catheters would reliably penetrate the pleural space in only 75% of patients [108]. Due to the apparent increased proportion of obese patients requiring medical care, some emergency medical services (EMS) systems have reportedly adopted the use of 7-cm catheters. Alternatively, some authors have found that needle decompression may be more successful when the catheter is placed in the anterior or midaxillary line [110, 111]. In tube thoracostomy, tube length is not the limiting difficulty for morbidly obese patients, but the space between the scapula and the underlying ribs can create confusion. This can be avoided by blunt dissection and finger decompression of the pleural space prior to chest tube insertion [112]. Once this is performed, it reduces the urgency and allows time for the subsequent placement of an appropriate chest tube.

Drug dosing

The physiologic changes of obesity also alter both the hepatic and renal clearance and the volume of distribution of many drugs. Fixed amount dosing regimens may result in underdosing, and, likewise, total body weight (TBW) dosing may result in overdosing. Several body weight definitions, such as TBW, actual body weight, ideal body weight, and lean body weight, have variable use and sometimes unclear definitions. Glomerular filtration rate and creatinine clearance are affected by obesity, and standard calculations for these values are less accurate in the obese population [113]. Obese patients not only have an obviously increased amount of adipose tissue weight, but also concomitantly have a greater amount of lean body weight to physically and metabolically compensate for the increased tissue burden. Over 99% of drug metabolism occurs in lean tissues [114]. While there are few clear and consistent dosing guidelines for obese patients, there seems to be a trend in the recommendations for weight-based dosing to be based on the lean body weight. Lean body weight calculators, based on the derivation of Janmahasatian et al. are available online (http://www.medcalc.com/body.html and ePocrates®

medical calculation applications MedMath and CardioMath). Considerations for dosing adjustments for obese patients appear in Table 11.1 above.

Sociologic and medicolegal risks of obesity

Obese patients are highly stigmatized, and weight bias has increased with the growing recognition of obesity as a medical issue. Research shows that physicians, nurses and medical students associate negative attitudes towards obese patients, including beliefs that they are noncompliant, lazy, and lack discipline [121]. Such beliefs may translate to the caregiver's notion that any treatment for an obese person's condition may be futile. Obese patients may avoid seeking preventive or early medical care for fear of receiving disrespectful treatment, unsolicited advice to lose weight, or being embarrassed by using gowns or equipment intended for normal weight patients [122, 123]. Despite these patient- and physician-focused obstacles to caring for obese patients, emergency physicians are duty bound to provide the best possible acute care to any patient population regardless of prejudice.

Failure of diagnosis, drug dosing errors due to incorrect weight estimation and ineffective medical devices, such as airway equipment or imaging modalities, are just a few examples in which the clinical manifestations of obesity may expose care providers to increased medicolegal risk. Obesity also has the potential to cause increased risk for patients and ED care providers unrelated to the presenting complaint. For instance, most medical equipment, such as stretchers, transport boards, and radiology tables, were not designed for morbidly obese patients and may be at risk of mechanical failure. Inadequate equipment, staff assistance, and training of health care providers may result in personal injury claims such as back injuries. Appropriate risk management and investment in capital equipment to manage obese patients may prevent unnecessary claims; however, it is unclear whether hospitals will be expected to have invested in equipment designed for bariatric patients. Very few ED have the equipment to image patients > 450 lbs, and although some veterinary schools and zoos are sometimes equipped with large CT scanners, most have policies prohibiting the imaging of humans [1].

The next five years

Landmark trials evaluating life saving emergency treatments have often excluded obese patients from the study populations or have not recorded BMI [124]. There is a paucity of data specifically addressing obese critically ill patients, and future studies will need to address this "minority" population and include them in clinical trials.

Most likely, the proportion of obese patients presenting to the ED will continue to grow. Obesity is a multibillion dollar market ready and waiting for device developers to catch up to fill an enormous unmet need. Medical device developers have already identified as a prime market opportunity the invention and adaptation of advanced technologies and devices specifically catered to the obese patient. An obvious need lies in the realm of imaging modalities such as CT, MRI, ultrasound, and even plain radiography. At its most basic level, the medical profession is in need of longer needles, airway devices, such as an indicator-guided percutaneous emergency cricothyrotomy adjunct, elevation pillows, imaging devices, scales, transfer boards, beds, and mobility aids (crutches, wheelchairs, scooters) to care for the obese patient.

As in many medical conditions, an increasing number of patients parallels an increasing number of pharmaceuticals targeting that process. The same is true with obesity in both the prescription and over-the-counter (OTC) drug arenas. Any pharmacy, grocery, or nutritional supplement store contains several agents purported to promote weight loss. Several companies produce OTC or herbal/all natural weight loss supplements that have no proven clinical efficacy, may have dangerous side effects or interactions, and are not approved by the FDA. The FDA determined and recently released news about the presence of sibutramine, fenproporex, fluoxetine, bumetanide, furosemide, phenytoin, rimonabant, cetilistat, and phenolphthalein in weight loss products being sold OTC under a variety of names [125]. One of the first mainstream medications targeting obesity, "Fen-Phen" (fenfluramine, phentermine, dexfenfluramine), was found to cause significant cardiac valvular complications that resulted in it being taken off the market in 1997. Since that time emerging agents are under intense regulatory scrutiny [126]. The FDA recently pulled sibutramine from the market citing an increased risk of myocardial infarction and stroke with prolonged use [127]. Despite being removed from the market, many of these agents can still be found internationally and on the Internet. The potential for millions of individuals to be taking prescription and OTC medications for obesity is immense. While emergency physicians are unlikely to prescribe these agents, they should realize the potential for complications and overdoses from this set of agents and consider including queries of such medication use in their history and physical.

Conclusion

Obesity is a clinical condition that affects nearly every disease process and population emergency physicians serve. Obesity in isolation is often not solely responsible for a poor prognosis, but is likely the contributing factor of difficulty in performing procedures, physical examination, and obtaining adequate imaging. Insulin resistance, increase in infection rate, and other co-morbidities also account for morbidity associated with the obese condition. For now, in the absence of definitive evidence, emergency physicians must continue to extrapolate from available literature and clinical experiences when managing the obese patient. There is currently a charge in the medical and surgical literature to identify diagnostic and treatment strategies for the obese. Emergency physicians need to identify and consider obesity as a clinical condition, rather than a social stigma, and combine this with the knowledge of associated co-morbidities to appropriately manage this challenging patient population.

References

1. Ginde AA, Foianini A, Renner DM, Valley M, Camargo CA, Jr. The challenge of CT and MRI imaging of obese individuals who present to the emergency department: a national survey. *Obesity (Silver Spring)* 2008; 16(11): 2549–2551.
2. Flegal KM, Carroll MD, Ogden CL, Curtin LR. Prevalence and trends in obesity among US adults, 1999–2008. *JAMA* 2010; 303(3): 235–241.
3. Raebel MA, Malone DC, Conner DA, Xu S, Porter JA, Lanty FA. Health services use and health care costs of obese and non-obese individuals. *Arch Intern Med* 2004; 164(19): 2135–2140.
4. Wang Y, Beydoun MA, Liang L, Caballero B, Kumanyika SK. Will all Americans become overweight or obese? Estimating the progression and cost of the US obesity epidemic. *Obesity (Silver Spring)* 2008; 16(10): 2323–2330.
5. Malnick SD, Knobler H. The medical complications of obesity. *QJM* 2006; 99(9): 565–579.
6. Flegal KM, Graubard BI, Williamson DF, Gail MH. Cause-specific excess deaths associated with underweight, overweight, and obesity. *JAMA* 2007; 298(17): 2028–2037.
7. Chatterjee TK, Stoll LL, Denning GM, et al. Proinflammatory phenotype of perivascular adipocytes: influence of high-fat feeding. *Circ Res* 2009; 104(4): 541–549.
8. Blomkalns AL, Chatterjee T, Weintraub NL. Turning ACS outside in: linking perivascular adipose tissue to acute coronary syndromes. *Am J Physiol Heart Circ Physiol* 2010; 298(3): H734–H735.
9. Arslanian-Engoren C, Patel A, Fang J, et al. Symptoms of men and women presenting with acute coronary syndromes. *Am J Cardiol* 2006; 98(9): 1177–1181.
10. Franklin K, Goldberg RJ, Spencer F, et al. Implications of diabetes in patients with acute coronary syndromes. The global registry of acute coronary events. *Arch Intern Med* 2004; 164(13): 1457–1463.
11. Park HS, Song YM, Cho SI. Obesity has a greater impact on cardiovascular mortality in younger men than in older men among non-smoking Koreans. *Int J Epidemiol* 2006; 35(1): 181–187.
12. McGill HC, Jr, McMahan CA, Herderick EE, et al. Obesity accelerates the progression of coronary atherosclerosis in young men. *Circulation* 2002; 105(23): 2712–2718.

13. Amsterdam EA, Kirk JD, Bluemke DA, et al. Testing of low-risk patients presenting to the emergency department with chest pain. A scientific statement from the American Heart Association. *Circulation* 2010; 122(17): 1756–1776.

14. Duvall WL, Croft LB, Corriel JS, et al. SPECT myocardial perfusion imaging in morbidly obese patients: image quality, hemodynamic response to pharmacologic stress, and diagnostic and prognostic value. *J Nucl Cardiol* 2006; 13(2): 202–209.

15. Elhendy A, Schinkel AF, van Domburg RT, et al. Prognostic stratification of obese patients by stress 99mTc-tetrofosmin myocardial perfusion imaging. *J Nucl Med* 2006; 47(8): 1302–1306.

16. Alkadhi H, Scheffel H, Desbiolles L, et al. Dual-source computed tomography coronary angiography: influence of obesity, calcium load, and heart rate on diagnostic accuracy. *Eur Heart J* 2008; 29(6): 766–776.

17. Husmann L, Leschka S, Boehm T, et al. Influence of body mass index on coronary artery opacification in 64-slice CT angiography. *Rofo* 2006; 178(10): 1007–1013.

18. Mehta L, Devlin W, McCullough PA, et al. Impact of body mass index on outcomes after percutaneous coronary intervention in patients with acute myocardial infarction. *Am J Cardiol* 2007; 99(7): 906–910.

19. Wienbergen H, Gitt AK, Juenger C, et al. Impact of the body mass index on occurrence and outcome of acute ST-elevation myocardial infarction. *Clin Res Cardiol* 2008 ; 97(2): 83–88.

20. Kenchaiah S, Evans JC, Levy D, et al. Obesity and the risk of heart failure. *N Engl J Med* 2002; 347(5): 305–313.

21. Uppot RN, Sahani DV, Hahn PF, Kalra MK, Saini SS, Mueller PR. Effect of obesity on image quality: fifteen-year longitudinal study for evaluation of dictated radiology reports. *Radiology* 2006; 240(2): 435–439.

22. Mehra MR, Uber PA, Park MH, et al. Obesity and suppressed B-type natriuretic peptide levels in heart failure. *J Am Coll Cardiol* 2004; 43(9): 1590–1595.

23. Taub PR, Gabbai-Saldate P, Maisel A. Biomarkers of heart failure. *Congest Heart Fail* 2010; 16(1 Suppl.): S19–S24.

24. Daniels LB, Clopton P, Bhalla V, et al. How obesity affects the cut-points for B-type natriuretic peptide in the diagnosis of acute heart failure. Results from the breathing not properly multinational study. *Am Heart J* 2006; 151(5): 999–1005.

25. Curtis JP, Selter JG, Wang Y, et al. The obesity paradox: body mass index and outcomes in patients with heart failure. *Arch Intern Med* 2005; 165(1): 55–61.

26. Borch KH, Hansen-Krone I, Braekkan SK, et al. Physical activity and risk of venous thromboembolism. The Tromso study. *Haematologica* 2010; 95(12): 2088–2094.

27. Ageno W, Becattini C, Brighton T, Selby R, Kamphuisen PW. Cardiovascular risk factors and venous thromboembolism: a meta-analysis. *Circulation* 2008; 117(1): 93–102.

28. Stein PD, Beemath A, Olson RE. Obesity as a risk factor in venous thromboembolism. *Am J Med* 2005; 118(9): 978–980.

29. Coche EE, Hamoir XL, Hammer FD, Hainaut P, Goffette PP. Using dual-detector helical CT angiography to detect deep venous thrombosis in patients

with suspicion of pulmonary embolism: diagnostic value and additional findings. *AJR Am J Roentgenol* 2001; 176(4): 1035–1039.

30. Garg K, Kemp JL, Wojcik D, et al. Thromboembolic disease: comparison of combined CT pulmonary angiography and venography with bilateral leg sonography in 70 patients. *AJR Am J Roentgenol* 2000; 175(4): 997–1001.

31. Inge TH, Donnelly LF, Vierra M, Cohen AP, Daniels SR, Garcia VF. Managing bariatric patients in a children's hospital: radiologic considerations and limitations. *J Pediatr Surg* 2005; 40(4): 609–617.

32. Newell MA, Bard MR, Goettler CE, et al. Body mass index and outcomes in critically injured blunt trauma patients: weighing the impact. *J Am Coll Surg* 2007; 204(5): 1056–1061; discussion 62–64.

33. Christmas AB, Reynolds J, Wilson AK, et al. Morbid obesity impacts mortality in blunt trauma. *Am Surg* 2007; 73(11): 1122–1125.

34. Sharma OP, Oswanski MF, Joseph RJ, et al. Venous thromboembolism in trauma patients. *Am Surg* 2007; 73(11): 1173–1180.

35. Neville AL, Brown CV, Weng J, Demetriades D, Velmahos GC. Obesity is an independent risk factor of mortality in severely injured blunt trauma patients. *Arch Surg* 2004; 139(9): 983–987.

36. Forman J, Lopez-Valdes FJ, Lessley D, Kindig M, Kent R, Bostrom O. The effect of obesity on the restraint of automobile occupants. *Annu Proc Assoc Adv Automot Med* 2009; 53: 25–40.

37. Kent RW, Forman JL, Bostrom O. Is there really a "cushion effect"?: a biomechanical investigation of crash injury mechanisms in the obese. *Obesity (Silver Spring)* 2010; 18(4): 749–753.

38. Viano DC, Parenteau CS, Edwards ML. Crash injury risks for obese occupants using a matched-pair analysis. *Traffic Inj Prev* 2008; 9(1): 59–64.

39. Zhu S, Layde PM, Guse CE, et al. Obesity and risk for death due to motor vehicle crashes. *Am J Public Health* 2006; 96(4): 734–739.

40. Brown CV, Neville AL, Rhee P, Salim A, Velmahos GC, Demetriades D. The impact of obesity on the outcomes of 1,153 critically injured blunt trauma patients. *J Trauma* 2005; 59(5): 1048–1051; discussion 51.

41. Chesser TJ, Hammett RB, Norton SA. Orthopaedic trauma in the obese patient. *Injury* 2010; 41(3): 247–252.

42. Arbabi S, Wahl WL, Hemmila MR, Kohoyda-Inglis C, Taheri PA, Wang SC. The cushion effect. *J Trauma* 2003 ; 54(6): 1090–1093.

43. Wang SC, Bednarski B, Patel S, et al. Increased depth of subcutaneous fat is protective against abdominal injuries in motor vehicle collisions. *Annu Proc Assoc Adv Automot Med* 2003; 47: 545–559.

44. Ryb GE, Dischinger PC. Injury severity and outcome of overweight and obese patients after vehicular trauma: a crash injury research and engineering network (CIREN) study. *J Trauma* 2008; 64(2): 406–411.

45. Tagliaferri F, Compagnone C, Yoganandan N, Gennarelli TA. Traumatic brain injury after frontal crashes: relationship with body mass index. *J Trauma* 2009; 66(3): 727–729.

46. Cormier JM. The influence of body mass index on thoracic injuries in frontal impacts. *Accid Anal Prev* 2008; 40(2): 610–615.

47. Zarzaur BL, Marshall SW. Motor vehicle crashes obesity and seat belt use: a deadly combination? *J Trauma* 2008; 64(2): 412–419; discussion 9.

48. Boulanger BR, Milzman D, Mitchell K, Rodriguez A. Body habitus as a predictor of injury pattern after blunt trauma. *J Trauma* 1992; 33(2): 228–232.

49. Bansal V, Conroy C, Lee J, Schwartz A, Tominaga G, Coimbra R. Is bigger better? The effect of obesity on pelvic fractures after side impact motor vehicle crashes. *J Trauma* 2009; 67(4): 709–714.

50. Maheshwari R, Mack CD, Kaufman RP, et al. Severity of injury and outcomes among obese trauma patients with fractures of the femur and tibia: a crash injury research and engineering network study. *J Orthop Trauma* 2009; 23(9): 634–639.

51. Spaine LA, Bollen SR. 'The bigger they come ...': the relationship between body mass index and severity of ankle fractures. *Injury* 1996; 27(10): 687–689.

52. Reiff DA, Davis RP, MacLennan PA, McGwin G, Jr, Clements R, Rue LW, 3rd. The association between body mass index and diaphragm injury among motor vehicle collision occupants. *J Trauma* 2004; 57(6): 1324–1328; discussion 8.

53. Poulain M, Doucet M, Major GC, et al. The effect of obesity on chronic respiratory diseases: pathophysiology and therapeutic strategies. *CMAJ* 2006; 174(9): 1293–1299.

54. Grant P, Newcombe M. Emergency management of the morbidly obese. *Emerg Med Australas* 2004; 16(4): 309–317.

55. Diaz JJ, Jr, Norris PR, Collier BR, et al. Morbid obesity is not a risk factor for mortality in critically ill trauma patients. *J Trauma* 2009; 66(1): 226–231.

56. Hakala K, Stenius-Aarniala B, Sovijarvi A. Effects of weight loss on peak flow variability, airways obstruction, and lung volumes in obese patients with asthma. *Chest* 2000; 118(5): 1315–1321.

57. Ma J, Strub P, Camargo CA, Jr, et al. The breathe easier through weight loss lifestyle (BE WELL) intervention: a randomized controlled trial. BMC Pulm Med 2010; 10: 16.

58. Stenius-Aarniala B, Poussa T, Kvarnstrom J, Gronlund EL, Ylikahri M, Mustajoki P. Immediate and long term effects of weight reduction in obese people with asthma: randomised controlled study. *BMJ* 2000; 320(7238): 827–832.

59. Todd DC, Armstrong S, D'Silva L, Allen CJ, Hargreave FE, Parameswaran K. Effect of obesity on airway inflammation: a cross-sectional analysis of body mass index and sputum cell counts. *Clin Exp Allergy* 2007; 37(7): 1049–1054.

60. Saint-Pierre P, Bourdin A, Chanez P, Daures JP, Godard P. Are overweight asthmatics more difficult to control? *Allergy* 2006; 61(1): 79–84.

61. Ma J, Xiao L, Knowles SB. Obesity, insulin resistance and the prevalence of atopy and asthma in US adults. *Allergy* 2010; 65(11): 1455–1463.

62. Peters-Golden M, Swern A, Bird SS, Hustad CM, Grant E, Edelman JM. Influence of body mass index on the response to asthma controller agents. *Eur Respir J* 2006; 27(3): 495–503.

63. Brandao DC, Lima VM, Filho VG, et al. Reversal of bronchial obstruction with bi-level positive airway pressure and nebulization in patients with acute asthma. *J Asthma* 2009; 46(4): 356–361.

64. Guerra S, Sherrill DL, Bobadilla A, Martinez FD, Barbee RA. The relation of body mass index to asthma, chronic bronchitis, and emphysema. *Chest* 2002; 122(4): 1256–1263.

65. Carrera M, Marin JM, Anton A, et al. A controlled trial of noninvasive ventilation for chronic obstructive pulmonary disease exacerbations. *J Crit Care* 2009; 24(3): 473, e7–e14.

66. Brochard L, Mancebo J, Wysocki M, et al. Noninvasive ventilation for acute exacerbations of chronic obstructive pulmonary disease. *N Engl J Med* 1995; 333(13): 817–822.

67. Series F. Upper airway muscles awake and asleep. *Sleep Med Rev* 2002; 6(3): 229–242.

68. Resta O, Foschino-Barbaro MP, Legari G, et al. Sleep-related breathing disorders, loud snoring and excessive daytime sleepiness in obese subjects. *Int J Obes Relat Metab Disord* 2001; 25(5): 669–675.

69. Winfield RD, Delano MJ, Dixon DJ, et al. Differences in outcome between obese and non-obese patients following severe blunt trauma are not consistent with an early inflammatory genomic response. *Crit Care Med* 2010; 38(1): 51–58.

70. Olson AL, Zwillich C. The obesity hypoventilation syndrome. *Am J Med* 2005; 118(9): 948–956.

71. Kessler R, Chaouat A, Schinkewitch P, et al. The obesity-hypoventilation syndrome revisited: a prospective study of 34 consecutive cases. *Chest* 2001; 120(2): 369–376.

72. Sullivan CE, Issa FG, Berthon-Jones M, Eves L. Reversal of obstructive sleep apnoea by continuous positive airway pressure applied through the nares. *Lancet* 1981; 1(8225): 862–865.

73. Winfield RD, Delano MJ, Lottenberg L, et al. Traditional resuscitative practices fail to resolve metabolic acidosis in morbidly obese patients after severe blunt trauma. *J Trauma* 2010; 68(2): 317–330.

74. Oliveros H, Villamor E. Obesity and mortality in critically ill adults: a systematic review and meta-analysis. *Obesity (Silver Spring)* 2008; 16(3): 515–521.

75. Garrouste-Orgeas M, Troche G, Azoulay E, et al. Body mass index. An additional prognostic factor in ICU patients. *Intensive Care Med* 2004; 30(3): 437–443.

76. Akinnusi ME, Pineda LA, El Solh AA. Effect of obesity on intensive care morbidity and mortality: a meta-analysis. *Crit Care Med* 2008; 36(1): 151–158.

77. Shenkman Z, Shir Y, Brodsky JB. Perioperative management of the obese patient. *Br J Anaesth* 1993; 70(3): 349–359.

78. Dossett LA, Dageforde LA, Swenson BR, et al. Obesity and site-specific nosocomial infection risk in the intensive care unit. *Surg Infect (Larchmt)* 2009; 10(2): 137–142.

79. Winiarsky R, Barth P, Lotke P. Total knee arthroplasty in morbidly obese patients. *J Bone Joint Surg Am* 1998 ; 80(12): 1770–1774.

80. Namba RS, Paxton L, Fithian DC, Stone ML. Obesity and perioperative morbidity in total hip and total knee arthroplasty patients. *J Arthroplasty* 2005; 20(7 Suppl. 3): 46–50.

81. Lorenz MW, Graf M, Henke C, et al. Anthropometric approximation of body weight in unresponsive stroke patients. *J Neurol Neurosurg Psychiatry* 2007; 78(12): 1331–1336.

82. Crandall CS, Gardner S, Braude DA. Estimation of total body weight in obese patients. *Air Med J* 2009 ; 28(3): 139–145.

83. Mortimore IL, Marshall I, Wraith PK, Sellar RJ, Douglas NJ. Neck and total body fat deposition in non-obese and obese patients with sleep apnea compared with that in control subjects. *Am J Respir Crit Care Med* 1998; 157(1): 280–283.

84. El-Solh AA, Aquilina A, Pineda L, Dhanvantri V, Grant B, Bouquin P. Noninvasive ventilation for prevention of post-extubation respiratory failure in obese patients. *Eur Respir J* 2006; 28(3): 588–595.

85. Budweiser S, Riedl SG, Jorres RA, Heinemann F, Pfeifer M. Mortality and prognostic factors in patients with obesity-hypoventilation syndrome undergoing noninvasive ventilation. *J Intern Med* 2007; 261(4): 375–383.

86. Gaszynski T. Anesthetic complications of gross obesity. *Curr Opin Anaesthesiol* 2004; 17(3): 271–276.

87. Brodsky JB, Lemmens HJ, Brock-Utne JG, Saidman LJ, Levitan R. Anesthetic considerations for bariatric surgery: Proper positioning is important for laryngoscopy. *Anesth Analg* 2003; 96(6): 1841–1842; author reply 2.

88. Neligan PJ, Porter S, Max B, Malhotra G, Greenblatt EP, Ochroch EA. Obstructive sleep apnea is not a risk factor for difficult intubation in morbidly obese patients. *Anesth Analg* 2009; 109(4): 1182–1186.

89. Rich JM. Use of an elevation pillow to produce the head-elevated laryngoscopy position for airway management in morbidly obese and large-framed patients. *Anesth Analg* 2004; 98(1): 264–265.

90. Ndoko SK, Amathieu R, Tual L, et al. Tracheal intubation of morbidly obese patients: a randomized trial comparing performance of Macintosh and AirtraqTM laryngoscopes. *Br J Anaesth*; 100(2): 263–268.

91. Tan BH, Liu EH, Lim RT, Liow LM, Goy RW. Ease of intubation with the GlideScope or Airway Scope by novice operators in simulated easy and difficult airways—a manikin study. *Anaesthesia* 2009; 64(2): 187–190.

92. Dhonneur G, Abdi W, Ndoko S, et al. Video-assisted versus conventional tracheal intubation in morbidly obese patients. *Obesity Surgery* 2009; 19(8): 1096–1101.

93. Sifri ZC, Kim H, Lavery R, Mohr A, Livingston DH. The impact of obesity on the outcome of emergency intubation in trauma patients. *J Trauma* 2008; 65(2): 396–400.

94. Gong MN, Bajwa EK, Thompson BT, Christiani DC. Body mass index is associated with the development of acute respiratory distress syndrome. *Thorax* 2010; 65(1): 44–50.

95. Costantino TG, Parikh AK, Satz WA, Fojtik JP. Ultrasonography-guided peripheral intravenous access versus traditional approaches in patients with difficult intravenous access. *Ann Emerg Med* 2005; 46(5): 456–461.

96. Mills CN, Liebmann O, Stone MB, Frazee BW. Ultrasonographically guided insertion of a 15-cm catheter into the deep brachial or basilic vein in patients with difficult intravenous access. *Ann Emerg Med* 2007; 50(1): 68–72.

97. Merrer J, De Jonghe B, Golliot F, et al. Complications of femoral and subclavian venous catheterization in critically ill patients: a randomized controlled trial. *JAMA* 2001 ; 286(6): 700–707.

98. Fujiki M, Guta CG, Lemmens HJ, Brock-Utne JG. Is it more difficult to cannulate the right internal jugular vein in morbidly obese patients than in non-obese patients? *Obes Surg* 2008; 18(9): 1157–1159.

99. Mallory DL, McGee WT, Shawker TH, et al. Ultrasound guidance improves the success rate of internal jugular vein cannulation: a prospective, randomized trial. *Chest* 1990 ; 98(1): 157–160.

100. Maecken T, Grau T. Ultrasound imaging in vascular access. *Crit Care Med* 2007; 35(5 Suppl.): S178–S185.

101. Ganeshan A, Warakaulle DR, Uberoi R. Central venous access. *Cardiovasc Intervent Radiol* 2007; 30(1): 26–33.

102. Miller AH, Roth BA, Mills TJ, Woody JR, Longmoor CE, Foster B. Ultrasound guidance versus the landmark technique for the placement of central venous catheters in the emergency department. *Acad Emerg Med* 2002; 9(8): 800–805.

103. Abe KK, Yamamoto LG, Itoman EM, Nakasone TA, Kanayama SK. Lumbar puncture needle length determination. *Am J Emerg Med* 2005; 23(6): 742–746.

104. Jayaraman L, Sethi N, Malhotra S, Sood J. Long length spinal needle in obese patients. *Internet J Anesthesiol* 2009; 19(1).

105. Ferre RM, Sweeney TW. Emergency physicians can easily obtain ultrasound images of anatomical landmarks relevant to lumbar puncture. *Am J Emerg Med* 2007; 25(3): 291–296.

106. Peterson MA, Abele J. Bedside ultrasound for difficult lumbar puncture. *J Emerg Med* 2005; 28(2): 197–200.

107. Britten S, Palmer SH. Chest wall thickness may limit adequate drainage of tension pneumothorax by needle thoracocentesis. *J Accid Emerg Med* 1996; 13(6): 426–427.

108. Givens ML, Ayotte K, Manifold C. Needle thoracostomy: implications of computed tomography chest wall thickness. *Acad Emerg Med* 2004; 11(2): 211–213.

109. Warner KJ, Copass MK, Bulger EM. Paramedic use of needle thoracostomy in the pre-hospital environment. *Prehosp Emerg Care* 2008; 12(2): 162–168.

110. Wax DB, Leibowitz AB. Radiologic assessment of potential sites for needle decompression of a tension pneumothorax. *Anesth Analg* 2007; 105(5): 1385–1388, table of contents.

111. Rawlins R, Brown KM, Carr CS, Cameron CR. Life threatening haemorrhage after anterior needle aspiration of pneumothoraces. A role for lateral needle aspiration in emergency decompression of spontaneous pneumothorax. *Emerg Med J* 2003; 20(4): 383–384.

112. Fitzgerald M, Mackenzie CF, Marasco S, Hoyle R, Kossmann T. Pleural decompression and drainage during trauma reception and resuscitation. *Injury* 2008; 39(1): 9–20.

113. Pai MP, Bearden DT. Antimicrobial dosing considerations in obese adult patients. *Pharmacotherapy* 2007; 27(8): 1081–1091.

114. Roubenoff R, Kehayias JJ. The meaning and measurement of lean body mass. *Nutr Rev* 1991; 49(6): 163–175.

115. Han PY, Duffull SB, Kirkpatrick CM, Green B. Dosing in obesity: a simple solution to a big problem. *Clin Pharmacol Ther* 2007; 82(5): 505–508.

116. Rondina MT, Wheeler M, Rodgers GM, Draper L, Pendleton RC. Weight-based dosing of enoxaparin for VTE prophylaxis in morbidly obese, medically-ill patients. *Thromb Res* 2010; 125(3): 220–223.

117. Duplaga BA, Rivers CW, Nutescu E. Dosing and monitoring of low-molecular-weight heparins in special populations. *Pharmacotherapy* 2001; 21(2): 218–234.

118. Lemmens HJ, Brodsky JB. The dose of succinylcholine in morbid obesity. *Anesth Analg* 2006; 102(2): 438–442.

119. Ingrande J, Brodsky JB, Lemmens HJ. Lean body weight scalar for the anesthetic induction dose of propofol in morbidly obese subjects. *Anesth Analg* 2010.

120. Casati A, Putzu M. Anesthesia in the obese patient: pharmacokinetic considerations. *J Clin Anesth* 2005; 17(2): 134–145.

121. Puhl R, Brownell KD. Bias, discrimination, and obesity. *Obes Res* 2001; 9(12): 788–805.

122. Wadden TA, Didie E. What's in a name? Patients' preferred terms for describing obesity. *Obes Res* 2003; 11(9): 1140–1146.

123. Reidpath DD, Crawford D, Tilgner L, Gibbons C. Relationship between body mass index and the use of healthcare services in Australia. *Obes Res* 2002; 10(6): 526–531.

124. Bernard GR, Vincent JL, Laterre PF, et al. Efficacy and safety of recombinant human activated protein C for severe sepsis. *N Engl J Med* 2001; 344(10): 699–709.

125. Food and Drug Administration. *Questions and Answers about FDA's Initiative Against Contaminated Weight Loss Products.* FDA; 2010; Available at: http://www.fda.gov/Drugs/ResourcesForYou/Consumers/QuestionsAnswers/ucm136187.htm, accessed October 11, 2010.

126. Food and Drug Administration. Fen-Phen Interim Safety Recommendations 2010; Available at: http://www.fda.gov/Drugs/DrugSafety/Postmarket DrugSafetyInformationforPatientsandProviders/ucm072820.htm, accessed October 10, 2010.

127. Reinberg S. Weight-Loss Drug Meridia Pulled From U.S. Market Bloomberg Business Week [serial on the Internet]. 2010; Available at: http://www.businessweek.com/print/lifestyle/content/healthday/644146.html, accessed October 11, 2010.

CHAPTER 12

The geriatric trauma patient

John M. O'Neill[1,2] and Elan Jeremitsky[1]
[1]Allegheny General Hospital, Pittsburgh, PA, USA
[2]Drexel University College of Medicine, Philadelphia, PA, USA

Introduction and epidemiology

With the aging of the general population [1], emergency physicians will encounter more geriatric patients who have suffered trauma. While the spectrum of trauma can vary from minor to major multisystem injuries, for the emergency physician, the geriatric trauma patient population requires a heightened awareness of complications that can arise and affect emergency department (ED) evaluation, management, and disposition. The combination of pre-existing medical conditions and prescribed medications can blunt the ability of the emergency physician to assess for the presence of worsening hemodynamic parameters in the geriatric trauma patient. As a result, disposition of the geriatric trauma patient can differ from younger trauma patients based on the need for more careful monitoring for physiological decompensation that may not manifest in the typically expected manner of trauma patients experiencing shock [2].

While the number of geriatric trauma patients is on the rise, the exact definition of what constitutes a geriatric patient is not standardized across the trauma literature. Some authors support the use of a functional status rather than age alone, contending that functional status can vary widely among the elderly [3]. There is considerable heterogeneity in the literature in the age ranges that are used to refer to geriatric trauma patients [4]. Ages as young as 45 to as old as 85 have been used to classify this patient population. One study of the Ohio trauma registry found that age 70 was the most appropriate transition point based on overall mortality [2]. Yet, no age or set of co-morbities has been standardized to define a patient as geriatric for the purposes of trauma evaluation.

Local prevalence of geriatric populations vary widely. Florida has 17.2% of its residents aged 65 or over, while Alaska has only 7.6% [5]. Japan's

Challenging and Emerging Conditions in Emergency Medicine, First Edition. Edited by Arvind Venkat.
© 2011 by John Wiley & Sons, Ltd. Published 2011 by Blackwell Publishing Ltd.

overall population is even older with 22.2% of the national population aged 65 or older [6]. A German study found that patients over the age of 60 accounted for 19% of trauma patients in 1996 and 25% of trauma patients in 2006 [7]. Overall, the populations of industrialized countries are aging. As populations age, a greater percentage of patients arriving with traumatic injury will be elderly.

Elderly patients have a greater burden of morbidity and mortality than their younger counterparts. Trauma is the ninth leading cause of death in patients over the age of 65 [8]. Geriatric patients who survive their traumatic events have a decreased life expectancy relative to their uninjured counterparts [9]. They also can account for a greater use of medical resources per capita [10]. The cost of hospitalizing an elderly trauma patient is generally greater than the costs incurred by younger patients [10]. A notable exception to this is in elderly patients with the most severe injuries. The high mortality rate in this cohort accounts for less use of resources [11]. The burden of this extra cost is likely to fall on hospitals as the elderly have relatively low reimbursement rates for trauma care [12, 13].

With this combination of increasing prevalence and potential morbidity and mortality, geriatric trauma represents an emerging and challenging patient population in the ED. This chapter discusses the evaluation and management of the geriatric trauma patient in the ED.

Patient co-morbidities that affect the evaluation of the geriatric trauma patient

As the general population ages, the prevalence of underlying chronic illness has increased [14]. Co-morbidities in the geriatric trauma patient may alter the goals of therapy. A patient's pre-existing conditions and level of function must be considered both in the evaluation of the patient in the ED and in the disposition of the patient. Patients with pre-existing medical conditions and a low baseline level of function are more likely to require placement in a long-term facility after their hospitalization [15]. They may also have a greater in-hospital mortality, suggesting the need for higher acuity monitoring relative to younger patients with similar injuries [16].

Chronic obstructive lung disease
Chronic obstructive lung disease (COPD) is a common disorder in the elderly. It is estimated that 13% of nursing home residents suffer from this ailment [17]. COPD has been associated with increased risk of nosocomial infection after trauma [18]. COPD also predisposes patients to more severe orthopedic injuries from lower energy traumatic mechanisms, as do the steroids, both systemic and inhaled, that may be used to treat this condition [19]. Bone density is reduced in patients with severe COPD [20], but it is not necessarily reduced in patients with moderate COPD [21]. While

published studies to date have not assessed the specific impact of COPD on geriatric trauma patients requiring ventilation, it is prudent to assume that a history of COPD may predispose this population to ventilator-related complications.

Dementia

As of 2007, there are an estimated 3.4 million patients with dementia in the United States [22]. Cognitively impaired geriatric patients fall frequently [23]. The causes of these falls are likely multifactorial. Some of these factors include the cognitive impairment itself, medication use, orthostatic changes, and environmental factors [23]. Many of these factors are not easily modifiable. Demented patients may also have difficulty providing a clear history and cooperating with physical examination in the ED. This causes the emergency physician to rely on imaging, monitoring, and laboratory findings more heavily than in cognitively intact patients.

Body habitus

As of 2008, 37% of men and 34% of women in the United States over the age of 60 were classified as clinically obese based on a body mass index (BMI) greater than 30 [24]. In-hospital mortality has been shown to be seven times higher for all obese adults admitted to the trauma intensive care unit [25]. Elevated BMI is also a risk factor for requiring mechanical ventilation after thoracic trauma [26]. Body habitus can also affect the risk of elderly trauma patient suffering orthopedic injuries. Low BMI has been associated with an increased risk of hip fractures and high BMI with an increased risk of humerus fractures in post-menopausal women [27]. Functional outcomes have not been well documented for the elderly obese trauma patient. Obese patients receiving hip arthroplasty have been found to be able to reach their functional goals as well as their non-obese counterparts, but at a greater cost and length of stay [28].

Diabetes mellitus

As the population ages and the prevalence of obesity increases, there has been a concomitant increase in the prevalence of diabetes mellitus [29]. Diabetes mellitus predisposes patients to injury in a variety of ways. In the later stages of the disease, many patients have decreased vision and decreased sensation in their feet. This loss of sensorium may lead patients to have greater difficulty navigating through their environment. Episodes of hyper- or hypoglycemia may lead patients to have alterations in consciousness or mental status that can lead to injury. Alterations in a diabetic patient's vasculature and immune function may lead to delayed healing or susceptibility to post-traumatic infection.

Hyperglycemia has been associated with poor outcome in trauma patients [30]. There has been considerable investigation in how to best manage the blood glucose in critically ill patients. In the past, intensive insulin therapy with tight glucose control has been the standard of care. This approach has not been shown to improve outcomes in the general critically ill population [31] nor in critically ill trauma patients [32,33]. Intensive insulin therapy has been shown to increase the frequency of hypoglycemia [31–33]. It is reasonable to avoid extremes in blood glucose in critically ill trauma patients.

Cardiovascular disease

Geriatric trauma patients with coronary artery disease or congestive heart failure present their own set of challenges to the emergency physician. Patients with congestive heart failure may have difficulty managing the large amount of intravenous fluids that trauma patients may receive. Patients with coronary artery disease may have difficulty adapting to the increased demand for cardiac output that the stress of a trauma may place on the body [34]. Patients over the age of 50 who have sustained blunt trauma to the chest wall are at a much higher risk for in-hospital mortality [35]. Patients with cardiovascular disease may also be on medications that alter coagulation, platelet aggregation, or the ability to appropriately elevate the heart rate. As such, geriatric trauma patients taking these medications may be predisposed to hemorrhagic injury from minor mechanisms and may also not manifest the typical vital sign abnormalities that accompany hypovolemic shock in younger patients [36].

Polypharmacy

Geriatric patients are more likely to be on numerous medications related to age-related illness. As alluded to above, these medications can affect the assessment and management of geriatric trauma patients. Table 12.1 outlines commonly prescribed medications in the elderly that can affect their ED trauma evaluation and management.

Substance abuse

Geriatric patients are not immune to the ills that plague other segments of society. Alcohol ingestion is not uncommon in geriatric trauma patients, and if a patient is found to have alcohol present in their system, they are likely to have levels above the legal limit for intoxication [43]. Alcohol screening by hospital staff using history and physical exam has been shown to be inaccurate [44]. Alcohol testing is not always universal in geriatric trauma patients, and using the data set of those who are tested may not be a reliable approximation of the population at large. Geriatric patients

Table 12.1 Commonly prescribed medications in the elderly that affect ED trauma evaluation and management

---

Beta-blockers/calcium-channel blockers/digoxin: Can blunt cardiac response to hypovolemia [36]

Platelet inhibitors: Bleeding complications, especially in head trauma [37]

Narcotic pain medications: Pre-trauma use can prevent adequate pain control without side effects

Statins: Possible protective effects concerning fractures; mixed effects on overall morbidity/mortality following major trauma [38–41]

Corticosteroids: May cause osteoporosis, delayed wound healing, and adrenal suppression [19]

Warfarin: Bleeding complications, especially in head trauma [37, 42]

---

who test positive for alcohol ingestion are more prone to falls [45]. A postmortem study of all fatal ground-level fall patients, regardless of age, found that alcohol changes the pattern, frequency, and severity of injury [46].

Depression and suicidal ideation

A retrospective review by Crandall et al. of the National Trauma Data Bank examined risk factors and outcomes for patients over the age of 65 admitted to the trauma service for attempted suicide. Geriatric trauma patients who present with suicide attempts are likely to be white males, insured, use a firearm, and have at least one medical co-morbidity. They are commonly found to be positive for alcohol or illicit drugs, though less commonly than younger patients who attempt suicide. They are unlikely to have a history of pre-existing psychiatric illness. Their injury severity score is likely to be high. Geriatric suicide attempt patients are twice as likely to die, and those who survive are half as likely to be discharged home [47].

Delirium

Acute delirium is not uncommon in geriatric trauma patients. The etiology of this is likely multifactorial. The trauma itself, necessary interventional procedures and the chaotic environment of the ambulance, helicopter, or ED trauma bay are factors that are not easily modifiable. Acute delirium may be exacerbated by benzodiazepines or opiates [48]. Trauma physicians often request the assistance of other services in treating pain in geriatric patients [49]. The emergency physician should likewise assist the trauma service in the balance of treating the patient's pain while being mindful of the effects that the medications may have on the patient's mental status. Nerve blocks, fostering a calm environment, anchoring the patient with direct communication with the staff or family, avoidance of overstimulation, and judicious use of systemic medications all may help in preventing delirium in the elderly trauma patient [50].

Emergency department management of the geriatric trauma patient

Prehospital management

The earliest interventions in the care of the geriatric trauma patient occur on scene and en route to the hospital. These interventions are provided by local emergency medical services (EMS). Counterintuitively, elderly patients are less likely to be brought to a level-1 trauma center or have the trauma team activated than their younger counterparts with equal severity of injury [51, 52]. One potential cause of this disparity is that the vital signs that younger patients can mount in the presence of severe physical stress may be blunted in older patients. In patients over the age of 65, blood pressure and heart rate have not been shown to predict severe injury [51]. A chronically hypertensive patient may be physiologically hypotensive despite a normal blood pressure reading. Those taking β-blockers or other medications that cause bradycardia may not be able to mount a tachycardic response despite significant volume loss [53, 54]. In order to curtail the frequency of geriatric patients being under triaged, the National Expert Panel on Field Triage includes age greater than 55 as a special criteria to consider when evaluating a patient. EMS providers may up-triage an older patient who does not meet the physiologic, anatomic, or mechanistic criteria for treatment at a level-1 trauma center. Proper triage is especially important in the elderly. Under-triaged patients over the age of 65 have a significantly higher rate of in-hospital mortality, disability, and overall complications [52].

Airway management

For many geriatric patients, a major trauma requires the placement of a definitive airway. Geriatric patients might be wearing dentures, which may be helpful in establishing a seal during bag-valve mask ventilation as long as they are properly secured and not dislodged by the procedure. Dentures should be removed prior to intubation, so that the physician's view is not obstructed by them. Care should be taken in positioning and stabilizing the cervical spine during intubation of the geriatric trauma patient. Degenerative changes may be present that make the patient more vulnerable to spinal injury, more difficult to properly position, and less tolerant of motion. The combination of age and limited cervical spine mobility is a predictor for difficult intubation [55]. Decreased mouth size and an anteriorly positioned glottis may also be encountered.

When intubating a geriatric trauma patient, the emergency physician should consider the medications and dosing used. Vecuronium or other relatively long-acting paralytics may have prolonged effects. A shorter acting agent such as succinylcholine or rocuronium may be a better choice for paralytic agent during rapid sequence intubation, and no age-based dose adjustments are needed [56]. Defasciculating doses of non-depolarizing agents should not be used when using succinylcholine as they have been shown to decrease oxygen saturation in elderly patients prior to intubation [57]. The doses of etomidate or benzodiazepines may be reduced in the geriatric patient and still achieve appropriate levels of sedation [56]. The effects of ketamine may be prolonged in geriatric trauma patients [56]. In the authors' experience, etomidate and succinylcholine are an effective induction combination with predictable effects on the geriatric trauma patient. Midazolam in small boluses or in a drip may then be used to keep the patient sedated while on the ventilator.

Vital signs assessment and determination of need for further resuscitation

Trauma resuscitation has classically relied heavily on vital signs to guide the need for intervention and to define resuscitative end points. A seminal article by Scalea et al. posited that since vital signs are not always indicative of underlying shock in geriatric multiple system blunt trauma patients, and that early invasive monitoring can better guide the resuscitation [58]. A combination of laboratory markers, such as lactate levels and arterial base deficit, in addition to invasive monitoring for cardiac output and oxygen delivery, should be used to direct the resuscitation [59].

Initial arterial base deficit and lactate levels can be used to indicate that the geriatric trauma patient needs further resuscitation. These markers may also be used to assess the patient's response to the resuscitative interventions and potential prognosis. Use of changes in the base deficit over time in addition to the initial sample strengthens the marker's ability to predict outcome in geriatric trauma patients [59].

The arterial base deficit may be altered by most factors that affect the anion gap, which must be taken into account when interpreting the results [59]. A patient may have a hyperchloremic non-anion gap acidosis from resuscitation with normal saline, dropping the total bicarbonate, and increasing the base deficit. The presence of alcohol intoxication decreases the test's specificity as the initial base deficit may be elevated from intoxication alone [59].

Use of invasive monitoring to assess cardiac output and oxygen delivery has been shown to be of more value in assisting in patient prognosis rather than as a tool to guide therapy. Supranormal levels, rather than simply attaining normal levels, of cardiac output and oxygen delivery have been shown to increase the trauma patient's chance of survival. This is only true if the patient is able to reach these supranormal levels on their own with standard supportive care. Interventions designed to cause the patient to reach these levels have not been shown to improve patient outcome. Mixed venous oxygen saturation has been shown to be a useful marker to guide resuscitation in septic patients, but it has not been shown to be helpful in trauma patients [59]. Proposed triggers for the initiation of early invasive monitoring in geriatric trauma patients include any sign of shock, an elevated arterial base deficit greater than 11 in patients with elevated injury severity scores or the presence of pre-existing cardiac disease or cardiac risk factors [60]. Other markers such as tissue or subcutaneous oxygenation have been studied with inconclusive results [59].

Physical examination

As with vital signs, there are limitations to the utility of the physical examination in the assessment of the geriatric trauma patient. Tenderness on examination may be reduced in geriatric trauma patients. The reduced reliablitiy of the physical exam compels the physician to rely more on imaging to exclude the presence of injury. Serial FAST examinations, especially in the presence of hypotension, are useful in rapidly determining whether acute surgical intervention is required in a geriatric trauma patient [61].

Imaging evaluation

CT imaging is useful in the geriatric trauma patient as it is in the general population. However, its use should be weighed by the emergency physician in the context of risk factors that accompany this testing. Deunk et al. found that age greater than 55 alone was not an independent predictor for intra-abdominal injury to be diagnosed on CT [62]. Intravenous contrast allows imaging of the vasculature and better defines injuries to solid and hollow organs, but it does carry some risk. Geriatric patients have an increased frequency of contrast-induced nephropathy (CIN). In one study, CIN was present in 1 in 5 patients over the age of 75, though none of these patients died or needed in-hospital dialysis [63]. A patient's age, presence of diabetes, heart failure, or other pre-existing conditions should be taken into account when making the decision to use intravenous contrast [64].

Cervical spine evaluation requires special attention in geriatric trauma patients [65]. The Canadian C-spine Rule excludes patients over the age of 65 from clinical clearance. The NEXUS criteria do not have any age cutoff, but care should still be taken when foregoing cervical spine imaging in those over the age of 65 [66]. CT imaging is the evaluation method of choice, and it may be appropriate to obtain such imaging even in geriatric patients with low-energy traumatic mechanisms. Cervical spine fractures in the elderly, whether isolated or associated with other injuries, have a high level of associated morbidity and mortality [65]. The atlanto–occipital complex and the upper cervical spine is especially vulnerable to injury in patients over the age of 75 or those who fall from standing [67].

Assessment of the geriatric trauma patient on anticoagulation

An area of special consideration when assessing geriatric trauma patients is whether the individual is taking anticoagulation medications. Evidence on the effect of anticoagulation on trauma outcome is somewhat contradictory. Multitrauma patients on warfarin, aspirin, or clopidogrel do not have increased mortality in the absence of an intracranial injury [68]. Kirsch et al. showed that warfarin use in geriatric orthopedic trauma patients was associated with prolonged hospital stay, number of units of transfused blood products given, and longer delays to surgery [69]. Intracranial injury in the presence of warfarin is a strong predictor of mortality [42]. For all head trauma patients, age greater than 70 and elevated International Normalized Ratio (INR) is associated with increased mortality [42]. A study of patients on anticoagulation and/or antiplatelet therapy with minor head trauma (GCS 15) showed results disparate from studies that included minor and major head trauma. In patients suffering only minor head trauma, external evidence of head injury, age, type of medication (warfarin or clopidogrel), and INR were not predictive of intracranial hemorrhage. Loss of consciousness was a significant marker and had a high positive predictive value, but the absence of a loss of consciousness could not be used to rule out the presence of intracranial bleeding [37]. A study by Cohen et al. found that INR elevation was a predictor of delayed or occult intracranial bleeding. The authors recommend that all patients on warfarin with any kind of head trauma receive a head CT and that those with supratherapeutic levels be admitted for a period observation and possible repeat head CT at 12–18 hours, but this has not been validated in general ED practice [70]. While the degree of risk posed by the use of warfarin in geriatric patients who have suffered head injury is debated, it does seem prudent based on this evidence for emergency physicians to have a low threshold for obtaining CT imaging in this patient population. The determination of whether to admit the geriatric trauma patient on anticoagulation with no evidence of intracranial injury on CT is one that should be based on the specific characteristics of the individual and their social support.

Patients on warfarin who require rapid reversal of their anticoagulated state can be treated in several ways. Fresh frozen plasma (FFP) may be used but it requires a large volume, usually dosed at 15 mL/kg. FFP also needs to be thawed prior to use, and many centers do not have pre-thawed FFP available for immediate use. Factor IX may not be adequately replaced by standard dosing of FFP. For these reasons, prothrombin complex concentrate (PCC), a combination of factors II, VII, IX, and X, is often used and in limited studies has been shown to be superior to FFP [71, 72]. Recombinant factor VIIa has also been used in combination with FFP to reverse warfarin. Large studies still need to be done to compare the relative efficacy and safety profile of FFP versus PCC versus recombinant factor VIIa [73]. Head injury patients with an intracranial hemorrhage and on antiplatelet therapy have been shown to be at increased risk of mortality [74]. Downey et al. found no improvement in mortality by the administration of platelets to geriatric trauma patients receiving antiplatelet medications who have suffered head injuries [75].

When faced with an injured patient who is on anticoagulation or antiplatelet therapy and is not to be admitted to the hospital, the emergency physician must consider the risk and benefits of continuing the therapy. Factors to be considered include the mechanism of injury and whether it might recur, the patient's behavior or home environment and the likely benefits from continued therapy. Consultation with the physician originally prescribing these medications is imperative if discontinuation of these therapies is to be considered.

Disposition of the geriatric trauma patient from the ED

When a geriatric trauma patient has been determined to be fit for discharge from the ED, the emergency physician must consider the type of facility and resources to which the patient has access. If the patient is to return to the home environment, many factors must first be considered (Table 12.2). The types of facilities used to house the elderly are varied, and the patient should be discharged to a facility that can provide the appropriate level of care. Facilities range from minimal intervention and monitoring to long-term acute care facilities that provide services similar to a standard hospital. The emergency physician should be familiar with the resources that the local facilities have and clarify with the facility when unsure.

Table 12.2 Factors to consider before a geriatric trauma patient can be discharged from the ED

Does the patient need someone to get needed items (food, toiletries, etc.) from outside the home?

Are there steps or other physical impediments in the home?

Has the patient's level of function changed such that they are no longer able to safely operate their mobility equipment (crutches, walker, wheelchair, scooter)?

Is the patient able to access the bathroom or commode in a safe manner?

Does the patient need to be monitored or assisted by a caregiver in any other way?

During what portion of the day will the patient need a caregiver?

Can the family or social services meet this need?

End of life care of the geriatric trauma patient

Other types of disease may have varying time courses that allow a patient and their family to make end of life decisions over time. The instantaneous, violent nature of major trauma often precludes such consideration. The patient and family suddenly find themselves in a situation that they did not expect and for which they are not prepared. End of life issues and decisions about withdrawal of care may arise in the ED in the severely injured geriatric trauma patient. Unfortunately, the patient's direct wishes are often not known or well documented [76]. Emergency physicians must be mindful that the way they portray the patient's physical condition and prognosis goes a long way towards directing the course of action that the patient or their family decides to take.

Mechanisms of trauma and injury patterns in geriatric trauma patients

Falls

Falls are extremely common in the geriatric population. A study by Sterling et al. found that for patients over the age of 65, injury severity and the mortality rate was much higher for all types of falls when compared to the younger cohort. This was especially true in ground-level falls. The types of injury were also different, with head, chest, and pelvis injuries overrepresented in the geriatric group [77]. Geriatric patients with even minor fall mechanisms should be assessed for the presence of serious internal injury.

In order to decrease the number of geriatric falls, many groups have devised strategies for fall prevention in the elderly. The Centers for Disease Control has published a collection of some of the most efficacious strategies. Exercise, home safety evaluation, and multifaceted interventions are discussed [78]. One of the simplest things an emergency physician can do after seeing a geriatric patient who has fallen or is at risk of falling is to refer the patient to one of these types of programs. Be mindful that though there are many effective interventions, there are others that have not been shown to be [79]. Further research needs to be conducted to assess whether and what type of interventions the emergency physician can use to prevent the recurrence of falls.

Motor vehicle accidents

The patterns of injury sustained in a motor vehicle accident can vary widely based on the point of impact, intrusion into the vehicle, and the type of safety devices installed. According to the National Household Travel Survey, elderly drivers are more likely to be driving older cars, which are less likely to have the modern safety features installed. It is a common misconception that larger, heavier, older cars are generally safer than modern vehicles [80].

Studies show that patients over the age of 65 who sustain a major trauma from a motor vehicle accident are more likely to have head and chest injuries than younger patients [81]. Blunt thoracic aortic injury has been shown to be more common and occur with less forceful impacts than in younger patients [82]. The frequency of lower extremity injury patterns were not found to be associated with age in one study, but younger patients under the age of 35 or older patients over the age of 65 were found to have more hip and thigh fractures and less foot and ankle fractures than their middle-aged counterparts [83].

Working with elderly drivers injured in motor vehicle accidents may lead one to speculate on the wisdom of elderly persons driving. Should licensing authorities restrict the ability of older patients to drive? What kind of interventions should the emergency physician take? A review of the National Household Travel Survey found that the very elderly, those over the age of 85, are disproportionally more likely to die in a fatal car accident when driving, per mile driven. Most vulnerable are drivers who drive infrequently and take short trips. They are much more likely to cause their own fatality than kill others involved in the accident. Young inexperienced drivers are much more likely to cause harm to others on the road [84]. The overall odds of death in patients over the age of 85, regardless of who was driving, are 11 times greater than younger patients aged 25–44 [85]. The emergency physician should take all these facts into account when counseling geriatric patients and their families on the risks of continued driving after trauma.

Pedestrian struck

There have been many safety advances in car design to prevent injuries to pedestrians since this first entered the public consciousness in 1965 [86]. Alterations to the angling of the bumpers and placement of the light fixtures, emblems, and wipers have been made to lessen the injury if a pedestrian is struck by the front of the vehicle. Crosswalks and pedestrian lights at intersections have been placed to help keep down the number of pedestrian injuries. Demetriades et al. found that head, chest, abdomen, and pelvic injuries are all more common in patients over the age of 65 struck by a motor vehicle. Injury severity and mortality was also greatly elevated in this group with a total mortality of 25% [87].

Burns

Elderly burn patients are difficult to manage for a variety of reasons. Skin thickness is often reduced in the elderly, and poor skin turgor may lead to increased skin edema [88]. Cardiovascular reserve may also be reduced in geriatric trauma patients, and they have difficulty meeting the increased physiologic demand [89]. This combination of increased fluid demands, due to increased third spacing in the skin, and the decreased ability of the cardiovascular system to tolerate the large volume of fluids required may lead geriatric burn patients to require early ventilator support [89]. Geriatric burn patients who arrive to the ED intubated, independent of the reason for intubation, have a high rate of mortality [90]. Elderly trauma patients in general are prone to nosocomial infections, and burn patients should be monitored closely for this complication [91].

Hospital length of stay over percentage of body surface area burned is much longer for patients over the age of 65. Mortality is also much higher in patients over the age of 65. Elderly burn patients, like their younger counterparts, most frequently die from lung injury or sepsis. A large percentage of elderly patients also die from cardiac events and renal failure [89]. Aggressive fluid resuscitation, early interventions for cardiovascular and ventilatory support, and efforts to minimize superinfection should be implemented in the ED.

Subdural hematoma

Elderly patients with head trauma are vulnerable to subdural hemorrhage (Figure 12.1). The pathologic explanation for this is the increased length

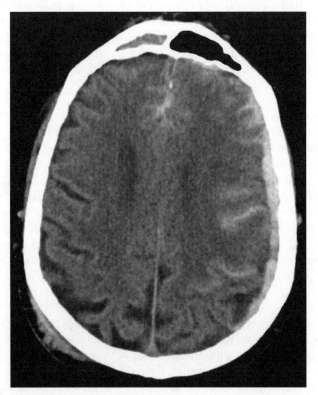

Figure 12.1 CT image of subdural hematoma.

of the bridging veins as the brain atrophies with age and is pulled further from the inner surface of the skull [92]. Acute subdural hematomas often occur in the presence of other injuries. For isolated subdural hemorrhage alone, the most important factors affecting prognosis are the size of any midline shift rather than the size of the bleed itself [92]. Elderly patients may have increased cerebral atrophy that may allow for a larger volume of hemorrhage prior to a parenchymal shift [93].

Spinal fracture

Geriatric patients may have vertebral structural deficiencies that leave them more vulnerable in the face of trauma to injury due to a multitude of factors. Osteoporosis, metastatic changes, and degenerative changes may all alter the structure of the spine. There have been no clinical rules even for young patients to assess the stability of the thoracic or lumbar spine. Any elderly patient with a mechanism of injury that places the thoracolumbar spine at risk should be evaluated both clinically and radiographically.

Elderly trauma patients frequently injure their cervical spine (Figure 12.2). The upper cervical spine is more frequently injured than the lower. Falls and motor vehicle collisions are the most common mechanisms of injury [67]. Cervical spine injuries carry a heavy burden of morbidity and

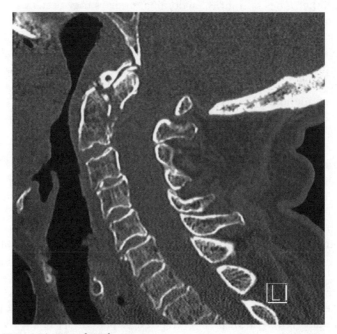

Figure 12.2 CT image of C2 fracture.

mortality [94]. Definitive treatment is more often surgical in patients over the age of 65 as these patients often respond poorly to the halo-vest immobilization [95].

Rib fracture

The chest wall becomes less compliant with age. Thoracic trauma in these patients may lead to rib fractures. Rib fractures in those over the age of 65 show an increased hospital length of stay, pneumonia risk, and overall mortality. This is especially true for isolated rib fractures that are rarely fatal to younger patients, but have been found to have mortality rates of 15% for patients over the age of 65. These patients are more likely to die of respiratory failure or sepsis than their younger counterparts [96]. Measurement of geriatric rib fracture patients' forced vital capacity at presentation and before intervention has been shown to be associated with length of hospital stay [97]. These measurements should be taken before any interventions, such as bronchodilators or bilevel positive airway pressure (BiPAP), are initiated. Patients over the age of 65 must be worked up aggressively for rib fractures as even a low-energy trauma can result in fractures and the potential for morbidity and mortality that comes with them.

Blunt abdominal trauma

As with other types of injuries, abdominal injuries may occur with lower impact trauma in the elderly. In the past, geriatric trauma patients were thought to respond worse than younger patients when treated non-operatively for solid organ injury. Management of intra-abdominal traumatic injuries in geriatric patients no longer differs significantly from that of the population at large. Markers of significant injury on CT scan or FAST examination, signs of hemodynamic instability, and response to non-operative management all play a role in deciding when these patients should go to the operating room [98].

Penetrating trauma

Penetrating trauma only accounts for 5%–10% of elderly trauma patients [99, 100]. Patients over the age of 65 who sustain penetrating traumatic injuries have poorer outcomes than do younger patients, though the excess morbidity and mortality is less than that of blunt trauma [101]. The worsening in outcomes may be due to pre-existing co-morbidities as well as age itself [100, 101]. Requirements of intensive care and overall length of stay is increased in older patients [100]. Still, most elderly penetrating trauma patients recover to the point where they can be discharged home [100]. This combination of factors suggests that emergency physicians should view geriatric penetrating trauma patients as a high-risk population requiring aggressive intervention and surgical consultation.

Extremity fracture

Fractures of the wrist and ankle are most common in patients over the age of 65 and under the age 70. As patients age beyond 70, hip fractures begin to predominate. Proximal humerus fractures are also common. Caucasian patients have a greater frequency of fractures than African-American patients. Patients sustaining a humerus or radius fracture over the age of 50 are at an increased risk of a future hip fracture [102].

Lacerations

Elderly patients with thin skin are at risk of skin tears. Skin tears are classified into three different categories. Category I, in which there is no tissue loss, can be reapproximated using steri-strips or similar type of surgical tape. Wound adhesives may also be used. Stitching or stapling these wounds is usually not effective, in that the skin will tear around the sutures. In category II wounds, a portion of tissue is lost. In category III, all of the skin has been removed, and the wound cannot be completely approximated. There are a variety of absorbent dressings, such as petroleum jelly or silicone dressings, which can be used. The dressings should be placed in layers with daily dressing changes of the outer layers and weekly of the inner [103].

The next five years

As the population ages over time, the frequency of geriatric trauma will surely increase. Trauma guidelines for their care in the field and the ED must adapt to care for this vulnerable group. The Eastern Association for the Surgery of Trauma Guidelines for Geriatric Trauma care was last updated in 2001 and will likely be revised in the near future [104]. Regional EMS guidelines vary, but guidelines specifically designed for the care of the geriatric trauma patient are now in place or in development in different regions.

In response to this change in population, how we teach physicians and other care providers must evolve as well. There is now a consensus proposal for the addition of specific geriatric core competencies, including care of geriatric trauma, to the emergency medicine residency core curriculum [105]. The Advanced Trauma Life Support course provided by the American College of Surgeons includes a section devoted to the care of geriatric trauma patients [106]. The National Highway Traffic and Safety Administration has created a Geriatric Education for EMS course, which includes a section on geriatric trauma [107]. With the dissemination of these teaching tools, awareness and treatment of geriatric trauma will likely increase and be more standardized, respectively.

Future research should be undertaken with more uniform definitions for what defines a geriatric patient. Further work in the areas of prognostic indicators, markers for effectiveness of resuscitation measures, and trauma prevention strategies will also likely progress geriatric trauma care. The treatment of geriatric trauma patients using a multidisciplinary approach from scene to final disposition is becoming better defined, and emergency physicians will play a vital role in the management of these patients.

Conclusion

With the aging of the general population, ED care of the elderly will become more common. Geriatric trauma represents a growing subset of care of the elderly that requires close consideration of the pre-injury medical conditions, prescribed medications, and differences in presentation and prognosis from the young. Close collaboration between emergency physicians, primary care providers, and trauma surgeons will aid in the careful management of this emerging and challenging patient population.

References

1. World population aging 2007. UN department of Economic and Social Affairs, Population division.
2. Martin JT, Alkhoury F, O'Connor JA, Kyriakides TC, Bonadies JA. 'Normal' vital signs belie occult hypoperfusion in geriatric trauma patients. *Am Surg* 2010; 76(1): 65–69.
3. Ensrud KE, Ewing SK, Cawthon PM, et al. A comparison of frailty indexes for the prediction of falls, disability, fractures, and mortality in older men. *J Am Geriatr Soc* 2009 ; 57(3): 492–498.
4. Caterino JM, Valasek T, Werman HA. Identification of an age cutoff for increased mortality in patients with elderly trauma. *Am J Emerg Med* 2010; 28(2): 151–158.
5. US Census Bureau GCT-T4-R. Percent of the total population who are 65 years and over (geographies ranked by estimate) Data Set: 2009 Population Estimates.
6. CIA World Factbook. https://www.cia.gov/library/publications/the-world-factbook/geos/ja.html, July 2010 Est, accessed October 1, 2010.
7. Wutzler S, Lefering R, Laurer HL, Walcher F, Wyen H, Marzi I. Changes in geriatric traumatology. An analysis of 14,869 patients from the German Trauma Registry. *Unfallchirurg* 2008; 111(8): 592–598.
8. Heron M. Deaths: leading causes for 2006. *National Vital Statistics Reports* 2010; 58(14): 1–100.
9. Gubler K, Davis R, Koepsell T, Soderberg R, Maier R, Rivara F. Long-term survival of elderly trauma patients. *Arch Surg* 1997; 132(9): 1010–1014.
10. McKevitt EC, Calvert E, Ng A, et al. Geriatric trauma: resource use and patient outcomes. *Can J Surg* 2003; 46(3): 211.
11. Taylor MD, Tracy JK, Meyer W, Pasquale M, Napolitano LM. Trauma in the elderly: intensive care unit resource use and outcome. *J Trauma* 2002; 53(3): 407–414.

12. Sartorelli KH, Rogers FB, Osler TM, Shackford SR, Cohen M, Vane DW. Financial aspects of providing trauma care at the extremes of life. *J Trauma* 1999; 46(3): 483–487.

13. Newell M, Rotondo M, Toschlog E, Waibel B, Sagraves S, Schenarts P, Bard M, Goettler C. The elderly trauma patient: an investment for the future? *J Trauma* 2009; 67(2): 337–340.

14. Vogeli C, Shields AE, Lee TA, et al. Multiple chronic conditions: prevalence, health consequences, and implications for quality, care management, and costs. *J Gen Intern Med* 2007; 22(3 Suppl.): 391–395.

15. Aitken LM, Burmeister E, Lang J, Chaboyer W, Richmond TS. Characteristics and outcomes of injured older adults after hospital admission. *J Am Geriatr Soc* 2010; 58(3): 442–449.

16. Grossman M, Miller D, Scaff D, Arcona S. When is an elder old? Effect of pre-existing conditions on mortality in geriatric trauma. *J Trauma* 2002; 52(2): 242–246.

17. Center for disease Control and Prevention. Available at: http://www.cdc.gov/nchs/data/nnhsd/Estimates/nnhs/Estimates_Diagnoses_Tables.pdf#Table33b, accessed June 2009.

18. Bochicchio G, Joshi M, Knorr K, Scalea, T. Impact of nosocomial infections in trauma: does age make a difference? *J Trauma* 2001; 50(4): 612–619.

19. Hubbard R, Tattersfield A, Smith C, West J, Smeeth L, Fletcher A. Use of inhaled corticosteroids and the risk of fracture. *Chest* 2006; 130(4): 1082–1088.

20. Vrieze A, de Greef M, Wýkstra P, Wempe J. Low bone mineral density in COPD patients related to worse lung function, low weight and decreased fat-free mass. *Osteoporosis Int* 2007; 18(9): 1197–1202.

21. Karadag F, Cildag O, Yurekli Y, Gurgey O. Should COPD patients be routinely evaluated for bone mineral density? *J Bone Miner Metab* 2003; 21(4): 242–246.

22. Plassman BL, Langa KM, Fisher GG, et al. Prevalence of dementia in the United States: the aging, demographics, and memory study. *Neuroepidemiology* 2007; 29(1–2): 125–132.

23. Kallin K, Gustafson Y, Sandman PO, Karlsson S. Factors associated with falls among older, cognitively impaired people in geriatric care settings: a population-based study. *Am J Geriatr Psychiatry* 2005; 13(6): 501–509.

24. Flegal K, Carroll M, Ogden C, Curtin L. Prevalence and trends in obesity among US adults, 1999–2008. *JAMA* 2010; 303(3): 235–241.

25. Bochicchio GV, Joshi M, Bochicchio K, Nehman S, Tracy JK, Scalea TM. Impact of obesity in the critically ill trauma patient: a prospective study. *J Am Coll Surg* 2006; 203(4): 533–538.

26. Reiff DA, Hipp G, McGwin G Jr, Modjarrad K, MacLennan PA, Rue LW 3rd. Body mass index affects the need for and the duration of mechanical ventilation after thoracic trauma. *J Trauma* 2007; 62(6): 1432–1435.

27. Gnudi S, Sitta E, Lisi L. Relationship of body mass index with main limb fragility fractures in post-menopausal women. *J Bone Miner Metab* 2009; 27(4): 479–484.

28. Vincent HK, Weng JP, Vincent KR. Effect of obesity on inpatient rehabilitation outcomes after total hip arthroplasty. *Obesity (Silver Spring)* 2007; 15(2): 522–530.

29. Sloan FA, Bethel MA, Ruiz D Jr, Shea AM, Feinglos MN. The growing burden of diabetes mellitus in the US elderly population. *Arch Intern Med* 2008; 168(2): 192–199.

30. Wahl WL, Taddonio M, Maggio PM, Arbabi S, Hemmila MR. Mean glucose values predict trauma patient mortality. *J Trauma* 2008; 65(1): 42–47.

31. Marik PE, Preiser JC. Toward understanding tight glycemic control in the ICU: a systematic review and metaanalysis. *Chest* 2010; 137(3): 544–551.

32. Coester A, Neumann CR, Schmidt MI. Intensive insulin therapy in severe traumatic brain injury: a randomized trial. *J Trauma* 2010; 68(4): 904–911.

33. Aldawood AS, Tamim HM, Alsultan MA, Rishu AH, Arabi YM. Intensive insulin therapy versus conventional insulin therapy for critically ill trauma patients admitted to ICU. *Middle East J Anesthesiol* 2010; 20(5): 659–666.

34. Chong CP, Lam QT, Ryan JE, Sinnappu RN, Lim WK. Incidence of postoperative troponin I rises and 1-year mortality after emergency orthopaedic surgery in older patients. *Age Ageing* 2009; 38(2): 168–174.

35. Harrington DT, Phillips B, Machan J, et al. Factors associated with survival following blunt chest trauma in older patients: results from a large regional trauma cooperative. *Arch Surg* 2010; 145(5): 432–437.

36. Arbabi S, Campion EM, Hemmila MR, et al. Beta-blocker use is associated with improved outcomes in adult trauma patients. *J Trauma* 2007; 62(1): 56–61.

37. Brewer ES, Reznikov B, Liberman RF, Baker RA, Rosenblatt MS, David CA, Flacke S. Incidence and predictors of intracranial hemorrhage after minor head trauma in patients taking anticoagulant and antiplatelet medication. *J Trauma* 2010. [Epub ahead of print]

38. Bauer DC, Mundy GR, Jamal SA, et al. Use of statins and fracture: results of 4 prospective studies and cumulative meta-analysis of observational studies and controlled trials. *Arch Intern Med* 2004; 164(2): 146–152.

39. Neal MD, Cushieri J, Rosengart MR, Alarcon LH, Moore EE, Maier RV. Preinjury statin use is associated with a higher risk of multiple organ failure after injury: a propensity score adjusted analysis. *J Trauma* 2009; 67(3): 476–482.

40. Redelmeier DA, Naylor CD, Brenneman FD, Sharkey PW, Juurlink DN. Major trauma in elderly adults receiving lipid-lowering medications. *J Trauma* 2001; 50(4): 678–683.

41. Efron DT, Sorock G, Haut ER, et al. Preinjury statin use is associated with improved in-hospital survival in elderly trauma patients. *J Trauma* 2008; 64(1): 66–73.

42. Mina AA, Bair HA, Howells GA, Bendick PJ. Complications of preinjury warfarin use in the trauma patient. *J Trauma* 2003; 54(5): 842–847.

43. Selway JS, Soderstrom CA, Kufera JA. Alcohol use and testing among older trauma victims in Maryland. *J Trauma* 2008; 65(2): 442–446.

44. Gentilello LM, Villaveces A, Ries RR, et al. Detection of acute alcohol intoxication and chronic alcohol dependence by trauma center staff. *J Trauma* 1999 ; 47(6): 1131–1135.

45. Zautcke JL, Coker SB Jr, Morris RW, Stein-Spencer L. Geriatric trauma in the State of Illinois: substance use and injury patterns. *Am J Emerg Med* 2002; 20(1): 14–17.

46. Thierauf A, Preuss J, Lignitz E, Madea B. Retrospective analysis of fatal falls. *Forensic Sci Int* 2010; 198(1–3): 92–96.

47. Crandall M, Luchette F, Esposito TJ, West M, Shapiro M, Bulger E. Attempted suicide and the elderly trauma patient: risk factors and outcomes. *J Trauma* 2007; 62(4): 1021–1027.

48. Pandharipande P, Cotton BA, Shintani A, et al. Prevalence and risk factors for development of delirium in surgical and trauma intensive care unit patients. *J Trauma* 2008; 65(1): 34–41.

49. Fallon WF Jr, Rader E, Zyzanski S, et al. Geriatric outcomes are improved by a geriatric trauma consultation service. *J Trauma* 2006; 61(5): 1040–1046.

50. Robinson S, Vollmer C, Jirka H, Rich C, Midiri C, Bisby D. Aging and delirium: too much or too little pain medication? *Pain Manag Nurs* 2008; 9(2): 66–72.

51. Lehmann R, Beekley A, Casey L, Salim A, Martin M. The impact of advanced age on trauma triage decisions and outcomes: a statewide analysis. *Am J Surg* 2009; 197(5): 571–574.

52. Sasser SM, Hunt RC, Sullivent EE, et al. Guidelines for field triage of injured patients: Recommendations of the National Expert Panel on Field Triage. *MMWR Recomm Rep* 2009; 58(RR-1): 1–35.

53. Wonisch M, Hofmann P, Fruhwald FM, Kraxner W, Hödl R, Pokan R, Klein W. Influence of beta-blocker use on percentage of target heart rate exercise prescription. *Eur J Cardiovasc Prev Rehabil* 2003; 10(4): 296–301.

54. Taniguchi T, Kurita A, Yamamoto K, Inaba H. Effects of carvedilol on mortality and inflammatory responses to severe hemorrhagic shock in rats. *Shock* 2009; 32(3): 272–275.

55. Mashour GA, Stallmer ML, Kheterpal S, Shanks A. Predictors of difficult intubation in patients with cervical spine limitations. *J Neurosurg Anesthesiol* 2008; 20(2): 110–115.

56. Lewis MC, Abouelenin K, Paniagua M. Geriatric trauma: special considerations in the anesthetic management of the injured elderly patient. *Anesthesiol Clin* 2007; 25(1): 75–90.

57. Aziz L, Jahangir SM, Choudhury SN, Rahman K, Ohta Y, Hirakawa M. The effect of priming with vecuronium and rocuronium on young and elderly patients. *Anesth Analg* 1997; 85(3): 663–666.

58. Scalea TM, Simon HM, Duncan AO, et al. Geriatric blunt multiple trauma: improved survival with early invasive monitoring. *J Trauma* 1990; 30(2): 129–134.

59. Tisherman SA, Barie P, Bokhari F, et al. Clinical practice guideline: endpoints of resuscitation. *J Trauma* 2004; 57(4): 898–912.

60. Friese RS, Shafi S, Gentilello LM. Pulmonary artery catheter use is associated with reduced mortality in severely injured patients: a National Trauma Data Bank analysis of 53,312 patients. *Crit Care Med* 2006; 34(6): 1597–1601.

61. Callaway DW, Wolfe R. Geriatric trauma. *Emerg Med Clin North Am* 2007; 25(3): 837–860.

62. Deunk J, Brink M, Dekker HM, et al. Predictors for the selection of patients for abdominal CT after blunt trauma: a proposal for a diagnostic algorithm. *Ann Surg* 2010; 251(3): 512–520.

63. Hipp A, Desai S, Lopez C, Sinert R. The incidence of contrast-induced nephropathy in trauma patients. *Eur J Emerg Med* 2008; 15(3): 134–139.

64. Goldenberg I, Matetzky S. Nephropathy induced by contrast media: pathogenesis, risk factors and preventive strategies. *CMAJ* 2005; 172(11): 1461–1471.

65. Golob JF Jr, Claridge JA, Yowler CJ, Como JJ, Peerless JR. Isolated cervical spine fractures in the elderly: a deadly injury. *J Trauma* 2008; 64(2): 311–315.

66. Stiell IG, Clement CM, McKnight RD, Brison R, Schull MJ, Rowe BH. The Canadian C-spine rule versus the NEXUS low-risk criteria in patients with trauma. *N Engl J Med* 2003; 349(26): 2510–2518.

67. Lomoschitz FM, Blackmore CC, Mirza SK, Mann FA. Cervical spine injuries in patients 65 years old and older: epidemiologic analysis regarding the effects of age and injury mechanism on distribution, type, and stability of injuries. *AJR Am J Roentgenol* 2002; 178(3): 573–577.

68. Ott MM, Eriksson E, Vanderkolk W, Christianson D, Davis A, Scholten D. Antiplatelet and anticoagulation therapies do not increase mortality in the absence of traumatic brain injury. *J Trauma* 2010; 68(3): 560–563.

69. Kirshch MJ, Vrabec GA, Marley RA, et al. Preinjury warfarin and geriatric orthopedic trauma patients: a case-matched study. *J Trauma* 2004; 57(6): 1230–1233.

70. Cohen DB, Rinker C, Wilberger JE. Traumatic brain injury in anticoagulated patients. *J Trauma* 2006; 60(3): 553–557.

71. Dickneite G, Pragst I. Prothrombin complex concentrate vs fresh frozen plasma for reversal of dilutional coagulopathy in a porcine trauma model. *Br J Anaesth* 2009; 102(3): 345–354.

72. Demeyere R, Gillardin S, Arnout J, Strengers PF. Comparison of fresh frozen plasma and prothrombin complex concentrate for the reversal of oral anticoagulants in patients undergoing cardiopulmonary bypass surgery: a randomized study. *Vox Sang* 2010; 99(3): 251–260.

73. Leissinger CA, Blatt PM, Hoots WK, Ewenstein B. Role of prothrombin complex concentrates in reversing warfarin anticoagulation: a review of the literature. *Am J Hematol* 2008; 83(2): 137–143.

74. Ohm C, Mina A, Howells G, Bair H, Bendick P. Effects of antiplatelet agents on outcomes for elderly patients with traumatic intracranial hemorrhage. *J Trauma* 2005; 58(3): 518–522.

75. Downey DM, Monson B, Butler KL, et al. Does platelet administration affect mortality in elderly head-injured patients taking antiplatelet medications? *Am Surg* 2009 ; 75(11): 1100–1103.

76. Trunkey D, Cahn R, Lenfesty B, Mullins R. Therapy withdrawal decision making. *Arch Surg* 2000; 135: 34–38..

77. Sterling DA, O'Connor JA, Bonadies J. Geriatric falls: injury severity is high and disproportionate to mechanism. *J Trauma* 2001; 50(1): 116–119.

78. Stevens J, Sogolow E. *Preventing Falls: What Works. A CDC Compendium of Effective Community-based Interventions from Around the World.* Georgia: National Center for Injury Prevention and Control Atlanta; 2008.

79. Weatherall M. Prevention of falls and fall-related fractures in community-dwelling older adults: a meta-analysis of estimates of effectiveness based on recent guidelines. *Intern Med J* 2004; 34(3): 102–108.

80. National Household Travel Survey. Older drivers safety implications. NHTSA Brief. May 2006.

81. Bauzá G, LaMorte WW, Burke PA, Hirsch EF. High mortality in elderly drivers is associated with distinct injury patterns: analysis of 187,869 injured drivers. *J Trauma* 2008; 64(2): 304–310.

82. McGwin G, Reiff D, Moran S, Rue L. Incidence and characteristics of motor vehicle collision-related Blunt thoracic aortic injury according to age. *J Trauma* 2002; 52(5): 859–866.

83. Chong M, Sochor M, Ipaktchi K, Brede C, Poster C, Wang S. The interaction of 'occupant factors' on the lower extremity fractures in frontal collision of motor vehicle crashes based on a level I trauma center. *J Trauma* 2007; 62(3): 720–729.

84. Eberhard J. Older drivers' "high per-mile crash involvement": the implications for licensing authorities. *Traffic Inj Prev* 2008; 9(4): 284–290.

85. Hanrahan RB, Layde PM, Zhu S, Guse CE, Hargarten SW. The association of driver age with traffic injury severity in Wisconsin. *Traffic Inj Prev* 2009; 10(4): 361–367.

86. Nader R. *Unsafe at Any Speed The Designed-In Dangers of The American Automobile.* New York: Grossman Publishers; 1965: LC # 65-16856

87. Demetriades D, Murray J, Martin M, et al. Pedestrians injured by automobiles: relationship of age to injury type and severity. *J Am Coll Surg* 2004; 199(3): 382–387.

88. West MD. The cellular and molecular biology of skin aging. *Arch Dermatol* 1994; 130: 87–95.

89. Pereira CT, Barrow RE, Sterns AM, et al. Age-dependent differences in survival after severe burns: a unicentric review of 1,674 patients and 179 autopsies over 15 years. *J Am Coll Surg* 2006; 202(3): 536–548.

90. Pomahac B, Matros E, Semel M, et al. Predictors of survival and length of stay in burn patients older than 80 years of age: does age really matter? *J Burn Care Res* 2006; 27(3): 265–269.

91. Bochicchio GV, Joshi M, Knorr KM, Scalea TM. Impact of nosocomial infections in trauma: does age make a difference? *J Trauma* 2001; 50(4): 612–617.

92. Yamashima T, Friede RL. Why do bridging veins rupture into the virtual subdural space? *J Neurol Neurosurg Psychiatry* 1984 ; 47(2): 121–127.

93. Fogelholm R, Heiskanen O, Waltimo O. Chronic subdural hematoma in adults. Influence of patient's age on symptoms, signs, and thickness of hematoma. *J Neurosurg* 1975; 42(1): 43–46.

94. Golob JF Jr, Claridge JA, Yowler CJ, Como JJ, Peerless JR. Isolated cervical spine fractures in the elderly: a deadly injury. *J Trauma* 2008; 64(2): 311–315.

95. Tashjian RZ, Majercik S, Biffl WL, Palumbo MA, Cioffi WG. Halo-vest immobilization increases early morbidity and mortality in elderly odontoid fractures. *J Trauma* 2006; 60(1): 199–203.

96. Bergeron E, Lavoie A, Clas D, et al. Elderly trauma patients with rib fractures are at greater risk of death and pneumonia. *J Trauma* 2003; 54(3): 478–485.

97. Bakhos C, O'Connor J, Kyriakides T, Abou-Nukta F, Bonadies J. Vital capacity as a predictor of outcome in elderly patients with rib fractures. *J Trauma* 2006; 61(1): 131–134.

98. Bala M, Menaker J. Torso trauma in the elderly. *Clin Geriatr* 2010; 18(3): 18–24.

99. Ottochian M, Salim A, DuBose J, Teixeira PG, Chan LS, Margulies DR. Does age matter? The relationship between age and mortality in penetrating trauma. *Injury* 2009; 40(4): 354–357.

100. Nagy KK, Smith RF, Roberts RR, Joseph KT, An GC, Bokhari F, Barrett J. Prognosis of penetrating trauma in elderly patients: a comparison with younger patients. *J Trauma* 2000; 49(2): 190–193.

101. Perdue PW, Watts DD, Kaufmann CR, Trask AL. Differences in mortality between elderly and younger adult trauma patients: geriatric status increases risk of delayed death. *J Trauma* 1998; 45(4): 805–810.

102. Baron JA, Barrett JA, Karagas MR. The epidemiology of peripheral fractures. *Bone* 1996; 18(3 Suppl.): 209S–213S.

103. Singer AJ, Dagum AB. Current management of acute cutaneous wounds. *N Engl J Med* 2008; 359(10): 1037.

104. Jacobs DG, Plaisier BR, Barie PS, et al. Practice management guidelines for geriatric trauma: the EAST Practice Management Guidelines Work Group. *J Trauma* 2003; 54(2): 391–416.

105. Hogan TM, Losman ED, Carpenter CR, et al. Development of geriatric competencies for emergency medicine residents using an expert consensus process. *Acad Emerg Med* 2010; 17(3): 316–324.

106. American College of Sugeons. *ATLS: Advanced Trauma Life Support for Doctors.* 8 Pap/DVD ed. American College of Surgeons; 2008.

107. Christmas C. *Geriatric Education for Emergency Medical Services (GEMS).* 1st ed. Sudbury, MA, USA: Jones and Bartlett Publishers, Inc.; 2003.

CHAPTER 13

Children with intestinal failure and complications from visceral transplant

Melissa A. Vitale[1,2], Jeffrey A. Rudolph[1,2] and Richard A. Saladino[1,2]
[1]Children's Hospital of Pittsburgh of UPMC, Pittsburgh, PA, USA
[2]University of Pittsburgh School of Medicine, Pittsburgh, PA, USA

Introduction and epidemiology

Intestinal failure is a physiological state defined as a critical reduction of functional gut mass below the minimal amount necessary for adequate digestion and absorption to satisfy body nutrient and fluid requirements in adults or growth in children [1]. Historically, intestinal failure has been used to describe children with the "short gut syndrome," a consequence of surgical resection of intestine after an intra-abdominal catastrophe (such as midgut volvulus). Children with short gut syndrome comprise the majority of the intestinal failure population. However, recognition of intestinal failure as a functional rather than anatomical diagnosis has led to the inclusion of children with full anatomical length but dysfunctional intestine. Regardless of cause, these patients require total or partial parenteral nutrition (TPN). Common diagnoses that may lead to intestinal failure are provided in Table 13.1 [2].

The incidence and prevalence of children with intestinal failure is not well defined as a result of the large number of associated diagnoses. The incidence of short gut syndrome has been estimated to be between 3 and 25 per 100,000 births [3, 4]. This range is in part due to a definition of short gut syndrome that is based on anatomical length. In addition, advances in surgical, neonatal, and anesthetic techniques, as well as the

Challenging and Emerging Conditions in Emergency Medicine, First Edition. Edited by Arvind Venkat.
© 2011 by John Wiley & Sons, Ltd. Published 2011 by Blackwell Publishing Ltd.

Table 13.1 Selected Diagnoses Leading to Intestinal Failure

Surgical Causes	Mixed Surgical/ Functional Causes	Functional Causes
Surgical Necrotizing Enterocolitis	Gastroschisis	Total Intestinal Aganglionosis
Complicated Gastroschisis*	Long-segment Hirschsprung's Disease	Chronic Intestinal Pseudo-obstruction
Isolated Intestinal Atresia		Megacystis–Microcolon Hypoperistalsis Syndrome
Malrotation/Volvulus		Microvillus Inclusion Disease
Trauma		Tufting Enteropathy
Surgical Debulking of Abdominal Tumors		
Vascular Thrombosis		

*Gastroschisis with associated atresia, ischemia, or volvulus.

success of parenteral nutrition and small bowel transplantation as therapies have likely led to an increase in the prevalence of such patients [5].

Patients with intestinal failure and short gut syndrome will present to the emergency department (ED) with any number of problems resulting from the primary medical or surgical diagnosis or with problems attendant to parenteral nutrition and the presence of a central catheter. Likewise, patients who have had intestinal transplantation are at risk for delayed surgical and post-transplantation medical complications.

This chapter outlines the various emergent presentations of patients with intestinal failure or intestinal transplantation, with an emphasis on specific problems encountered in the acute setting including electrolyte and fluid management, bowel obstruction, liver failure, central venous catheter complications, enteral feeding device complications, and infection.

Descriptions of surgical or procedural interventions

Central venous catheters

Patients with intestinal failure uniformly require TPN to maintain adequate fluid, electrolyte, and caloric balance. TPN requires central venous access, most often a tunneled catheter made from a silastic material that makes it more pliable and softer than the non-tunneled versions [6].

Tunneled catheters have a longer in situ duration potential, but are predisposed to stretching, thinning, or the formation of blebs in the catheter over time, all of which may result in malfunction of the line. In addition, importantly, tunneled catheters are at risk for becoming infected, particularly in the patient with intestinal failure.

Enteral feeding devices

Enteral feeding devices are common in patients with intestinal failure. Temporary tubes placed via the nares can be either nasogastric or nasojejunal. Gastrostomies are created for placement of long-term feeding tubes via surgical, endoscopic, or interventional radiographic techniques. Once the fistula tract has matured, a skin-level button device is commonly placed. While some buttons have an intra-gastric balloon to anchor the site in place, other models have discs or other soft plastic appendages. A working knowledge of which type of tube is in place is essential prior to manipulating any enteric feeding device. Dislodgement of feeding tubes is a frequent reason for ED care.

Abdominal surgery

Patients with short gut syndrome or small intestine transplantation have undergone major abdominal surgical intervention. As with any patient with prior abdominal surgery, these patients are at risk for either partial or complete obstruction due to adhesions, bands, volvulus, or stricture at the anastomotic site.

Regardless of surgical anatomy, electrolyte disturbances may occur in patients after intestinal resection or transplantation. High-end ostomies may be associated with increased output of intestinal contents due to the lack of absorptive capacity of the proximal small intestine. Patients are, therefore, predisposed to dehydration, hyponatremia, and acidosis due to bicarbonate losses. Lower ostomies and bowel re-anastamosed to colon take advantage of the absorptive capacity of the lower intestine, but these patients can still be at risk for electrolyte disturbances.

Emergent complications in pediatric intestinal failure patients

Altered fluid and electrolyte balance

Children who are dependent on parenteral nutrition may become dehydrated with seemingly minor increases in enteral fluid output. Increased output may be the result of enteral infection or oral intake in amounts greater than the intestines can process. Acute dehydration in the patient

Table 13.2 Initial Laboratory Evaluation and Management of the Pediatric Intestinal Failure Patient with Dehydration

Ancillary Test	Typical Abnormalities	Essential Management
Basic metabolic panel	Hypoglycemia	Dextrose: 0.5–1 g/kg IV bolus
	Hyponatremia-Seizure	3% saline
	Hyponatremia-Asymptomatic	Normal saline bolus therapy
	Hypokalemia	Slow correction via IV K^+
Electrocardiogram	Flattened T-waves (low K^+)	Slow correction via IV K^+
	Peaked T-waves (high K^+)	Calcium infusion, Insulin, Glucose, Sodium polystyrene

with intestinal failure can lead to altered serum electrolyte concentrations, most notably low sodium and potassium [7].

Patients presenting with acute dehydration will most often report a history of diarrhea. They may have increased thirst, decreased activity level, and irritability. Those with severe hyponatremia (sodium <120 mEq/L) may present with seizure activity, while those with severe hypokalemia may have complaints of weakness. On physical examination, the clinician should pay particular attention to heart rate and blood pressure. Additional examination findings suggestive of dehydration include decreased energy level, lethargy, dry mucous membranes, poor skin turgor, and prolonged capillary refill time. A patient with severe dehydration may present in hypovolemic shock, with tachycardia and hypotension.

The diagnosis of acute dehydration is based on history and physical examination. An initial laboratory evaluation and management strategy is suggested in Table 13.2. The initial goal of treatment is to normalize heart rate, perfusion, and blood pressure with rapid administration of an isotonic fluid (normal saline or lactated ringer's solution) as 20 mL/kg fluid boluses. Intravenous fluids should be given even if the patient can tolerate enteral fluids [7]. Fluid boluses can be repeated to a maximum of 60–80 mL/kg, at which point a continuous infusion of a pressor (e.g., epinephrine) should be considered in the patient with fluid-refractory shock [8]. Of note, in the patient with ECG changes secondary to hypokalemia in whom more rapid correction of potassium is desired, intravenous potassium chloride, 0.2–0.3 mEq/kg/h, may be given [9]. Admission to an inpatient unit should be considered for patients with electrolyte abnormalities or for those with significant dehydration that requires ongoing fluid replacement. Patients with mild dehydration and normal electrolytes whose vital signs normalize after administration of intravenous fluids can be considered for discharge to home with close outpatient follow-up.

Intestinal obstruction

Patients who have had intra-abdominal surgery (e.g., bowel resection or transplant) are at increased risk of bowel obstruction secondary to adhesions [10]. These patients classically present with acute onset of abdominal pain, bilious vomiting, and distension. Peritoneal signs may be present if the bowel has perforated. Imaging is the test of choice to establish the diagnosis of bowel obstruction. Plain radiographs are fairly sensitive and should be performed in the upright and supine positions (Figure 13.1). A cross-table lateral or a decubitus view may also be helpful in visualizing intra-peritoneal free air. Additional findings on plain film suggestive of bowel obstruction are dilated, stacked loops of bowel and air-fluid levels prior to the point of obstruction [10]. Patients with suspected bowel obstruction should be made nil per os (NPO) and have intravenous fluids initiated. Bolus fluid therapy is indicated in the setting of unstable vital signs. Placement of a nasogastric tube should be considered for decompression of the stomach. Surgical consultation should be obtained for all patients. Hospital admission is required for patients with bowel obstruction. Surgical intervention may be needed for some, but many will recover with conservative measures such as bowel rest, decompression, and intravenous hydration. Optimal care of patients with complications of intestinal failure or transplantation is achieved by transfer to a tertiary referral center familiar with such patients.

Hepatobiliary complications associated with intestinal failure

Patients with intestinal failure who require long-term TPN are at risk of hepatobiliary dysfunction (reported rates vary between 40%–60%) [11]. Three hepatobiliary complications are most commonly associated with long-term TPN therapy: (1) steatosis; (2) cholestasis; and (3) gallbladder stones or sludging [12, 13]. Steatosis is more common in adults than children and is usually asymptomatic. Cholestasis may be initially asymptomatic, but is heralded by stereotypical lab abnormalities such as elevated conjugated bilirubin, transaminases, alkaline phosphatase, and gamma glutamyl transpeptidase. Cholestasis must be detected early, as failure to do so may result in liver cirrhosis and failure.

Cholelithiasis and cholecystitis

Patients who develop cholelithiasis or cholecystitis may present acutely to the ED. These patients usually present with biliary colic, characterized by mid-upper and right-sided abdominal pain that begins after a meal, builds in intensity and lasts up to several hours. The pain is intense, causing the patient to be very restless. It can be accompanied by nausea, vomiting, fever, and jaundice. On physical examination, the patient may display a Murphy's sign. Laboratory investigation to support the diagnosis reveals elevated transaminases, alkaline phosphatase, and bilirubin levels.

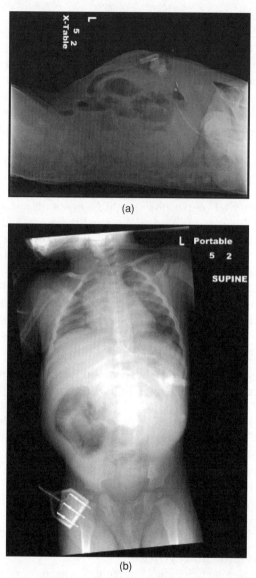

(a)

(b)

Figure 13.1 Plain radiograph of the abdomen of a 4-year-old boy with ischemic distal intestine as a result of torsion of his intestine allograft causing obstruction. (a) Cross-table lateral image demonstrates abdominal distension with dilated bowel loops. (b) Upright radiograph demonstrates dilated bowel loops and the absence of air in the distal intestine. (Courtesy of George Mazariegos, MD.)

Diagnosis is best made via abdominal ultrasound that may demonstrate gallstones, dilated bile ducts, thickened gallbladder wall, and biliary sludge. Febrile patients should have a blood culture sent. In the ED setting, once the diagnosis of cholecystitis is made, the patient should be made NPO, placed on intravenous fluids and given pain control. Surgical consultation is also warranted, and antibiotics should be initiated, especially in the setting of fever. Ampicillin–sulbactam provides appropriate coverage for Gram-negative pathogens as well as *Enterococcus*. All patients with cholecystitis should be admitted to the hospital for further management [14].

Esophageal variceal bleeding

Portal hypertension in the setting of liver failure leads to esophageal varices that may bleed acutely. Patients usually present to the ED with melena or hematochezia. Diagnosis should be suspected based on history and examination. In the stable patient, the level of bleeding can be assessed via nasogastric lavage [14]. Patients who present with unstable vital signs due to hemorrhage require rapid fluid resuscitation, with care being given not to expand the intravascular volume too rapidly as this may lead to rebleeding [14, 15]. Isotonic crystalloid solutions (normal saline or lactated ringer's solution) can be given initially in small boluses, such as 10 mL/kg, with consideration for the administration of packed red blood cells. If volume resuscitation does not stabilize the patient, an infusion of octreotide should be started at a rate of 1–2 µg/kg/h [15, 16]. Consultation with a gastroenterologist should be obtained to facilitate endoscopy to identify and stop the source of bleeding. Severe bleeding that cannot be controlled by the above measures requires general surgical consultation for possible operative interventions. All patients with esophageal variceal bleeding should be admitted to the hospital, and any patient with unstable vital signs should be monitored in the intensive care setting.

Encephalopathy

Patients with hepatobiliary disease secondary to TPN are at risk for the eventual development of frank liver failure and subsequent encephalopathy. Early symptoms may include fatigue, nausea, vomiting, abdominal pain, and jaundice, all of which may lead the patient to seek care in an ED. In more advanced stages of liver disease, manifestations of hepatic encephalopathy may develop as a result of elevated ammonia levels. Patients may be excessively somnolent or lethargic, or they may be confused, agitated, combative, or unresponsive. The diagnostic evaluation of a patient with suspected liver failure should include a physical examination with a thorough neurological assessment. Laboratory investigations should include ammonia level, liver function tests, coagulation factors, fibrinogen, glucose level, albumin level, electrolytes, and blood culture. Lactulose is the mainstay of treatment for hepatic encephalopathy in children [15]. In children, lactulose is given as 40–90 mL, divided 3–4 times, daily with the goal of achieving 2–3 soft stools per day. Additional lab abnormalities should also be addressed, including hypoglycemia and hypoalbuminemia. Intravenous vitamin K is indicated for coagulopathy. Most patients with worsening hepatic function or encephalopathy should be admitted for supportive care. Liver transplant remains the only definitive therapy.

Complications associated with central venous catheters

Central venous catheter occlusion

Several potential complications may occur related to *in situ* central venous catheters, many of which necessitate timely medical attention (Table 13.3). The most common complication is line occlusion. A central venous catheter may become partially occluded, wherein the line will infuse but not draw back, or may become completely occluded. Line occlusion may be thrombotic (60% of cases) or non-thrombotic in nature [17, 18].

The diagnostic approach to a patient presenting with central venous catheter occlusion should start with careful inspection of the catheter to rule out mechanical obstruction. Function should be confirmed by attempting to aspirate and flush the line, ascertaining whether function changes with line position. Plain radiographs may be considered to confirm that the line is not kinked and is still in good position. If a mechanical obstruction is not suspected, consideration should be given to the presence of a drug precipitate or lipid residue by taking a careful history of what was last infused into the line prior to the line occlusion. Once these types of obstruction have been excluded, thrombotic obstruction can be assumed. If there is concern for a deep vein thrombosis, evaluation via ultrasound should be pursued.

Table 13.3 Central Venous Catheter Occlusion

Thrombotic Occlusions	
Fibrin sheath at catheter tip	Typically develops 1–2 weeks after line placement
Intra-luminal clot	Often a complete occlusion
Mural thrombus	Typically occludes the tip of the catheter
Deep vein thrombosis	Often in an upper extremity catheter
Non-thrombotic Occlusions	
Mechanical obstruction	Examples: kink in a catheter, tight stabilizing suture, tubing clamp in place
Drug or mineral precipitates	Typically a result of incompatible infusates
Lipid residue	Residues of parenteral nutrition components

The treatment of a central venous catheter occlusion is dependent upon the suspected etiology. External mechanical occlusions can usually be easily and quickly remedied. If the line is kinked or broken internally or has migrated to a less than ideal position, the line may need to be repaired via interventional radiology or replaced altogether. Central venous catheters can become occluded by drugs that have low solubility or are incompatible with TPN. Interestingly, studies have demonstrated that an acidic drug precipitate can be treated with a hydrochloric acid solution and a basic drug precipitate with a sodium bicarbonate solution [17–19]. Calcium phosphate crystals (e.g., due to parenteral nutrition with high levels of calcium and phosphorus) can also be treated with hydrochloric acid [17–19]. However, the practicality of using these solutions in an ED setting is low given the clinician will not likely know the pH of most medications. Finally, a lipid residue can occlude and central venous catheter secondary to intralipid infusion. To dissolve this, a 70% ethanol solution can be injected into the line [17–19]. A maximum dose of 3 mL or 0.55 mL/kg (whichever is greater) is recommended [19].

The mainstay of treatment for central venous catheter occlusion secondary to thrombus is recombinant tissue plasminogen activator (rt-PA). Several studies have demonstrated both efficacy and safety in the use of rt-PA for children. Although treatment protocols vary, most authors recommend instillation of 2 mg of rt-PA in children weighing more than 30 kg and 110% of the catheter volume to a maximum of 2 mg in children weighing less than 30 kg. Dwell times are 60–120 minutes before testing the patency of the line. Treatment may be repeated once if the first attempt fails [20–23]. Patients with a central venous catheter may develop an associated deep vein thrombosis (up to 12% of children), which usually presents with pain, swelling, warmth, and tenderness most often in the upper extremity where the central venous catheter is located [17]. An ultrasound can be helpful in diagnosing deep vein thrombosis. Although management of catheter-related deep vein thrombosis in children is controversial, anticoagulation with heparin or low molecular weight heparin is recommended.

Patients with central venous catheter occlusions who are treated successfully during their ED visit can be discharged to home and instructed to use their line as usual. Patients with an occluded catheter that fail treatment should have peripheral intravenous access placed until central venous access is reestablished.

Central venous catheter infection

All children with a central venous catheter are at risk for line infection. Central venous catheters can be colonized with bacteria within 24 hours of placement. Sources of colonization include migration of bacteria from the skin surrounding the outer surface of the catheter and the introduction of bacteria into the catheter lumen when the line is accessed. A hallmark of central line infection is unexplained fever. Other symptoms include chills and malaise. Pulse may be elevated and signs of shock may be present in patients who are more ill. There also may be indicators of infection around the catheter site such as erythema, swelling, and drainage.

An elevated peripheral white blood cell count may be helpful in making the diagnosis of line infection, but may be normal in many patients. Blood cultures sent from the central venous catheter along with a peripheral blood culture are the gold standard for diagnosis. Common causative organisms include *Staphylococcus epidermidis*, *Staphylococcus aureus* (including methacillin-resistant *Staphylococcus aureus*), and *Enterococcus spp* [24–26], as well as many Gram-negative organisms and fungi. One study reported that 23% of infections evaluated in their case series ($n = 47$) were polymicrobial [26]. Empiric broad-spectrum antibiotics are initiated until culture results are known, and specific choice of antibiotics should be based on regional microbiological susceptibilities. Common recommendations in most settings include vancomycin and piperacillin–tazobactam. Empiric treatment of fungal infection should be considered in more ill or unstable patients or those known to have past fungal central venous catheter infections. Current preferred antifungal agents in this setting include amphotericin B and caspofungin. Patients with a suspected line infection should be admitted for parenteral antibiotics. An uncommon exception may be the patient with stable vital signs and additional symptoms suggestive of a source for fever (e.g., a mild upper respiratory infection) with reassuring peripheral blood counts. With close follow-up, these patients may be eligible for discharge to home.

Complications associated with enteral feeding device

Several complications associated with gastrostomy tubes may result in patients seeking emergency care, the most common of which is tube dislodgement [27–30]. Other common complications related to the tube itself include tube obstruction, tube leakage, gastric ulceration, and gastric outlet obstruction. Complications may also occur at the stoma site and include skin irritation, skin infection, and granulation tissue.

Gastrostomy tube dislodgement

A gastrostomy tube may become dislodged secondary to trauma (e.g., the tube is pulled out accidentally without balloon deflation) or secondary to accidental deflation or rupture of the anchoring balloon. A careful history should include the date of the operation to create the stoma and place the gastrostomy tube and how long the tube has been displaced. Patients may present with a benign appearing stoma or have bleeding from the site, depending on the mechanism of dislodgement.

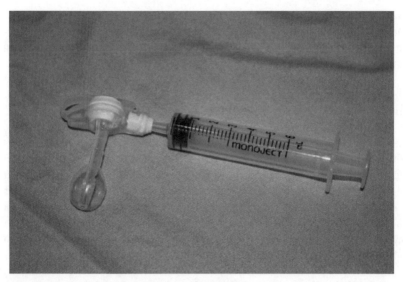

Figure 13.2 Mic-key button gastrostomy tube with 5-mL syringe attached at the gastrostomy tube valve. The balloon is inflated prior to placement to ensure competence. (Courtesy of Melissa Vitale, MD.)

Reinsertion is generally straightforward (Figure 13.2). However, consultation with a pediatric surgeon is recommended if the gastrostomy stoma is new, that is, if the stoma was created within the previous 4–8 weeks. Recently placed enteral tubes must be handled with caution due to the possibility of an immature tract and subsequent tract disruption. While generally considered safe after 90 days, tract disruption has been described up to 5 months after placement [31]. Replacement of new tubes should be confirmed radiographically and in most cases with close surgical supervision. Otherwise, the emergency physician should attempt reinsertion as soon as possible. Many caregivers will bring a replacement tube with them to the ED. Typically, if the gastrostomy tube has been out for more than 3–4 hours, the stoma may have constricted and the clinician will feel resistance when attempting reinsertion. In this case, a Foley catheter one to two sizes smaller than the gastrostomy tube can be inserted in order to dilate the stoma. Each Foley catheter is left in place for 10 minutes prior to placement of the next size tube. A plain radiograph demonstrating proper placement upon instillation of radio-opaque dye (a "dye study") should be performed after reinsertion of a gastrostomy tube. Patients with a new tube in place that is functioning properly can be safely discharged to home. If tube replacement is unsuccessful, a smaller catheter may be left in place to keep the existing stoma patent until surgical replacement of the proper size gastrostomy tube. These patients most often are admitted to a surgical service for definitive care.

Gastrostomy tube obstruction and leakage

Obstruction of a gastrostomy tube commonly occurs as a result of dried formula clogging the tube or simply a kink in the tube. Simple repositioning and a flush with warm water may suffice to relieve the obstruction [30]. If flushing and aspiration of the tube is unsuccessful, the gastrostomy tube should be replaced. Once the obstruction is removed, or the tube replaced, the patient may be discharged to home.

Fluid leakage from the gastrostomy tube suggests that the gastrostomy tube is not intact, and the tube should be replaced. The presence of purulent drainage from the tube or around the stoma should alert the medical practitioner to possible infection. Surgical consultation and the initiation of antibiotics are warranted. Common first-line treatment is cefazolin for coverage of skin flora. Drainage of gastric contents from the stoma is an indication for placement of a larger tube. Most patients who present with leakage from a gastrostomy tube or from the stoma can be discharged to home once the source is identified and rectified.

Gastric ulceration and gastric outlet obstruction

A gastrostomy tube that is too long may irritate the gastric mucosa resulting in the formation of an ulcer. Patients may report abdominal pain, bloody emesis, or blood in the stool. Saline lavage through the gastrostomy tube should be completed to assess for active bleeding. If the aspirate is non-bloody, H-2 blockers, antacids and carafate are prescribed [30]. The tube should also be replaced with one that is shorter in length. These patients may be discharged to home with close follow-up. If a brisk gastrointestinal bleed is suspected, peripheral intravenous access should be established for the administration of resuscitative fluids, including blood, when necessary.

Gastric outlet obstruction is a rare complication associated with a gastrostomy tube. Obstruction results from migration of the tube tip into the pylorus. Outlet obstruction is suspected in the patient who presents with acute onset of vomiting and a dilated stomach on abdominal radiographs. There may only be retching if the patient has previously undergone a Nissen fundoplication. An attempt to alleviate symptoms can be made by pulling back on the gastrostomy tube to attain a better position. If this is unsuccessful, the tube should be removed. A shorter tube may be considered for replacement. Patients whose symptoms are resolved with tube repositioning may be discharged to home.

Stoma site complications

Leakage of fluid around the gastrostomy tube is common and often leads to skin irritation. Red skin around the stoma site with vesicular lesions is suggestive of irritant dermatitis [30] and should be treated with a barrier cream. The area should be kept as dry as possible, and the source of leaking should be addressed.

Cellulitis is an uncommon complication of irritated skin from fluid leakage and presents classically with erythema, warmth, tenderness to palpation, and swelling around the stoma site. Fever may also be present. If cellulitis is suspected, oral antibiotics directed against both *Streptococcus* and *Staphylococcus* species should be initiated. As long as the patient is otherwise well appearing, they may be discharged to home with close follow-up.

Fungal infection may also develop on the skin surrounding the stoma site and presents as erythematous pustules or papules that typically coalesce into beefy red plaques around the stoma site. The area should be kept as dry as possible. The application of topical antifungal agents usually leads to resolution [30].

Granulation tissue commonly develops around the stoma of gastrostomy tube sites. This appears as deep red extraneous tissue protruding from the stoma border (Figure 13.3). Patients usually come to medical attention because of bleeding from the granulation tissue. Small areas of bleeding can be cauterized with silver nitrate. Once the bleeding has been controlled, these patients can be safely discharged to home.

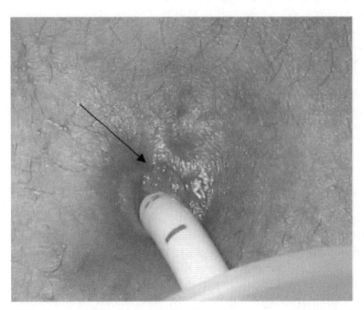

Figure 13.3 Granulation tissue at the site of a gastrostomy stoma. Note the beefy red tissue protruding from the stoma (arrow). (Photo courtesy of Julia Warner, RN.)

Emergent care of the patient with intestinal transplantation

Children with intestinal failure may undergo isolated small intestine transplantation alone or in combination with liver transplantation or multivisceral transplantation. Regardless of the differences in procedures, all patients are at risk of complications after transplantation that may require emergent care. Infection is one of the most common causes of post-transplantation complications and includes both bacterial and viral etiologies. Transplant rejection can also lead to significant graft dysfunction and complications.

The etiologies of infection after organ transplantation are many. During small intestine transplantation in particular, the bowel mucosa may be injured, altering the protective barrier of the gut mucosa and allowing for bacterial translocation. In addition, immunosuppressive therapies after transplantation place the child at increased risk of infection.

Evaluation for infection in a patient after transplantation includes determination of the date of the transplantation. In the first month after transplantation, patients are most susceptible to bacterial infections that are common to all patients who undergo major surgery [32, 33] including wound, urinary tract and intra-abdominal infections, pneumonia, and central venous catheter infection. One to six months after transplantation, the patient is maximally immunocompromised and susceptible to viral infections (cytomegalovirus (CMV) or Epstein–Barr virus (EBV)) and opportunistic infections (e.g., *Pneumocystis jiroveci*) [32, 33]. During this time, the patient may acquire a new strain of viral infection, acquire a viral infection from the donor organ or have reactivation of a latent virus. Beyond 6 months post-transplantation, patients who are doing well acquire the same community infections as immunocompetent children. Patients who have not done well post-transplant are more susceptible to chronic infection and opportunistic infection [32, 33].

Evaluation for bacterial infections

Bacterial infections are most common during the first month after transplant. The majority of these infections will present while the patient is still hospitalized. However, the emergency physician should include bacterial infection on the differential diagnosis of any transplant patient with fever. Intestinal transplant patients are particularly susceptible to bacteremia and intra-abdominal infection (peritonitis) [34].

In addition to fever, the transplant patient with a bacterial infection may present with a wide spectrum of signs and symptoms, including hemodynamic instability and shock. Review of systems should focus on symptoms that may be related to bacteremia, peritonitis, pneumonia, and urinary tract infection. A thorough physical examination, with special attention paid to pulse, perfusion, blood pressure, and mental status should be performed.

Any transplant patient for whom infection is suspected should have a blood culture sent and complete blood count performed. Additional studies should be guided by symptoms and may include urinalysis/urine culture as well as chest and abdominal radiographs.

Resuscitation of shock is paramount, and empiric broad-spectrum antibiotics should be administered to cover for *Staphylococcus* and *Streptococcus* species as well as Gram-negative gut flora [35]. Vancomycin and piperacillin–tazobactam are common first-line antibiotics. Virtually all transplant patients with a fever are admitted to the hospital for intravenous antibiotics and monitoring.

Evaluation for viral infections

CMV may be acquired as a new infection (primary infection), either from the environment or the transplant donor, or may occur from reactivation of latent infection (secondary infection). Prior to age 20, only about half of the population has had CMV infection; therefore, many patients who have had intestinal transplantation have not had prior exposure [33].

The majority of patients with CMV infection will present within 1–6 months after transplantation and may present as either CMV syndrome or CMV tissue invasive disease [33]. Children with CMV syndrome usually present with fever in association with leukopenia, thrombocytopenia, and atypical lymphocytosis. There is no evidence of specific organ involvement [33, 35]. Those with CMV tissue invasive disease present with signs and symptoms of end-organ injury, the most common of which is enteritis [35]. Other presentations include those consistent with pneumonitis, hepatitis, myocarditis, and encephalitis.

EBV, similarly to CMV, may be acquired as a primary or secondary infection post-transplant. Many patients present with a mononucleosis-type illness, including fever, malaise, pharyngitis, and lymphadenopathy, and specific organ disease, such as hepatitis or enteritis may be present. Post-transplantation lymphoproliferative disorder (PTLD) may also be a consequence of EBV infection, particularly in the patient with small intestine transplantation [32]. In the intestinal transplant patient, the transplanted organ is often involved, and thus patients with evolving PTLD can often present with gastrointestinal symptoms such as diarrhea, as well as non-specific constitutional symptoms [36, 37].

Evaluation of the post-transplantation patient with fever who is at risk of disease from CMV or EBV should include ancillary testing such as blood culture, complete blood count, basic metabolic panel, liver function tests, and chest radiographs. CMV and EBV viral loads (by polymerase chain reaction) can be sent to initiate the evaluation for viral infection [36, 37]. However, further evaluation for CMV or EBV, which includes tissue biopsy, should be completed as an inpatient on a transplant surgical service [32, 33].

Both CMV and EBV infection may be difficult to differentiate from a bacterial infection. The primary goal of the emergency physician is to treat unstable vital signs and start empiric broad-spectrum antibiotics. If the diagnosis of CMV infection has already been made or is strongly suspected, treatment should include intravenous ganciclovir. This is rarely indicated in the ED and more typically started in the inpatient setting. Reduction in immunosuppression is the mainstay of treatment for EBV once a definitive diagnosis has been made [36, 37]. All patients with fever and possible CMV or EBV infection should be admitted to a tertiary care center on a transplant service.

Graft rejection

Patients who have had small intestine transplantation are at highest risk of graft rejection during the first year and most especially within the first 6 months [34]. The most common symptoms of graft rejection include fever, increase in stoma output, and gastrointestinal symptoms such as abdominal pain, bleeding, vomiting, and diarrhea [34,38]. It is, therefore, difficult to differentiate rejection from infection. ED evaluation of patients presenting with symptoms of rejection should include blood culture, complete blood count, and a basic metabolic panel. Clinical presentation should dictate additional lab testing. Initial treatment of the patient with possible graft rejection should include fluid resuscitation and correction of electrolyte abnormalities. Empiric broad-spectrum antibiotics should be initiated in the setting of fever. Consultation is mandatory, as the only way to diagnose rejection is to biopsy the transplanted organ. All patients with suspected graft rejection should be admitted to a tertiary care center on a transplant surgical service for further management, which usually includes treatment with steroids.

The next five years

During the past decade, management of patients with intestinal failure has begun to evolve, largely focusing on the prevention and treatment of the two major complications of TPN-associated care: (1) infection; and (2) parenteral nutrition-associated liver disease. While the prevention of catheter-associated bloodstream infections will always consist of aseptic techniques while handling central catheters, management using new technologies such as the chlorhexidine impregnated patch [39], anti-microbial coated catheters [40], and "line-lock therapy" are beginning to come into vogue. Preventative line-lock therapy using the antimicrobial properties of ethanol is one particular example [41].

The prevention of parenteral nutrition-associated liver disease has also advanced. Soy-based lipid emulsions, a staple in TPN management because of their relatively high caloric content, have been theorized to be hepatotoxic due to the generation of phytosterols and resultant cholestasis [42]. Strategies such as lipid minimalization and investigational omega-3-based lipid preparations are being used to prevent cholestasis. While these strategies appear to decrease direct hyperbilirubinemia [43], a marker for cholestasis, it is unknown whether they ultimately prevent fibrosis and eventual cirrhosis in patients requiring TPN [44].

As the field of intestinal transplantation evolves, there will be a population shift to long-term survival. While data is limited, the overall long-term survival in post-transplant patients has begun to increase. One relatively new concept in intestinal transplantation is the development of chronic rejection [45], which can present with more subtle symptoms, but can be just as devastating as acute cellular rejection.

Conclusion

Evolution of the management of patients with intestinal failure and small intestinal transplantation will impact care in the ED. Vigilant attention to the details of each patient's history and current status, including the presence of a central catheter and feeding tube, is necessary to provide optimal care to these patients. Rapid response to signs of infection and shock is paramount, and careful evaluation for other of potential complications of intestinal failure and transplantation is imperative. The care of most patients with intestinal failure and small bowel transplantation will include consultation with gastrointestinal and transplantation specialists and may require transfer to a tertiary care center.

References

1. Thompson JS. Overview of etiology and management of intestinal failure. *Gastroenterology* 2006; 130: S3–S4.
2. Nucci A, Burns RC, Armah T, et al. Interdisciplinary management of pediatric intestinal failure: a 10-year review of rehabilitation and transplantation. *J Gastrointest Surg* 2008; 12: 429–435; discussion 35–36.
3. Wales PW, de Silva N, Kim J, Lecce L, To T, Moore A. Neonatal short bowel syndrome: population-based estimates of incidence and mortality rates. *J Pediatr Surg* 2004; 39: 690–695.
4. Wallander J, Ewald U, Lackgren G, Tufveson G, Wahlberg J, Meurling S. Extreme short bowel syndrome in neonates: an indication for small bowel transplantation? *Transplant Proc* 1992; 24: 1230–1235.
5. Rudolph JA, Squires R. Current concepts in the medical management of pediatric intestinal failure. *Curr Opin Organ Transplant* 2010; 15: 324–329.
6. Chung DH, Ziegler MM. Central venous catheter access. *Nutrition* 1998; 14: 119–123.
7. Kaufman SS, Fennelly EM. Management of complex fluid and electrolyte disturbances. In: Langnas AN, Goulet O, Quigley EMM, Tappenden KA (eds.)

Intestinal Failure: Diagnosis, Management and Trasnplantation. Massachusetts: Blackwell Publishing Inc; 2008: pp. 185–190.

8. Brierley J, Carcillo JA, Choong K, et al. Clinical practice parameters for hemo-dynamic support of pediatric and neonatal septic shock. *Crit Care Med* 2009; 37: 666–688.

9. Cronan KM, Kost SI. Renal and electrolyte emergencies. In: Fleisher GR, Ludwig S, Henretig FM (eds.) *Textbook of Pediatric Emergency Medicine.* 5th ed. Philadelphia: Lippincott Williams & Wilkins; 2006: pp. 873–919.

10. Bachur RG, Kost SI. Abdominal emergencies. In: Fleisher GR, Ludwig S, Henretig FM (eds.) *Textbook of Pediatric Emergency Medicine.* 5th ed. Philadelphia: Lippincott Williams & Wilkins; 2006: pp. 1605–1629.

11. Gupte GL, Beath SV, Kelly DA, Millar AJW, Booth IW. Current issues in the management of intestinal failure. *Arch Dis Child* 2006; 91: 259–264.

12. Kumpf VJ. Parenteral nutrition-associated liver disease in adult and pediatric patients. *Nutr Clin Pract* 2006; 21: 279–290.

13. Kelly DA. Intestinal failure–associated liver disease: what do we know today? *Gastroenterology* 2006; 130: S70–S77.

14. Durbin DR, Liacouras CA. Gastrointestinal emergencies. In: Fleisher GR, Ludwig S, Henretig FM (eds.) *Textbook of Pediatric Emergency Medicine.* 5th ed. Philadelphia: Lippincott Williams & Wilkins; 2006:pp. 1087–1112.

15. Leonis MA, Balistreri WF. Evaluation and management of end-stage liver disease in children. *Gastroenterology* 2008; 134: 1741–1751.

16. Kelly DA. Managing liver failure. *Postgrad Medical J* 2002; 78: 660–667.

17. Baskin JL, Pui C-H, Reiss U, et al. Management of occlusion and thrombosis associated with long-term indwelling central venous catheters. *Lancet* 2009; 374: 159–169.

18. Kerner JA, Garcia-Careaga MG, Fisher AA, Poole RL. Treatment of catheter occlusion in pediatric patients. *J Parenter Enteral Nutr* 2006; 30: S73–S81.

19. Werlin SL, Lausten T, Jessen S, et al. Treatment of central venous catheter occlusion with ethanol and hydrochloric acid. *J Parenter Enteral Nutr* 1995; 19: 416–418.

20. Choi M, Massicotte P, Marzinotto V, Chan AKC, Holmes JL, Andrew M. The use of alteplase to restore patency of central lines in pediatric patients: a cohort study. *J Peds* 2001; 139: 152–156.

21. Jacobs BR, Haygood M, Hingl J. Recombinant tissue plasminogen activator in the treatment of central venous catheter occlusion in children. *J Peds* 2001; 139: 593–596.

22. Shen V, Li A, Murdock M, Resnansky L, McCluskey E, Semba CP. Recombinant tissue plasminogen activator (Alteplase) for restoration of function to occluded central venous catheters in pediatric patients. *J Pediatr Hematol Oncol* 2003; 25: 38–45.

23. Blaney M, Shen V, Kerner JA, et al. Alteplase for the treatment of central venous catheter occlusion in children: results of a prospective, open-label, single-arm study (The Cathflo Activase Pediatric Study). *J Vasc Interv Radiol* 2006; 17: 1745–1751.

24. de Jonge RCJ, Polderman KH, Gemke JBJ. Central venous catheter use in the pediatric patient: mechanical and infectious complications. *Pediatr Crit Care Med* 2005; 6: 329–339.

25. Hodge D, Puntis JW. Diagnosis, prevention, and management of catheter re-
    lated bloodstream infection during long term parenteral nutrition. *Arch Dis
    Child Fetal Neonatal Ed* 2002; 87: F21–F24.

26. Marra AR, Opilla M, Edmond MB, Kirby DF. Epidemiology of bloodstream
    infections in patients receiving long-term total parenteral nutrition. *J Clin Gas-
    troenterol* 2007; 41: 19–28.

27. Crosby J, Duerksen D. A retrospective survey of tube-related complications
    in patients receiving long-term home enteral nutrition. *Dig Dis Sci* 2005; 50:
    1712–1717.

28. Friedman JN, Ahmed S, Connolly B, Chait P, Mahant S. Complications associ-
    ated with image-guided gastrostomy and gastrojejunostomy tubes in children.
    Pediatrics 2004; 114: 458–461.

29. Saavedra H, Losek JD, Shanley L, Titus MO. Gastrostomy tube-related com-
    plaints in the pediatric emergency department: identifying opportunities for
    improvement. *Pedatr Emerg Care* 2009; 25: 728–732.

30. Fein JA, Cronan KM, Posner JC. Approach to the care of the technology-
    assisted child. In: Fleisher GR, Ludwig S, Henretig FM (eds.) *Textbook of Pediatric
    Emergency Medicine*. 5th ed. Philadelphia: Lippincott Williams & Wilkins; 2006:
    pp. 1737–1758.

31. Romero R, Martinez FL, Robinson SY, Sullivan KM, Hart MH. Complicated
    PEG-to-skin level gastrostomy conversions: analysis of risk factors for tract dis-
    ruption. *Gastrointest Endosc* 1996; 44: 230–234.

32. Allen U, Green M. Prevention and treatment of infectious complications af-
    ter solid organ transplantation in children. *Pediatr Clin North Am* 2010; 57:
    459–479.

33. Fonseca-Aten M, Michaels MG. Infections in pediatric solid organ transplant
    recipients. *Semin Pediatr Surg* 2006; 15: 153–161.

34. Fryer JP. Intestinal transplantation: current status. *Gastroenterol Clin North Am*
    2007; 36: 145–159.

35. Freifeld A, Kalil A. Infections in small bowel transplant recipients. In: Langnas
    AN, Goulet O, Quigley EMM, Tappenden KA (eds.) *Intestinal Failure: Diagnosis,
    Management and Trasnplantation*. Massachusetts: Blackwell Publishing Inc; 2008:
    pp. 297–304.

36. Bakker NA, van Imhoff GW, Verschuuren EA, van Son WJ. Presentation and
    early detection of post-transplant lymphoproliferative disorder after solid organ
    transplantation. *Transpl Intl* 2007; 20: 207–218.

37. Gross TG, Savoldo B, Punnett A. Post-transplant lymphoproliferative diseases.
    Pediatr Clin of North Am 2010; 57: 481–503.

38. Avitzur Y, Grant D. Intestine transplantation in children: update 2010. *Pediatr
    Clin of North Am* 2010; 57: 415–431.

39. Garland JS, Alex CP, Mueller CD, et al. A randomized trial comparing
    povidone-iodine to a chlorhexidine gluconate-impregnated dressing for pre-
    vention of central venous catheter infections in neonates. *Pediatrics* 2001; 107:
    1431–1436.

40. Ramritu P, Halton K, Collignon P, et al. A systematic review comparing the
    relative effectiveness of antimicrobial-coated catheters in intensive care units.
    Am J Infect Control 2008; 36: 104–117.

41. Jones BA, Hull MA, Richardson DS, et al. Efficacy of ethanol locks in reducing central venous catheter infections in pediatric patients with intestinal failure. *J Pediatr Surg* 2010; 45: 1287–1293.

42. Clayton PT, Whitfield P, Iyer K. The role of phytosterols in the pathogenesis of liver complications of pediatric parenteral nutrition. *Nutrition* 1998; 14: 158–164.

43. Gura KM, Lee S, Valim C, et al. Safety and efficacy of a fish-oil-based fat emulsion in the treatment of parenteral nutrition-associated liver disease. *Pediatrics* 2008; 121: e678–e686.

44. Soden JS, Lovell MA, Brown K, Partrick DA, Sokol RJ. Failure of resolution of portal fibrosis during omega-3 fatty acid lipid emulsion therapy in two patients with irreversible intestinal failure. *J Peds* 2010; 156: 327–331.

45. Mazariegos GV, Steffick DE, Horslen S, et al. Intestine transplantation in the United States, 1999–2008. *Am J Transplant* 2010; 10: 1020–1034.

CHAPTER 14

Family violence

Daniel M. Lindberg[1,2] and Esther K. Choo[3,4]
[1]Brigham and Women's Hospital, Boston, MA, USA
[2]Harvard Medical School, Boston, MA, USA
[3]Rhode Island Hospital and The Miriam Hospital, Providence, RI, USA
[4]Warren Alpert Medical School of Brown University, Providence, RI, USA

Introduction and epidemiology

The medical community's approach to child abuse (defined here as physical abuse of a minor), and intimate partner violence (IPV) (defined here as physical abuse of a spouse or significant other), together referred to here as family violence, has dramatically changed in the last several decades. Child physical abuse was only recognized in the medical literature in the mid-twentieth century [1], but has recently been designated as the newest subspecialty of pediatrics. IPV, once considered a problem best addressed by police and the courts, was redefined in the 1980s as a public health problem. But while awareness is increasing and tools are improving, clinicians continue to show uncertainty and variability in recognizing abuse, and reluctance in reporting [2–5].

Unlike other forms of trauma, emergency physicians may be reluctant to consider the diagnosis of family violence, likely because the topic threatens to change the typical patient–clinician dynamic. Under normal circumstances, the clinician, patient, and family are working toward a common goal; raising the possibility of abuse can make the clinician feel pitted in an adversarial role against the spouse or parent. Victims of abuse may have relatively minor injuries or no physical evidence of abuse at all, making the social aspects of care more central than typical medical treatments. Further, clinicians may feel that compared to their treatment of discrete medical issues, their efforts in addressing abuse are futile and that there is little chance for a good outcome. Finally, emergency physicians may feel overwhelmed and isolated by the challenge of facing a complex issue with little support.

Challenging and Emerging Conditions in Emergency Medicine, First Edition. Edited by Arvind Venkat.
© 2011 by John Wiley & Sons, Ltd. Published 2011 by Blackwell Publishing Ltd.

However, emergency physicians are not alone in dealing with violence, and the potential for improved outcomes is just as real as with other illnesses [6, 7]. Early recognition and best practices for management of family violence can improve outcomes not only for the presenting patient, but also for other family members affected by the violence. A rational and systematic approach, coupled with team effort and an understanding of the role of the emergency physician, has the potential to improve both the experience of the clinician and the short- and long-term outcomes of their patients.

Because victims of family violence are frequently unable, or unwilling, to speak out about their victimization [8] and because of poor clinician screening, documentation, and coding practices for IPV [9, 10], it is difficult to be precise in estimating the incidence or prevalence of family violence. Results of epidemiological studies for child abuse differ greatly depending on methodology and definitions of abuse [11, 12], but it is clear that the true scope of problem is much broader than most people suspect. The number of cases that are actually detected in the emergency department (ED) likely represents only a fraction of the true toll of the disease.

Child abuse

The estimated incidence of US children who suffer physical abuse annually is 2–5/1000, suggesting that hundreds of thousands of children are physically abused each year [11, 12]. The annual estimate of children killed by abuse or neglect (1740) [12] is strikingly similar to the number killed by road traffic collisions (1794) [13], and the number of infants who die from homicide is comparable to the number who die from sepsis [14]. But implementation of screening protocols for abuse continues to lag behind routine evaluation for sepsis or accidental trauma.

Abusive head trauma (AHT), formerly known as "Shaken Baby Syndrome" is the most lethal form of child abuse, with case-fatality ratios of approximately 20% and long-term disability in the majority of survivors. Estimates of AHT are 20–30 victims per 100,000 for infants and approximately half that for children between 12 and 24 months of age [15–18]. While reports of abusive head trauma have been published for older children, and even adults [19], the vast majority of patients are less than 3 years old.

The true rates of child abuse may be much higher than those cited above. In an anonymous phone survey of parents' disciplinary practices, 4.3% of parents reported using methods that would generally be considered abusive (e.g., burning, beating, kicking) as discipline and 2.6% of parents reported using shaking as discipline in children less than 2 years of age [20]. These rates are 40–150 times the rates of abuse recognized by medical professionals. Further, the vast majority of those with recognized abusive injury have moderate to severe injury, suggesting that emergency physicians are failing to recognize a large number of children with milder injuries.

Because physical abuse represents such a broad spectrum of injuries, many of which go unrecognized, it is impossible to speak broadly of the prognosis for abuse. However, the mere fact of witnessing or experiencing any abuse has been linked to long-term health deficits in adults throughout their lifetime [21].

Intimate partner violence

The National Violence Against Women survey estimated that IPV occurs in 25% of US women and 7.6% of men over their lifetimes and approximately 2 million women and 1 million men annually [22]. The health consequences of IPV are wide-ranging and profound. IPV adversely affects 8 of 10 of the leading health indicators identified by the Department of Health and Human Services and is responsible for an estimated $4.1 billion in direct medical and mental health care costs [23]. IPV occurs against both men and women, although the majority of violence, and the health sequelae of violence, occurs in women [24].

IPV is common in the ED population, among whom estimates for prevalence of past-year abuse range from 12%–19% (approximately 8–12 times that of the general population) and of lifetime abuse from 44%–54% (approximately 1.8–2.2 times that of the general population) [25–29]. There are over 500,000 visits to the ED per year for IPV-related injuries [30]. In one study of women who reported IPV to the police, 64% were seen in the ED within the previous year [31]. Another study of IPV homicides showed that 44% of victims had visited the ED within 2 years of their death [32]. The importance of the ED in recognizing abuse is compounded by the fact that victims of IPV often have poor access to primary care [33, 34].

While physical injuries from IPV often provide the most direct and striking evidence of abuse, it is becoming increasingly clear that IPV impacts every aspect of women's health. It is associated with risky health behaviors such as cigarette smoking, heavy alcohol use, and drug use [28, 35–37], as well as mental illness (depression, anxiety, post-traumatic stress disorder) and suicidality [38, 39]. IPV patients have poor maintenance of chronic medical conditions such as asthma, joint disease, peptic ulcer disease, and chronic pain syndromes [40–42]. Pregnant women who are victims of IPV tend to seek prenatal care late and are at risk for placental abruption, preterm delivery, and low infant birth weight [43]. IPV is responsible for most intentional injuries experienced by women [44] and constitutes 30%–50% of all female homicides in the United States each year [45].

Role of the emergency physician

Child abuse

With the most severe abuse, injuries are obvious and management is similar to standard trauma care, with the exception of notifying Child Protective Services (CPS). In these cases, the role of the emergency physician is relatively straightforward. However, physical abuse is often thought to become more violent over time, and early detection is considered key to improving outcomes [46]. The emergency physician is, therefore, charged with:

- identifying the early signs of inflicted injury (Table 14.1);
- initiating the process of screening for other injuries;
- preserving any appropriate evidence; and
- protecting the child and any other children at risk.

However, it is seldom possible and almost never necessary to come to the final diagnosis of abuse in the initial hours or days of the patient encounter. An ultimate determination that abuse has occurred often involves prolonged diagnostic testing, the exclusion of mimics of abuse, and careful social, and sometimes criminal, investigation. Emergency physicians should, therefore, seek collaboration with child abuse specialists and/or CPS before making definitive statements about the etiology of injuries and

Table 14.1 Red flags for child abuse [47]

History
  Serious injury from a short (<5 foot) fall [48]
  Serious injury attributed to a young sibling
  Traumatic injury without a report of trauma
  History that changes significantly over time or between caregivers
  Obvious injuries with unexplained delay in seeking care
Physical exam
  Bruising to infants not yet "cruising" [49]
  Bruising to the pinna, abdomen, genitalia, or neck
  Patterned bruises
  Bite marks
  Retinal hemorrhages
  Oral (labial, sublingual) frenulum tears
  Palatal petechiae or lacerations
  Circumferential burns of the hands or feet (stocking/glove pattern)
  Perineal burns (immersion pattern)
Radiology
  Classic metaphyseal fractures (corner "chip" or "bucket-handle" pattern) in infants
  Posterior rib fractures
  Fractures in various stages of healing

Source: Reference [47].

should refrain from specific accusations against any person. The following phrases can communicate concern for abuse in a neutral and non-accusatory manner:

- I'm concerned that someone might be hurting your child.
- The number of injuries we have found is more than we would expect in a child with this history. It is important that we make sure there isn't another reason (including another medical reason) for the findings we've identified.
- When we see injuries like this, we sometimes find other injuries that aren't obvious and it's important that we do testing to make sure we aren't missing something important.

Intimate partner violence

It is the role of the emergency physician to maintain a high level of suspicion for IPV among all patients, to be familiar with screening and management protocols at their facility, including human resources available to care for patients with IPV (such as social work or victim advocates) and to know what steps to take in the event that a patient divulges abuse.

Presenting signs and symptoms

Child abuse—seeing the red flags

Considering that (a) screening studies can detect subtle abusive injuries when children have a real chance for good recovery [50–52] and that (b) early intervention can prevent the most serious outcomes of physical abuse [5] and (c) current screening strategies fail to identify a significant fraction of abused children [5, 20], it is easy to reach the conclusion that *emergency physicians should be screening more for child physical abuse*. But *who* do we screen and *how*?

Demographic red flags

Risk factors such as poverty, substance abuse, and exposure to IPV have been found to be associated with increased rates of recognized child abuse [53]. In a retrospective study of child fatalities, the presence of an unrelated caregiver in the home (boyfriend, stepparent) dramatically increased the chance of a child dying from abuse [54]. Large studies of abuse incidence report different rates of substantiated abuse according to race, gender, and ethnicity [12]. These studies have supported a theory that abuse often results from the confluence of social stressors and a caretaker unable to cope.

However, while several studies have suggested that demographic factors are associated with abuse, the value of demographics to the emergency physician is questionable. Abuse has been documented in every population where it has been sought, by every type of perpetrator; at the same time, the vast majority of parents (of any demographic characteristic) do not abuse their children. Therefore, demographic characteristics should not be used to guide suspicion of abuse.

Historical red flags

The hallmark of child physical abuse is the presence of injuries unexplained by the given history. As such, one role of the emergency physician is to carefully document the initial history offered for any childhood injury. Injuries that may initially seem innocuous may seem more concerning with a history that is inconsistent over time or between caregivers, or if new injuries are identified [55]. Documentation for every injured child (regardless of the level of concern for abuse) should, at a minimum, include information about *when, where,* and *how* the injury occurred as well as *who* was present at the time of the injury.

Two specific histories should raise special concern when offered to explain serious injury to a pre-verbal child. Short falls (less than 5 feet) have been shown to be a rare source of serious injury [48]. Surprisingly, this even holds for children who fall down several steps [56, 57]. Similarly, serious injury attributable to another young (especially a pre-verbal) child is extremely rare and should prompt evaluation for abuse.

While delay in seeking care is often cited as a red flag for abuse, one study of abdominal injuries showed that, even in cases of non-inflicted injury, delay in seeking care was common when the injury mechanism was not clearly dangerous [58]. In the authors' experience, delay in seeking care is not uncommon in young infants with both accidental and inflicted skull or extremity fractures, which may be difficult to appreciate [59], or in some burns where the depth of the burn progresses with time. Ultimately, the foundation for concern is a caregiver who recognizes a dangerous situation, yet fails to act. Reports that a child was ill-appearing, unarousable, or even seizing for several hours while the caretaker avoided medical care are concerning.

While emergency physicians should be alert to histories that are inconsistent with the developmental abilities of the child (e.g., a not-yet-crawling infant is reported to have climbed up several steps), each child's developmental abilities are unique. One study showed that a surprising fraction of toddlers (e.g., 40% of 14-month olds) were capable of climbing into a bathtub to turn on scalding water [60].

Physical examination red flags

Children without a concerning history, and whose overall appearance may be reassuring, may be found on physical examination to have signs that are relatively specific for abuse. Because the vast majority of abused children with serious or fatal injuries are less than 4 years old [12], it is essential that all pre-verbal children seen in the ED undergo a thorough physical examination, including genitalia.

Bruises

While bruises are often considered the sine qua non of trauma, bruises are both less sensitive and less specific than many physicians believe. Large series of children with fractures, brain injury, or intra-abdominal injury demonstrate that bruises are absent in *the majority* of children with any of these injuries [50–52, 61]. Bruising should not, therefore, be relied on as a screen for occult trauma, and its absence should not have any implication for which testing ought to be pursued. The presence or absence of bruises cannot determine the force necessary to produce any given injury.

On the other hand, some bruising patterns are extremely concerning for abuse, even in isolation. Bruising is extremely uncommon in pre-mobile children, without a history of trauma. "If they don't cruise, they don't bruise" is a reasonable maxim for infants as shown by a large study that demonstrated a rate of less than 2.5% among more than 500 pre-cruising infants [49]. While bruises on the forehead, shins, and forearms are common among toddlers, bruising to the genitalia, cheeks, ears, and abdomen are rare and should raise concern for abuse [62].

Linear or patterned bruises are extremely concerning for abuse. While bruising can take the shape of the implement used to inflict the bruise, it can also take on an outline pattern, as capillaries rupture laterally from the impact. Two classic examples of this phenomenon are the "tram-track" appearance of loop marks, where parallel lines of ecchymoses or petechiae outline the path of a cord used to whip a child, and the parallel lines seen in the classic slap mark (Figure 14.1). Linear bruising about the wrists or ankles (ligature marks) can be seen when children are bound or about the corners of the mouth when children are gagged. The majority of bruises in

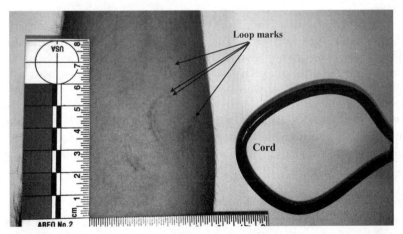

Figure 14.1 Loop marks that were the result of whipping with the pictured cord. Note the parallel or "tram-track" appearance of the petechiae, which results as capillaries rupture outwards from impact.

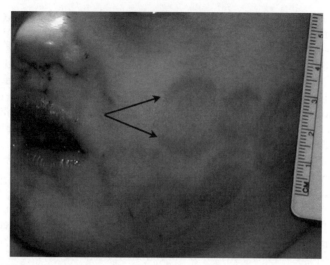

Figure 14.2 A young infant with multiple bite marks on the face. Note the symmetric, semilunar rows of box-shaped lesions. In conjunction with the history, the short maxillary intercanine distance was used to confirm that the biter had been a child (with primary teeth).

children with inflicted injuries follow no identifiable pattern. Faced with unpatterned bruises, some clinicians will describe small, oval bruises as "fingertip" bruising. Such descriptions should generally be avoided given the difficulty of demonstrating the etiology of these common bruises.

Bites

Bite marks are roughly symmetric, half-moon rows of rectangular bruises (Figure 14.2). The controversies surrounding the use of bite marks to identify a particular biter are beyond the scope of this chapter, but bear two comments. First, the maxillary intercanine distance has been used as a general method to differentiate primary teeth (child bites) from secondary teeth (adult bites). Second, the most specific method by which a biter can be identified is DNA isolation. When forensic evidence is collected, bite marks should be swabbed twice with cotton swabs (wet first, then dry) [63], and swabs should be submitted as when evidence is collected from sexual assault victims.

Burns

Burns were identified in nearly 10% of one large cohort of children evaluated for physical abuse [50]. In the authors' experience, abuse-related burns are often inflicted when a caretaker becomes frustrated in the process of toilet training. Some burn patterns are concerning for immersion, such as burns to the buttocks and perineum or burns in a stocking or glove distribution. While there is insufficient evidence to support a blanket statement of concern for burns without splash marks, deep burns in a circumferential pattern with clear lines of demarcation and no splash marks are concerning for a forced immersion. The relatively cool surface of a tub can cause central sparing if the palms, soles, or perineum are held down, a so-called "donut" pattern. This sparing, coupled with the sparing of skin folds or joint creases can, occasionally, be used to reconstruct the position of a child at the time of a scald burn [64]. While these reconstructions can sometimes be used to determine the credibility of an offered story, the simple presence of spared folds or creases does not itself imply an inflicted burn.

Oropharyngeal injuries

Oropharyngeal injuries are less well-known indicators of abuse. The soft palate, lingual and labial frenula, and inner surfaces of the lips should be examined in all children with concern for abuse [65]. Injuries have been associated with frustrated caretakers shoving fingers, bottles, spoons, or other objects into the mouths of children (Figure 14.3). Caustic ingestions may be a sign of neglect, especially in the setting of methamphetamine synthesis [66].

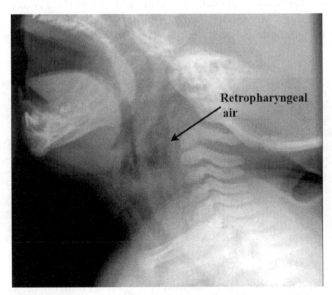

Figure 14.3 Pharyngeal injury in a young child referred for very mild oropharyngeal bleeding. The injury was ultimately thought to be the result of a frustrated caretaker shoving a spoon into the child's mouth.

Head injuries

Red flags are harder to find for abusive head injury. The neurological examination is more variable, and less sensitive in children who are preverbal and who cannot cooperate with the exam by following commands. Two studies of children at risk for abuse showed rates as high as 37% of occult head injury in children with normal neurological examinations and no external evidence of head injury [51,52]. While robust evidence is lacking, the presence of a bulging fontanel is often cited as a red flag for head injury in a child with nonspecific symptoms. As checking a fontanel is safe and easy, with a presumably low rate of false positives, we suggest this in all infants.

Fractures

In many ways, the field of child abuse pediatrics was started not by pediatricians, but by radiologists [1, 67]. Even today, some of the most specific findings for abuse remain radiographic findings. Perhaps the most specific of these is the so-called "classic metaphyseal fracture" (i.e., classic for abuse) definitively described by Paul Kleinman and others [68]. Sometimes called "chip", "corner," or "bucket-handle" fractures (Figure 14.4), these fractures can be subtle and difficult to appreciate, but when identified in infants, are extremely concerning for abuse and should always prompt further screening.

Similarly, while any unexpected fracture in a young child is concerning, fractures of the posterior ribs, near the costovertebral articulation are extremely uncommon in accidental injury and are very concerning for abuse

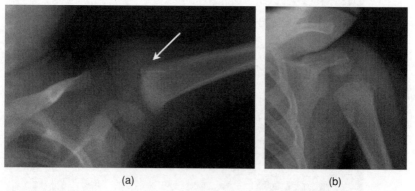

(a)   (b)

Figure 14.4 (a) Classic metaphyseal fracture of the proximal humerus in a 9-month-old child whose parents noticed decreased arm use. In this projection, the fracture appears as a chip on the lateral edge of the bone. (b) Follow-up film 12 days later. In this projection, and with increased healing and periosteal reaction, the same fracture now shows a "bucket handle" morphology.

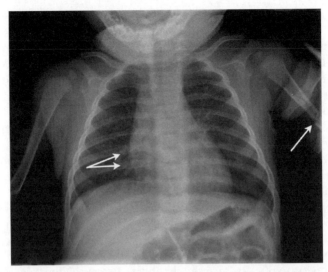

Figure 14.5 Posterior rib fractures in a 3-month-old child brought for arm pain (dual arrows). The history given by the parents, that the child was dropped and then caught by the arm, is a plausible explanation for the left humeral fracture (single arrow), but does not explain these fractures, which are very concerning for abuse.

(Figure 14.5). Traditional CPR rarely causes rib fractures of any kind, and has not been shown to cause posterior rib fractures [69]. Newer techniques of two-handed chest compressions have not been studied for their effect on rib fractures.

Myths
Research has shown that some findings once widely considered as red flags for abuse are less useful than previously thought. One well-known correlation linking the color of a bruise with its age has been discredited by studies showing that physicians have poor reliability when estimating the age of a bruise and rarely even agree about which colors are present in a bruise [70]. The appearance and color of a bruise can be affected by many factors in addition to age, including the child's complexion, depth of bleeding, and the way the bruise was inflicted.

Using the appearance of blood on CT to determine the age of a brain injury is another example of an idea that is widely taught but not well supported by evidence. Conventional teaching is that fresh bleeding is bright on CT, that dark collections must be chronic, and that collections with mixed density represent evidence of multiple episodes of trauma. Several theories have been advanced to explain why mixed density collections have been well described in children with a single traumatic episode, at both acute and more chronic stages of the injury [71, 72]. Hyperacute bleeding or re-bleeding into a chronic collection are two ways that mixed density subdural hematomas could result from a single injury, though the incidence of either finding is unknown and probably uncommon or rare [73]. The presence of CSF within a subdural hematoma could also result in either mixed density or in a darker appearance of an acute subdural hematoma. Regardless of the physiological explanation, the appearance of an intracranial injury on CT is not a reliable way to determine the age of the injury.

Finally, the spiral fracture continues to carry an overly dark reputation as being specific for abuse. Studies of fracture morphology in the upper [74] and lower [75] extremities disagree as to whether the spiral fracture is overrepresented among abused children, but agree that no fracture morphology (aside from the classic metaphyseal fracture) should be used in isolation to determine whether a fracture was inflicted. This is not to imply that spiral fractures need not be considered for the possibility of abuse. Rather the cause of a fracture should always be considered, regardless of morphology.

Intimate partner violence

As with child abuse, there are demographic and patient characteristics associated with the occurrence of IPV. IPV is associated with younger age, female gender, and low socioeconomic status [76]. It is also highly prevalent among those with mental health and alcohol and substance use problems [77]. Among ED patients, IPV victims tend to present to the ED during evening, overnight, and weekend hours [78]. However, again, using any of these characteristics as flags for IPV is problematic, as abuse occurs in patients of all backgrounds and all medical histories.

Clinical indicators

While there are "classic" injuries of IPV, including cigarette burns, ligature marks, strangulation marks, and defensive wounds [79], *any* injuries due to interpersonal violence should prompt questioning about IPV, particularly among women, who experience assault most often in the context of an intimate partner relationship [80]. Further, it is important to remember that IPV victims often present to the ED for reasons other than injury [31]. Although certain injury patterns (e.g., maxillofacial injuries, multiple injuries, extremity fractures) and non-injury complaints (e.g., nonspecific abdominal pain) have been studied for their ability to serve in screening algorithms for IPV [81, 82], to date, these have demonstrated limited predictive value [44]. It therefore seems reasonable to conclude that "routine screening"—asking *all* patients about abuse, regardless of race, gender, sexual orientation, or presenting compliant—is the most appropriate and effective approach to identify IPV.

Screening studies

Child abuse

In many cases, it will not be possible for the clinician to definitively determine whether the offered history is sufficient to explain the identified injury. In these cases, the identification of other occult injuries may be the most conclusive evidence that the offered history is inconsistent, and that the child is being abused. A handful of tests have been used commonly as part of an emerging standard of care to supplement a detailed history and physical examination in screening for occult injuries (Table 14.2).

Importantly, the forensic implications of abusive injuries make screening standards very different than for cases where there is no concern for abuse. Many abusive injuries are self-limited, require no treatment, and are unlikely themselves to be a source of morbidity. Rather, injuries like classic metaphyseal fractures, retinal hemorrhages, and hepatic contusions are more important for what they say about the mechanism or timing of an injury and the danger of a child's environment. The goal in diagnosing these injuries is not only to treat them, but also to prevent future injuries. Therefore, a normal examination or a well-appearing child should not be used as a reason to omit screening that is otherwise indicated.

Skeletal survey

The radiographic skeletal survey is the oldest screening test for abusive injuries and has the most support in the medical literature. Studies consistently show that 20% of infants referred for skeletal survey are found

Table 14.2 Testing protocols when suspecting child abuse

Test	Indication	Notes
Skeletal survey	All children <24 months Selected cases 24–60 months Rarely >60 months	Includes children with burns
Neuroimaging	Children with mental status change, evidence of head injury Children <6 months Infants with facial bruising, rib fractures, or multiple fractures	Consider MRI in stable children
Retinal examination	Traumatic brain injury Mental status change Facial bruising	Requires ophthalmologist using dilated pupil examination
Abdominal CT	AST or ALT > 80 IU Abdominal tenderness, bruising, or distention	Abdominal ultrasound and serial transaminases do not replace CT

to have occult fractures, and that the rate for children between 1–2 years of age runs between 10%–20% [83–85]. The American Academy of Pediatrics, therefore, considers the skeletal survey to be mandatory in all children less than 2 years of age when there is a concern for physical abuse [86]. Children above 5 years of age are unlikely to benefit from the skeletal survey and children between 2–5 years should be considered on a case-by-case basis. Factors that may suggest screening for children between 2 and 5 years include decreased mobility, communication difficulties, concerning history, or altered mental status due to brain injury.

Some clinicians have considered children with abusive burns to be an exception to the otherwise universal recommendation for skeletal survey in young children suspected to have suffered child abuse. While children who present with burns seem to have a lower rate of occult fractures than other children with concerns for abuse, the rate of occult fractures remains high enough to support routine skeletal survey [87, 88].

To be accurate, the skeletal survey requires specialized equipment and technique, and should be interpreted by a radiologist with experience with the skeletal survey [89]. Guidelines define the specific views and equipment required for a proper skeletal survey [90, 91]. In most EDs, the implication of these guidelines is that young children with concern for physical abuse will need to be transferred to an experienced center (usually a children's hospital) for a proper evaluation.

The skeletal survey is not a time-critical test and sensitivity may even increase as fractures begin the healing process (days to weeks). As such, it is reasonable to wait until a child is clinically stable rather than performing a suboptimal survey with portable equipment. In rare cases where a safe environment for the child can be assured (e.g., when abuse is suspected from a daycare provider), a skeletal survey could even be arranged as an outpatient study, assuming other serious injuries have been excluded. A follow-up skeletal survey performed in 10–14 days will frequently identify fractures missed by the initial survey and improve the interpretation of inconclusive findings [92]. Post-mortem skeletal surveys may identify injuries that would not be appreciated on autopsy. While radionuclide bone scans are occasionally used to supplement skeletal surveys, they are not a first-line study and are not commonly ordered by emergency physicians.

Neuroimaging

Because abusive head trauma is responsible for the vast majority of morbidity and mortality from abuse, neuroimaging is a core component in screening for abuse. As in children with accidental head injury, it seems reasonable to perform imaging with altered mental status, bulging fontanel, or evidence of injury to the head on physical examination. However, unlike adults, the infants and young children who are likely to be victims of abusive head trauma are unable to communicate the subtle signs of brain trauma, like headache, nausea, confusion, or paresthesias. Two studies have shown high rates of occult head injuries in children with concerns for abuse, even in the absence of physical examination findings [51, 52]. Therefore, it seems reasonable to use the criteria studied by Rubin et al. to determine which infants with suspicion of abuse but without clinical evidence of head injury should undergo imaging: age less than 6 months, multiple fractures, rib fractures, or facial injury [52].

The role of neuroimaging in children who present with an acute life-threatening event (ALTE) is unclear. While the incidence of child abuse quoted by one moderate-sized ($n = 128$) series of children with ALTE (2.3%) seems too low to recommend routine neuroimaging, it suggests that this group at least deserves careful consideration of the possibility of abuse [93].

As with the skeletal survey, the results of screening neuroimaging, while critical to the long-term health of the child, will not impact the immediate management of the stable child. With this in mind, and coupled with increasing concerns about the use of diagnostic radiation, MRI is a reasonable alternative to CT in stable children.

Retinal examination

While a number of conditions can cause retinal hemorrhages, certain patterns of retinal hemorrhages (multilayered, too numerous to count, extending to the ora serrata), or other retinal findings like retinoschisis (mechanical disruption of the layers of the retina leading to a cystic cavity, partially or completely filled with blood) are very specific for abusive head trauma [94]. The accuracy of examinations performed by non-ophthalmologists without a dilated pupil is poor [95]. While characteristic retinal hemorrhages have been reported in abused children with normal neuroimaging [96], this is rare and is usually associated with evidence of facial injury or altered mental status [97].

Abdominal injuries

Abdominal injuries are found in less than 10% of children evaluated for physical abuse [50, 98], and the majority of children with accidental abdominal trauma heal without intervention [99]. Yet abdominal trauma is second only to head injury as a source of mortality in abused children [54], and even as routine "trauma panels" for children with blunt injuries are being abandoned, most experts recommend routine laboratory or CT screening in children with concern for abuse [100, 101]. The fact that abdominal injuries from child abuse may be self-limited actually *increases* the urgency for the emergency physician since these injuries might not be detected if testing is left for the follow-up consultation.

Screening for abdominal injuries involves two types of testing: blood tests and imaging. Of all blood tests, hepatic transaminases (AST and ALT) have received the most attention. Two studies have shown that well-appearing children with transaminase elevations are likely to have abdominal injuries [50, 98] and support routine screening in children with concerns for abuse. Children with significant elevations of AST or ALT (a level of 80 IU/dL is one conservative threshold [50]) should undergo definitive testing such as CT, laparotomy, or autopsy, as clinically appropriate. It is clear that some abdominal injuries are missed by hepatic transaminases, regardless of the threshold used [50, 102]. Children with clinical signs of abdominal injury like abdominal bruising or tenderness, or a history of assault to the abdomen should undergo definitive testing, regardless of transaminase results.

Literature is scarce in support of other screening laboratory tests like amylase, lipase, and urinalysis for microscopic hematuria. While many experts recommend sending these studies routinely, practice varies in the absence of evidence-based guidelines [103, 104].

Because children with occult abdominal injuries are, by definition, well appearing, there is often reluctance to use CT as the initial imaging screening modality, in favor of abdominal ultrasound or serial transaminase measurements. However, professional guidelines agree that CT with IV contrast is the most appropriate first-line study [90, 105]. Abdominal ultrasound lacks sensitivity for several abusive injuries [102] and hepatic transaminases will almost universally trend to normal, regardless of whether an injury exists [106].

Siblings and contacts

Unfortunately, many abused children are only identified when symptoms are obvious and when treatments have limited efficacy (as in most cases of abusive head trauma). However, if family violence is indeed a disease that affects an entire household, siblings and contacts of abused children may represent a group that is especially likely to benefit from early intervention. To date, there are no evidence-based guidelines for screening the contacts (siblings and other at-risk children) of abused children and there is some variability among both medical experts and child protection workers [107]. In cases where there is serious concern for abuse, many experts would recommend, at a minimum, physical examination for all contact children and skeletal survey for contact children that are less than 2 years of age [107]. Though firm evidence is difficult to obtain, twins of abused children are thought to be at especially increased risk and warrant more screening [108].

Estimates of the co-occurrence of IPV and child abuse vary widely, but are certainly high (33%–77%) [109], supporting universal violence screening for all adults living in a household with an abused child.

Intimate partner violence

Screening for IPV remains a controversial issue. The United States Preventive Services Task Force (USPSTF) does not currently endorse screening for family violence. Its most recent recommendations state, "No studies have directly addressed the harms of screening and interventions for family and intimate partner violence ... the USPSTF could not determine the balance between the benefits and harms of screening for family and intimate partner violence ... " [110]. However, many physicians feel that sheer logic and the humanity of screening—of asking patients about a condition influential in virtually all aspects of their health and well-being and potentially fatal—is enough to justify the practice of screening [104]. Routine assessment of patients for violence has been mandated by the Joint Commission and supported by many major medical societies [111–113].

There are a variety of screening tools studied in the ED setting (Table 14.3) [114–116]. ED-based screening tools are designed to be brief and inclusive. They are not diagnostic, and should prompt notification of the treating clinician or a social worker to perform a full evaluation, which

Table 14.3 Screening tools for intimate partner violence

Screening tools	Questions	Topics covered
HITS (Hurt, Insult, Threaten, and Scream)	How often does your partner[†]: 1. Physically hurt you? 2. Insult you or talk down to you? 3. Threaten you with harm? 4. Scream or curse at you?	Physical and emotional abuse
PVS (Partner Violence Screen)[‡]	1. Have you been hit, kicked, punched, or otherwise hurt by someone within the past year? If so, by whom? 2. Do you feel safe in your current relationship? 3. Is there a partner from a previous relationship who is making you feel unsafe now?	Physical abuse and injury
STaT[*]	1. Have you ever been in a relationship where your partner has pushed or slapped you? 2. Have you ever been in a relationship where your partner threatened you with violence? 3. Have you ever been in a relationship where your partner has thrown, broken, or punched things?	Physical and emotional abuse

[†]Respondents are asked to respond on a 5-point Likert scale: never (1 point); rarely [2]; sometimes [3]; fairly often [4]; frequently [5]. Total scores >10 are positive.
[‡]A positive response to any question indicates abuse.
[*]Considering any affirmative response a positive screen provides the highest sensitivity.

should include more detailed questioning about the circumstances referred to in the screen and an assessment of safety. In the absence of screening protocols, or if there is suspicion of abuse that was not identified during triage screening, emergency physicians may ask directly about abuse, framing questions with statements such as "Because violence is so common in people's lives, I ask all my patients about it," or "I'm concerned that your symptoms may have been caused by someone hurting you" [117].

Treatment

Acute treatment for the injuries that result from family violence is no different than if the same injuries had occurred accidentally. But inflicted injuries invoke the potential for future injury and the duty to protect, or offer protection to, the patient. For children, this often means acting to protect the child in the short term and reporting concerns of abuse to agencies or groups charged with investigating abuse. For competent adults, this means ensuring that the patient has safe housing, a safety plan, and contact with law enforcement and community resources for counseling.

Children-mandated reporting

The actual process of reporting a child to CPS is much simpler than most physicians assume. Each state's CPS agency and associated child abuse hotline can be found using any standard Internet search engine. Filing a report usually involves a phone call, with or without a faxed, written report detailing the reason(s) for concern. CPS will determine the extent and timing of the investigation. Knowing the address where the abuse is thought to have occurred will help CPS assign a lead team to respond.

Important protections exist for reporters of child abuse and neglect. Physicians cannot be successfully sued for malpractice because of reporting in good faith, even if the concern for abuse is not ultimately substantiated. The HIPAA privacy regulations were specifically written so as not to limit the ability (or duty) to report concerns for abuse and neglect. Section 1178(b) of the statute specifically excludes reports for concerns of abuse from the scope of the law.

Intimate partner violence

Almost every state has some legal requirement for health care practitioners to report IPV in patients with injuries resulting from abuse. The exact laws vary from state to state [118]. States may require reporting of any partner violence treated by a clinician, or reporting only in the context of criminal acts, injuries by firearms or sharp weapons, potentially fatal injuries, burn injuries, or any injuries at all that result from partner violence (or some combinations of these).

Basic treatment for IPV involves four steps. First, an assessment should be performed to determine if the patient is at high risk for severe or lethal violence. There is no single accepted tool for assessing risk, but, in general, the patient should be asked about escalating violence, threats of lethal violence, threats to children in the household, perpetrator risk factors such as alcohol and drug use and the patient's subjective sense of safety. The option of relocating to a shelter or other housing for IPV victims should be discussed with women who report risk factors for violent abuse and who do not have alternate options. Second, women should be offered assistance in contacting law enforcement during their ED stay. Third, a safety plan should be discussed with the patient, emphasizing basic, immediate actions to improve safety, such as removing weapons from the house, creating and practicing a rapid escape plan, and teaching children how to get help. Making a long-term plan for increasing safety and coping with abuse (e.g., increasing financial independence, couples counseling) is also important, and should be discussed with in follow-up with community partner violence agencies and/or primary-care provider. Finally, victims should be referred to community partner violence programs where they can receive further counseling, support, and often legal and housing assistance. If local resources are unavailable or unknown, the National Domestic Violence Hotline (1-800-799-SAFE) provides 24-hour assistance and referrals to IPV victims. Many victims will not wish to leave their relationship immediately, and directing them to resources will assist them in improving their safety over the long term.

In some institutions, these functions—assessment, safety options, police engagement, and referral to community resources—may be performed by a specific staff member such as a social worker or case manager. In other circumstances, local community partner violence agencies may have advocates available to come to the hospital, meet with victims, and offer needed services and resources. At present, availability of these services is highly variable; thus, in many settings clinicians must become familiar with the standard treatment algorithm and management resources, such as intervention checklists and referral resources (the "Domestic Violence Packet") available in their ED.

Accurate and complete medical documentation of IPV is important for clinical, epidemiological, and legal reasons. Having IPV as part of the medical record allows other treating clinicians to understand the patient's health needs, reassess patient safety, and follow-up on need for IPV-related services. Coding of IPV is necessary for disease surveillance and appropriate allocation of resources. Finally, documentation and testimony based on documentation are valuable for victims seeking legal relief from abuse [119].

Documentation should be clear, concise, and objective. Emergency physicians should describe: all injuries and the medical treatment provided; the stated cause, timing, and mechanism of injuries (including any use of a weapon); the alleged perpetrator's name and relationship to the patient; observed behaviors of the victim to the alleged perpetrator;

whether photographs were taken; if police are involved, the name and contact details of the police officer; the referral and follow-up plans discussed with the patient; and the status of others in the home, including children.

Disposition

Child abuse

The majority of young children with concerns for physical abuse will require admission to the hospital—if only so that CPS can determine a safe place for the child to be discharged. Medically stable children can be discharged in cases where the immediate workup is complete and a safe environment has been identified. These cases usually involve an older child with cutaneous injuries attributed to a specific perpetrator or household. If the child is under the care of a different household (e.g., when one parent with joint custody alleges abuse by the other parent) or if the alleged perpetrator will not be near the child (as when CPS establishes a safety plan requiring the alleged perpetrator to live somewhere else), the investigation can continue in the outpatient setting.

Intimate partner violence

The majority of patients who are victims of IPV will be able to return home or to another safe situation—sometimes the home of a friend or family member. In exceptional circumstances, when risk for harm or fatality is high, shelter at an IPV facility is not available and women have no alternate safe housing with friends or family, the patient may need to be admitted to the hospital.

The next five years

Child abuse

At times, the medical approach to abused children can seem woefully primitive. There are no gold-standard diagnostic criteria for abuse, practices and opinions of experts can differ and estimates of the number of abused children can vary widely [2, 11, 12]. There are, as yet, no specific treatments for abusive injuries, and prevention is just starting to have an impact [120]. But it is worth noting that modern medicine did not even recognize child abuse as an entity until the mid-twentieth century [67]. Since then, the field has moved beyond raising awareness and measuring demographics into establishing best practices for screening and testing dogma to determine which indicators of abuse are reliable and which are merely myths [69, 70, 121].

With its establishment as a new subspecialty of pediatrics, the field of child abuse pediatrics has recently made an important transition within medicine. As fellowship training programs become accredited and continue to produce board-certified subspecialists, the field will be better equipped to take on the next challenges and improve the ability of doctors to protect children from abusive injury [122].

Current research is seeking to establish best-practice guidelines for screening and reporting in order to decrease variability in the evaluation of potentially abused children. As hospital-based, multidisciplinary child protection teams become both more common and better integrated into the public child protection system, reporting practices should continue to become more uniform between different hospitals and states. Prevention programs continue to gain acceptance and have shown some progress, while the goal of developing specific treatments for abusive injuries remains stubbornly elusive.

Intimate partner violence

The past 25 years have led to great advances in the understanding and awareness of the prevalence and sequelae of IPV. The mission over the near future for health professionals will be:

1. To correct the deficiencies in evidence noted in the 2004 USPSTF family violence screening statement. Further data on the outcomes of health care-based screening and intervention programs will allow us to provide evidence-based recommendations to providers.
2. To adequately address IPV beyond the education of individual emergency physicians. We need to identify the most effective and cost-effective resources for health care *systems* to support their clinicians in the identification and management of IPV.
3. To work with community IPV organizations to define meaningful outcomes and to design and test safe, effective interventions that can be initiated in the ED are priorities in the upcoming years.

Conclusion

Child abuse and intimate partner violence are challenging conditions that face emergency physicians on a regular basis. An understanding of the epidemiology, clinical management, and evolution of care of these patient populations and coordination with specialists and legal and community resources will aid the emergency physician in providing quality care to victims of family violence.

References

1. Kempe CH, Silverman FN, Steele BF, Droegemueller W, Silver HK. The battered-child syndrome. *JAMA* 1962; 181: 17–24.
2. Trokel M, Wadimmba A, Griffith J, Sege R. Variation in the diagnosis of child abuse in severely injured infants. *Pediatrics* 2006; 117(3): 722–728.

3. Flaherty EG, Sege RD, Griffith J, et al. From suspicion of physical child abuse to reporting: primary care clinician decision-making. *Pediatrics* 2008; 122(3): 611–619.

4. Jones R, Flaherty EG, Binns HJ, et al. Clinicians' description of factors influencing their reporting of suspected child abuse: report of the Child Abuse Reporting Experience Study Research Group. *Pediatrics* 2008; 122(2): 259–266.

5. Jenny C, Hymel KP, Ritzen A, Reinert SE, Hay TC. Analysis of missed cases of abusive head trauma. *JAMA* 1999; 281(7): 621–626.

6. Barlow KM, Thomson E, Johnson D, Minns RA. Late neurologic and cognitive sequelae of inflicted traumatic brain injury in infancy. *Pediatrics* 2005; 116(2): e174–e185.

7. Makoroff KL, Putnam FW. Outcomes of infants and children with inflicted traumatic brain injury. *Dev Med Child Neurol* 2003; 45(7): 497–502.

8. Sjoberg RL, Lindblad F. Limited disclosure of sexual abuse in children whose experiences were documented by videotape. *Am J Psychiatry* 2002; 159(2): 312–314.

9. Rhodes KV, Frankel RM, Levinthal N, Prenoveau E, Bailey J, Levinson W. "You're not a victim of domestic violence, are you?" Provider patient communication about domestic violence. *Ann Intern Med* 2007; 147(9): 620–627.

10. Rudman WJ. Coding and Documentation of Domestic Violence: Family Violence Prevention Fund; 2000.

11. Sedlak AJ, Mettenburg J, Besena M, et al. Fourth National Incidence Study of Child Abuse and Neglect (NIS-4): Report to Congress. Department of Health & Human Services; 2010.

12. US Department of Health and Human Services. Child Maltreatment 2008. Administration on Children Youth & Families; 2010.

13. NHTSA. Traffic Safety Facts 2006 Data – Children. In: *Transportation*, editor; 2010.

14. Heron M, Tejada-Vera B. Deaths: leading causes for 2005. *Natl Vital Stat Rep* 2009; 58(8): 1–97.

15. Keenan HT, Runyan DK, Marshall SW, Nocera MA, Merten DF, Sinal SH. A population-based study of inflicted traumatic brain injury in young children. *JAMA* 2003; 290(5): 621–626.

16. Barlow KM, Minns RA. Annual incidence of shaken impact syndrome in young children. *Lancet* 2000; 356(9241): 1571–1572.

17. Kelly P, Farrant B. Shaken baby syndrome in New Zealand,2000–2002. *Journal of Paediatrics and Child Health* 2008; 44(3): 99–107.

18. King WJ, MacKay M, Sirnick A. Shaken baby syndrome in Canada: clinical characteristics and outcomes of hospital cases. *CMAJ* 2003; 168(2): 155–159.

19. Carrigan TD, Walker E, Barnes S. Domestic violence: the shaken adult syndrome. *J Accid Emerg Med* 2000; 17(2): 138–139.

20. Theodore AD, Chang JJ, Runyan DK, Hunter WM, Bangdiwala SI, Agans R. Epidemiologic features of the physical and sexual maltreatment of children in the Carolinas. *Pediatrics* 2005; 115(3): e331–e337.

21. Felitti VJ, Anda RF, Nordenberg D, et al. Relationship of childhood abuse and household dysfunction to many of the leading causes of death in adults. The Adverse Childhood Experiences (ACE) study. *Am J Prev Med* 1998; 14(4): 245–258.

22. Tjaden P, Thoennes N. Full report on the prevalence, incidence, and consequences of violence against women. Washington, DC: U.S. Department of Justice; 2000. Report No.: NCJ 183781

23. Coker A, Smith P, Bethea L, King M, McKeown R. Physical health consequences of physical and psychological intimate partner violence. *Arch Fam Med* 2000; 9(5): 451–457.

24. Rennison CM WS. *Intimate Partner Violence*. Washington, DC: Bureau of Justice Statistics, U.S. Department of Justice; 2000. Report No.: NCJ 178247.

25. Brokaw J, Fullerton-Gleason L, Olson L, Crandall C, McLaughlin S, Sklar D. Health status and intimate partner violence: a cross-sectional study. *Ann Emerg Med* 2002; 39(1): 31–38.

26. Dearwater SR, Coben JH, Campbell JC, et al. Prevalence of intimate partner abuse in women treated at community hospital emergency departments. *JAMA* 1998; 280(5): 433–438.

27. El-Bassel N, Gilbert L, Krishnan S, et al. Partner violence and sexual HIV-risk behaviors among women in an inner-city emergency department. *Violence Vict* 1998; 13(4): 377–393.

28. Abbott J, Johnson R, Koziol-McLain J, Lowenstein SR. Domestic violence against women. Incidence and prevalence in an emergency department population. *JAMA* 1995; 273(22): 1763–1767.

29. Ernst AA, Nick TG, Weiss SJ, Houry D, Mills T. Domestic violence in an inner-city ED. *Ann Emerg Med* 1997; 30(2): 190–197.

30. National Consensus Guidelines. *On Identifying and Responding to Domestic Violence Victimization in Health Care Settings*. San Francisco, CA: Family Violence Prevention Fund; 2004.

31. Kothari CL, Rhodes KV. Missed opportunities: emergency department visits by police-identified victims of intimate partner violence. *Ann Emerg Med* 2006; 47(2): 190–199.

32. Wadman MC, Muelleman RL. Domestic violence homicides: ED use before victimization. *Am J Emerg Med* 1999; 17(7): 689–691.

33. Martino MA, Balar A, Cragun JM, Hoffman MS. Delay in treatment of invasive cervical cancer due to intimate partner violence. *Gynecol Oncol* 2005; 99(2): 507–509.

34. Brookoff D, O'Brien KK, Cook CS, Thompson TD, Williams C. Characteristics of participants in domestic violence. Assessment at the scene of domestic assault. *JAMA* 1997; 277(17): 1369–1373.

35. Weinsheimer RL, Schermer CR, Malcoe LH, Balduf LM, Bloomfield LA. Severe intimate partner violence and alcohol use among female trauma patients. *J Trauma* 2005; 58(1): 22–29.

36. El-Bassel N, Gilbert L, Witte S, et al. Intimate partner violence and substance abuse among minority women receiving care from an inner-city emergency department. *Women's Health Issues* 2003; 13(1): 16–22.

37. Najavits LM, Sonn J, Walsh M, Weiss RD. Domestic violence in women with PTSD and substance abuse. *Addict Behav* 2004; 29(4): 707–715.

38. Breiding MJ, Black MC, Ryan GW. Chronic disease and health risk behaviors associated with intimate partner violence—18 U.S. states/territories, 2005. *Ann Epidemiol* 2008; 18(7): 538–544.

39. Coker AL, Davis KE, Arias I, et al. Physical and mental health effects of intimate partner violence for men and women. *Am J Prev Med* 2002; 23(4): 260–268.

40. Coker AL, Smith PH, Bethea L, King MR, McKeown RE. Physical health consequences of physical and psychological intimate partner violence. *Arch Fam Med* 2000; 9(5): 451–457.

41. Breiding MJ, Black MC, Ryan GW. Prevalence and risk factors of intimate partner violence in eighteen U.S. states/territories, 2005. *Am J Prev Med* 2008; 34(2): 112–118.

42. Coker AL, Smith PH, Fadden MK. Intimate partner violence and disabilities among women attending family practice clinics. *J Women's Health (Larchmt)* 2005; 14(9): 829–838.

43. Mayer L, Liebschutz J. Domestic violence in the pregnant patient: obstetric and behavioral interventions. *Obstet Gynecol Surv* 1998; 53(10): 627–635.

44. Fanslow JL, Norton RN, Spinola CG. Indicators of assault-related injuries among women presenting to the emergency department. *Ann Emerg Med* 1998; 32(3 Pt 1): 341–348.

45. National Center for Injury Prevention and Control. *Costs of Intimate Partner Violence Against Women in the United States*. Atlanta, GA: Centers for Disease Control and Prevention; 2003.

46. Adamsbaum C, Grabar S, Mejean N, Rey-Salmon C. Abusive head trauma: judicial admissions highlight violent and repetitive shaking. *Pediatrics* 2010; 126(3): 546–555.

47. Lindberg D. Child abuse. In: Schutzman SA (ed.) *Essential Emergency Imaging*. Philadelphia, PA, USA: Lippincott (in press); 2011.

48. Chadwick DL, Bertocci G, Castillo E, et al. Annual risk of death resulting from short falls among young children: less than 1 in 1 million. *Pediatrics* 2008; 121(6): 1213–1224.

49. Sugar NF, Taylor JA, Feldman KW. Bruises in infants and toddlers: those who don't cruise rarely bruise. Puget Sound Pediatric Research Network. *Arch Peds Adolesc Med* 1999; 153(4): 399–403.

50. Lindberg D, Makoroff K, Harper N, et al. Utility of hepatic transaminases to recognize abuse in children. *Pediatrics* 2009; 124(2): 509–516.

51. Laskey AL, Holsti M, Runyan DK, Socolar RR. Occult head trauma in young suspected victims of physical abuse. *J Pediatrics* 2004; 144(6): 719–722.

52. Rubin DM, Christian CW, Bilaniuk LT, Zazyczny KA, Durbin DR. Occult head injury in high-risk abused children. *Pediatrics* 2003; 111(6 Pt 1): 1382–1386.

53. Kotch JB, Browne DC, Dufort V, Winsor J. Predicting child maltreatment in the first 4 years of life from characteristics assessed in the neonatal period. *Child Abuse & Neglect* 1999; 23(4): 305–319.

54. Schnitzer PG, Ewigman BG. Child deaths resulting from inflicted injuries: household risk factors and perpetrator characteristics. *Pediatrics* 2005; 116(5): e687–e693.

55. Hettler J, Greenes DS. Can the initial history predict whether a child with a head injury has been abused? *Pediatrics* 2003; 111(3): 602–607.

56. Chiaviello CT, Christoph RA, Bond GR. Stairway-related injuries in children. *Pediatrics* 1994; 94(5): 679–681.

57. Joffe M, Ludwig S. Stairway injuries in children. *Pediatrics* 1988; 82(3 Pt 2): 457–461.
58. Wood J, Rubin DM, Nance ML, Christian CW. Distinguishing inflicted versus accidental abdominal injuries in young children. *J Trauma* 2005; 59(5): 1203–1208.
59. Morris S, Cassidy N, Stephens M, McCormack D, McManus F. Birth-associated femoral fractures: incidence and outcome. *J Pediatr Orthop* 2002; 22(1): 27–30.
60. Allasio D, Fischer H. Immersion scald burns and the ability of young children to climb into a bathtub. *Pediatrics* 2005; 115(5): 1419–1421.
61. Peters ML, Starling SP, Barnes-Eley ML, Heisler KW. The presence of bruising associated with fractures. *Arch Peds Adolesc Med* 2008; 162(9): 877–881.
62. Carpenter RF. The prevalence and distribution of bruising in babies. *Arch Dis Childhood* 1999; 80(4): 363–366.
63. Sweet D, Lorente M, Lorente JA, Valenzuela A, Villanueva E. An improved method to recover saliva from human skin: the double swab technique. *J Forensic Sci* 1997; 42(2): 320–322.
64. Lenoski EF, Hunter KA. Specific patterns of inflicted burn injuries. *J Trauma* 1977; 17(11): 842–846.
65. Thackeray JD. Frena tears and abusive head injury: a cautionary tale. *Ped Emerg Care* 2007; 23(10): 735–737.
66. Farst K, Duncan JM, Moss M, Ray RM, Kokoska E, James LP. Methamphetamine exposure presenting as caustic ingestions in children. *Ann Emerg Med* 2007; 49(3): 341–343.
67. Caffey J. Multiple fractures in the long bones of infants suffering from chronic subdural hematoma. *Am J Roentgenol Radium Ther* 1946; 56(2): 163–173.
68. Kleinman PK, Marks SC, Blackbourne B. The metaphyseal lesion in abused infants: a radiologic–histopathologic study. *AJR* 1986; 146(5): 895–905.
69. Maguire S, Mann M, John N, Ellaway B, Sibert JR, Kemp AM. Does cardiopulmonary resuscitation cause rib fractures in children? A systematic review. *Child Abuse & Neglect* 2006; 30(7): 739–751.
70. Maguire S, Mann MK, Sibert J, Kemp A. Can you age bruises accurately in children? A systematic review. *Arch Dis Childhood* 2005; 90(2): 187–189.
71. Tung GA, Kumar M, Richardson RC, Jenny C, Brown WD. Comparison of accidental and non-accidental traumatic head injury in children on noncontrast computed tomography. *Pediatrics* 2006; 118(2): 626–633.
72. Vinchon M, Noule N, Tchofo PJ, Soto-Ares G, Fourier C, Dhellemmes P. Imaging of head injuries in infants: temporal correlates and forensic implications for the diagnosis of child abuse. *J Neurosurgery* 2004; 101(1 Suppl.): 44–52.
73. Hymel KP, Jenny C, Block RW. Intracranial hemorrhage and rebleeding in suspected victims of abusive head trauma: addressing the forensic controversies. *Child Maltreatment* 2002; 7(4): 329–348.
74. Strait RT, Siegel RM, Shapiro RA. Humeral fractures without obvious etiologies in children less than 3 years of age: when is it abuse? *Pediatrics* 1995; 96(4 Pt 1): 667–671.
75. Scherl SA, Miller L, Lively N, Russinoff S, Sullivan CM, Tornetta P, 3rd. Accidental and non-accidental femur fractures in children. *Clinical Orthopaedics and Related Research* 2000; 376: 96–105.

76. Thompson RS, Bonomi AE, Anderson M, et al. Intimate partner violence: prevalence, types, and chronicity in adult women. *Am J Prev Med* 2006; 30(6): 447–457.
77. Najavits L, Sonn J, Walsh M, et al. Domestic violence in women with PTSD and substance abuse. *Addict Behav* 2004; 29(4): 707–715.
78. Birnbaum A, Calderon Y, Gennis P, Rao R, Gallagher EJ. Domestic violence: diurnal mismatch between need and availability of services. *Acad Emerg Med* 1996; 3(3): 246–251.
79. Mitchell C, Anglin D. *Intimate Partner Violence: A Health-Based Perspective*. Oxford, New York: Oxford University Press; 2009.
80. Fanslow J, Norton R, Spinola C. Indicators of assault-related injuries among women presenting to the emergency department. *Ann Emerg Med* 1998; 32: 341–348.
81. Le BT, Dierks EJ, Ueeck BA, Homer LD, Potter BF. Maxillofacial injuries associated with domestic violence. *J Oral Maxillofac Surg* 2001; 59(11): 1277–1283; discussion 83–84.
82. Olson L, Anctil C, Fullerton L, Brillman J, Arbuckle J, Sklar D. Increasing emergency physician recognition of domestic violence. *Ann Emerg Med* 1996; 27(6): 741–746.
83. Merten DF, Radkowski MA, Leonidas JC. The abused child: a radiological reappraisal. *Radiology* 1983; 146(2): 377–381.
84. Ellerstein NS, Norris KJ. Value of radiologic skeletal survey in assessment of abused children. *Pediatrics* 1984; 74(6): 1075–1078.
85. Belfer RA, Klein BL, Orr L. Use of the skeletal survey in the evaluation of child maltreatment. *Am J Emerg Med* 2001; 19(2): 122–124.
86. Sane SM, Kleinman PK, Cohen RA, et al. Diagnostic imaging of child abuse. *Pediatrics* 2000; 105(6): 1345–1348.
87. Harris TL, Hicks RA, Laskey AL, Applegate K, Hibbard RA. Incidence of Occult Injury in Siblings and Other Children Living with Abused Children. Tucson, AZ: Helfer Society Annual Meeting; 2008.
88. DeGraw M, Hicks RA, Lindberg D. Incidence of fractures among children with burns with concern regarding abuse. *Pediatrics* 2010; 125(2): e295–e299.
89. Kleinman PL, Kleinman PK, Savageau JA. Suspected infant abuse: radiographic skeletal survey practices in pediatric health care facilities. *Radiology* 2004; 233(2): 477–485.
90. Kleinman PK, Di Pietro MA, Brody AS, et al. Diagnostic imaging of child abuse. *Pediatrics* 2009; 123(5): 1430–1435.
91. Applegate KE, Jr WRA, Black DA, Carlson RA, Cartland JP, Cawley KM, et al. ACR Practice Guideline for Skeletal Surveys in Children. *ACR Practice Guideline* 2006: 253–257.
92. Kleinman PK, Nimkin K, Spevak MR, et al. Follow-up skeletal surveys in suspected child abuse. *AJR* 1996; 167(4): 893–896.
93. Pitetti RD, Maffei F, Chang K, Hickey R, Berger R, Pierce MC. Prevalence of retinal hemorrhages and child abuse in children who present with an apparent life-threatening event. *Pediatrics* 2002; 110(3): 557–562.
94. Levin AV, Christian CW. The eye examination in the evaluation of child abuse. *Pediatrics* 2010; 126(2): 376–380.

95. Morad Y, Kim YM, Mian M, Huyer D, Capra L, Levin AV. Non-ophthalmologist accuracy in diagnosing retinal hemorrhages in the shaken baby syndrome. *J Pediatrics* 2003; 142(4): 431–414.

96. Morad Y, Avni I, Benton SA, et al. Normal computerized tomography of brain in children with shaken baby syndrome. *J AAPOS* 2004; 8(5): 445–450.

97. Thackeray JD, Scribano PV, Lindberg DM. Yield of retinal examination in suspected physical abuse with normal neuroimaging. *Pediatrics* 2010; 125: e1066–e1071.

98. Coant PN, Kornberg AE, Brody AS, Edwards-Holmes K. Markers for occult liver injury in cases of physical abuse in children. *Pediatrics* 1992; 89(2): 274–278.

99. Gross M, Lynch F, Canty T, Sr, Peterson B, Spear R. Management of pediatric liver injuries: a 13-year experience at a pediatric trauma center. *J Pediatr Surg* 1999; 34(5): 811–816; discussion 6–7.

100. Kellogg ND. Evaluation of suspected child physical abuse. *Pediatrics* 2007; 119(6): 1232–1241.

101. Herr S, Fallat M. Abusive abdominal and thoracic trauma. Clinical Pediatric Emergency Medicine *[Review]*. 2006; 7(3): 149–152.

102. Karam O, La Scala G, Le Coultre C, Chardot C. Liver function tests in children with blunt abdominal traumas. *Eur J Pediatr Surg* 2007; 17(5): 313–316.

103. Jenny C. Evaluating infants and young children with multiple fractures. *Pediatrics* 2006; 118(3): 1299–1303.

104. Lane WG, Dubowitz H, Langenberg P. Screening for occult abdominal trauma in children with suspected physical abuse. *Pediatrics* 2009; 124(6): 1595–1602.

105. Slovis TL, Smith W, Kushner DC, et al. Imaging the child with suspected physical abuse. American College of Radiology. ACR Appropriateness Criteria. *Radiology* 2000; 215 Suppl.: 805–809.

106. Baxter AL, Lindberg DM, Burke BL, Shults J, Holmes JF. Hepatic enzyme decline after pediatric blunt trauma: a tool for timing child abuse? *Child Abuse & Neglect* 2008; 32(9): 838–845.

107. Campbell KA, Bogen DL, Berger RP. The other children: a survey of child abuse physicians on the medical evaluation of children living with a physically abused child. *Arch Pediatr Adolesc Med* 2006; 160(12): 1241–1246.

108. Hansen KK. Twins and child abuse. *Arch Pediatr Adolesc Med* 1994; 148(12): 1345–1346.

109. Dubowitz H, Prescott L, Feigelman S, Lane W, Kim J. Screening for intimate partner violence in a pediatric primary care clinic. *Pediatrics* 2008; 121(1): e85–e91.

110. USPSTF. Screening for family and intimate partner violence: recommendation statement. *Ann Intern Med* 2004; 140(5): 382–386.

111. Joint Commission on Accreditation of Healthcare Organizations: 1996 Accreditation Manual for Hospitals. Oakbrook Terrace, IL: Joint Commission on Accreditation of Healthcare Organizations; 1995.

112. *Policy Statement: Domestic Family Violence.* Dallas, Texas: American College of Emergency Physicians; 2007 [updated 2007; cited 2009 February 3]; Available at: http://www.acep.org/practres.aspx?id=29184, accessed September 8, 2010.

113. Physicians' Obligations in Preventing, Identifying, and Treating Violence and Abuse. American Medical Association. Available at: https://ssl3.ama-assn.org/apps/ecomm/PolicyFinderForm.pl?site=www.ama-assn.org&uri=/ama1/pub/upload/mm/PolicyFinder/policyfiles/HnE/E-2.02.HTM, accessed July 20, 2010.

114. Sherin KM, Sinacore JM, Li XQ, Zitter RE, Shakil A. HITS: a short domestic violence screening tool for use in a family practice setting. *Fam Med* 1998; 30(7): 508–512.

115. Paranjape A, Liebschutz J. STaT: a three-question screen for intimate partner violence. *J Women's Health (Larchmt)* 2003; 12(3): 233–239.

116. Feldhaus KM, Koziol-McLain J, Amsbury HL, Norton IM, Lowenstein SR, Abbott JT. Accuracy of 3 brief screening questions for detecting partner violence in the emergency department. *JAMA* 1997; 277(17): 1357–1361.

117. Preventing Domestic Violence. *Clinical Guidelines on Routine Screening*. San Francisco, CA: Family Violence Prevention Fund; 1999.

118. Scalzo T. Reporting Requirements for Competent Adult Victims of Domestic Violence: The National Center for the Prosecution of Violence Against Women, American Prosecutors Research Institute; 2006.

119. Enos VP, Linden JA, Tieszen L, Bernstein J, Brown J. An intervention to improve documentation of intimate partner violence in medical records. U.S. Department of Justice; 2004.

120. Olds DL, Eckenrode J, Henderson CR, Jr, et al. Long-term effects of home visitation on maternal life course and child abuse and neglect. Fifteen-year follow-up of a randomized trial. *JAMA* 1997; 278(8): 637–643.

121. Maguire S, Mann MK, Sibert J, Kemp A. Are there patterns of bruising in childhood which are diagnostic or suggestive of abuse? A systematic review. *Arch Dis Childhood* 2005; 90(2): 182–186.

122. Ludwig S (ed.) *Child Abuse on the Launch Pad: T Minus Ten and Counting*. Philadelphia, PA: The Helfer Society; 2010 April.

CHAPTER 15

The intellectually disabled patient

Jonathan S. Anderson[1,2,3] and Shamai A. Grossman[1,3]
[1]Beth Israel Deaconess Medical Center, Boston, MA, USA
[2]Milton Hospital, Boston, MA, USA
[3]Harvard Medical School, Boston, MA, USA

Introduction

Intellectual disability, the preferred term for what was formerly called mental retardation, represents a complex conglomeration of cognitive and adaptive impairments. The American Association on Intellectual and Developmental Disabilities defines intellectual disability as impairments both of cognitive function and adaptive behavior, covering a wide range of social and practical skills, which must appear before the age of 18 [1]. This generally correlates to an IQ less than 75 [1]. It is difficult to ascertain the true incidence of intellectual disability. Experts from divergent fields, such as medicine and governmental agencies, state that the general prevalence rate of intellectual disability is between 1% and 3.5%, though up to half of these cases never receive a formal diagnosis [2–4]. The WHO estimates that 60 million people worldwide suffer from intellectual disability [5]. A recent survey in the United States reported that 0.6% of children carry a formal diagnosis of intellectual disability [6]. In mild forms of intellectual disability, males outnumber females by a ratio of 1.6:1, though in severe forms the prevalence is equal between the sexes [7].

In ancient Greece and Rome, infanticide was considered the appropriate solution to the birth of any deformed child. Sadly, the perception of intellectual disability as an untreatable and even evil condition continued for thousands of years. In the early nineteenth century, perceptions shifted, and intellectual disability was thought of as a form of mental illness. Later in that century, advances in care demonstrated that with education and

Challenging and Emerging Conditions in Emergency Medicine, First Edition. Edited by Arvind Venkat.
© 2011 by John Wiley & Sons, Ltd. Published 2011 by Blackwell Publishing Ltd.

medical treatment, many individuals with intellectual disability could begin or increase their functioning within society [8].

Throughout the early twentieth century educational testing for the intellectually disabled improved, accelerating the founding of many residential training schools [9]. These were widespread by mid-century, but many of the more severely handicapped were left in simple custodial status, with no therapeutic interventions. During the 1960s and 70s, advocacy groups encouraged improved treatment for persons with intellectual disability, and, in 1975, the United States Congress passed the Education for the Handicapped Act. This law guaranteed educational services for persons with physical and intellectual disabilities up to the age of 21 [9]. By the end of the twentieth century, with improved medical care, longevity among the intellectually disabled had increased. In the United States, Down Syndrome patients had an increased median age at death from 25 years in 1983 to 49 years in 1997 [10]. This resultant longevity was concomitantly associated with a strong trend towards deinstitutionalization via both the establishment of group homes and increasing numbers of patients staying with their biologic families [5].

With these changes in both longevity and residential settings for the intellectually disabled, governmental agencies have advocated for new approaches to the medical management of this patient population. In 2001, the WHO published a lengthy report encouraging improved health care for the intellectually disabled [5]. Their suggestions included that healthcare providers should adopt a lifespan approach that recognizes the progression or consequences of specific diseases and therapeutic interventions. In 2001, the US Surgeon General's Conference on Health Disparities and Mental Retardation opened their report with the statement that:

"Today, the life expectancy of people with conditions associated with Mental Retardation (MR) has lengthened into adulthood and middle age. People with MR are remaining in their communities. In ever-increasing numbers, people with MR either do not enter institutions, or they leave them to live with their families or in other community settings, and they are determined to understand and take charge of their health. But in most cases, neither the education and training of health professionals nor other elements of the nation's health system have been updated to reflect their progress." [2]

For emergency physicians, the combination of improved longevity and deinstitutionalization among the intellectually disabled has resulted in increased encounters with this patient population. At the same time, knowledge among emergency physicians of the intellectually disabled and their medical reasons for presentation is limited [11]. This chapter discusses the emergency department (ED) evaluation and management of patients with intellectual disability.

Etiologies

By identifying the underlying cause of intellectual disability, one may be able to predict the constellation of associated medical conditions that may cause patients with intellectual disability to present to an acute care setting such as the ED. However, despite advances in testing, only half of the intellectually disabled population has an identifiable etiology of their condition [11]. In cases where a cause is identified, it generally falls into one or more of the following categories: genetic, traumatic, environmental, metabolic, or infectious (Table 15.1).

Table 15.1 Causes of intellectual disability [11–21]

Category	Subcategory		Conditions	Estimated prevalence
Genetic	Chromosomal	Gross aberrations	Down Syndrome	1 in 800 births
			Turner Syndrome	1 per 3125
			Klinefelter Syndrome	1 in 500
		Microdeletions	Fragile X	1 in 4000
			DiGeorge Syndrome	1 in 4000
	Single gene		Neurofibromatosis	1 per 3000
			Tuberous sclerosis	1 per 10,000
			Phenylketonuria	1 per 15,500
	Multifactoral		Variety of familial disorders	Variable
Trauma			Traumatic brain injury	Unknown
			Cerebral palsy	1 per 500
Metabolic/ endocrine			Congenital hypothyroidism	1 per 150,000
			Reye Syndrome	1 per million
Infectious			Congenital toxoplasmosis	1 per 10,000
			Congenital syphilis	1 per 13,000

Source: References 11–21.

Genetic causes, which are often syndromic, can be grossly divided into chromosomal, single gene, and multifactoral types [22]. The most common of these subsets is chromosomal abnormalities, which account for up to a quarter of the total known causes [23]. Best known among these is Down Syndrome (Trisomy 21), but the category also includes Fragile X Syndrome, Klinefelter Syndrome, Prader–Willi Syndrome, and Cri-du-chat. Non-chromosomal conditions include Tay–Sachs disease, phenylketonuria, Hunter Syndrome, Hurler Syndrome, Lesch–Nyhan Syndrome, and tuberous sclerosis [11].

Environmental or teratogenic causes can be found in 5%–13% of cases, and another 2%–10% can be linked directly to the trauma of prematurity [24]. Brain injury, including hemorrhage, direct head trauma, and hypoxic injury, can all lead to cerebral palsy. Approximately two-thirds of patients with cerebral palsy have an intellectual disability [25]. Of the environmental factors, Fetal-Alcohol Syndrome deserves special note; it is the leading preventable cause of intellectual disability in the United States, affecting 1–10:1000 lives births [26]. Lead poisoning is also notable for its effects, which often occur after birth [20, 27].

Metabolic triggers of intellectual disability can be either genetic or situational and include congenital hypothyroidism, hypoglycemia, and Reye Syndrome. Infections, especially those in the prenatal period, are a final cause of intellectual disability. Examples include rubella, meningitis, CMV encephalitis, toxoplasmosis, and other CNS agents [11].

Organ system-based pathologies

While the intellectually disabled experience the same spectrum of disease as the general population, the prevalence of particular illnesses differs greatly from the non-intellectually disabled. Recent studies have demonstrated that intellectually disabled adults are more likely to present with digestive disorders and ill-defined symptoms versus a general population control group, and present less often with complaints related to pregnancy, psychiatry, trauma, or the musculoskeletal system [28]. Reduced mobility and tube feeding are both independent predictors of a large increase in mortality risk [29]. Many intellectually disabled patients have larger numbers of cardiovascular risk factors, higher mortalities, and more undiagnosed conditions than the general population [30]. They also have a higher rate of sensory organ dysfunction, which can interfere with access to care [31].

To aid in the focused evaluation of intellectually disabled patients who present to the ED, we present below an organ system-based review of the common pathologies afflicting this population.

Neurology

Seizures are the most frequent neurologic abnormality associated with the intellectually disabled. Some studies have estimated that about 15% of people with intellectual disability have concomitant epilepsy [32]. These seizures are more difficult to manage and frequently refractory to single-drug therapy than in the general epileptic population [11]. They also tend to be worse in patients with more severe forms of disability and decrease life expectancy by as much as two decades [32]. There are no specific changes in pharmacologic management in these patients; however, the physician should be prepared to use second- or third-line agents and for airway management as needed. The clinician must be careful not to misidentify the movement disorder side effects of neuroleptic drugs as seizures. Metoclopramide and neuroleptic medications can cause tardive dyskinesia, and stereotyped movements such as lip smacking, tongue darting, and upper extremity choreatic movements can be reported as "seizures" [33]. In cases where the emergency physician cannot distinguish between these possibilities, neurology consultation is indicated and at times an electroencephalogram may be necessary.

Psychiatry

Estimates of the prevalence of separate mental health disease in patients with intellectual disability are remarkably varied, with published studies in the United States noting a rate of 14%–60% [34]. This variability reflects the extreme difficulty in diagnosing these disorders in patients where communication can be difficult and features may overlap with their primary intellectual disability diagnosis. Providers should remember the possibility of a separate psychiatric condition when dealing with behavior concerns in patients with intellectual disability [34]. Recent research in the area of mental health in patients with intellectual disability laments the lack of a standardized form of assessment. Most authors suggest a multidisciplinary "biopsychosocial" approach to the possibility of psychiatric disease and that caregivers must understand the potential for mental health disease and refer for further assessment when indicated [35].

Suicidality is a problem that emergency physicians frequently encounter, and it is the 11th leading cause of death in the United States. Classic teaching held that patients with intellectual disability had a relative buffer to suicide, and there was rarely research aimed at this problem. Recently, researchers have challenged this maxim. While few studies have been performed, the data indicates that there is a significant rate of suicidality in the intellectually disabled. Practitioners should be aware that risk factors for suicidality in the intellectually disabled appear to mirror those in the general population, including history of prior psychiatric hospitalization, co-morbid physical disabilities, loneliness, sadness, depression, or anxiety [36].

Ear, nose, and throat

Sensory loss is common in patients with intellectual disability [31]. Chronic serous otitis media caused by facial hypoplasia and a subtle immune deficiency produces mild to moderate conductive hearing loss in 60%–90% of children with Down Syndrome [11]. In any disorder with facial dysmorphism, otitis media and sinusitis can be common causes of infection that can present in a subacute or non-specific manner. For similar reasons, obstructive sleep apnea can often present in patients with intellectual disability and can require surgical correction if they fail to tolerate positive airway pressure by mask [33].

Cardiac

Recent studies have noted the increasing prevalence of adults with congenital heart defects related to a genetic syndrome, likely due to increased survival thanks to advances in medical care [37]. Many of these syndromes are also associated with intellectual disability. While some patients retain medical providers at specialized children hospitals well into adulthood, many more are seen in the community for their day-to-day cardiovascular care. Table 15.2 provides a summary of the association between congenital heart disease and chromosomal abnormalities.

Down Syndrome is classically associated with atrio–ventricular canal defects, including complete defects, and sometimes less significant atrial septal defects (ASD) or ventricular septal defects (VSD). In infancy, these are often repaired aggressively. In adults, there can still be an ASD or VSD with the typical sequelae, including embolic events such as stroke and progressive heart failure due to right-sided overload. Secondary to prior surgical repair, there can be stenosis or reflux at the atrio–ventricular valves. These can present with palpitations, dyspnea, or simply as fatigue. Diagnosis can be made with careful physical exam, aided by chest X-ray or EKG; however, a formal echocardiogram is often required. Separately, there can be progressive heart block in Down Syndrome patients, often presenting as decreased exercise tolerance over weeks to months [37]. This is easily diagnosed with an EKG and can be treated with an implanted pacemaker. Rarely, this condition can present as a hemodynamically unstable third degree heart block, which may require emergent temporary pacing while cardiology is consulted for definitive management.

In patients with Down Syndrome but no prior congenital heart disease, there is a marked increase in the rate of mitral valve prolapse, with some increase in the rates of other valvular regurgitations [44]. There are also the occasional patients who have congenital heart disease, but never had a repair. They can present as adults with progressive Eisenmenger Syndrome with worsening cyanosis, pulmonary hypertension, subacute bacterial endocarditis, and stroke [37].

Table 15.2 Chromosomal abnormalities and their associated congenital heart disease prevalence and types [38–43]

Chromosomal disorder	Prevalence of congenital heart disease (%)	Types of congenital heart disease
Deletion 5p (Cri-du-chat)	30–60	Atrial and Ventricular Septal Defects (ASD, VSD), Patent Ductus Arteriosis (PDA)
Deletion 7q11.23 (Williams–Beuren Syndrome)	66	Supravalvar Aortic and Pulmonary Stenosis, Peripheral Pulmonary Stenosis, Stenosis of the Coronary Ostia
Trisomy 21 (Down Syndrome)	50	VSD, ASD, Tetrology of Fallot (TOF), Mitral Valve Prolapse (MVP), Progressive Heart Block
Deletion 22q11 (DiGeorge Syndrome)	75	Interrupted Aortic Arch, Truncus Arteriosus, Isolated Aortic Arch Anomalies, TOF, VSD
Monosomy X (Turner Syndrome)	30	Aortic Coarctation, Bicuspid Aortic Valve, Valvular Aortic Stenosis, Hypoplastic Left Heart Syndrome, Aortic Dissection
Klinefelter Syndrome (47, XXY)	50	MVP, Venous Thromboembolic Disease (predisposition), PDA, ASD

Source: References 38–43.

The 22q11.2 deletion is generally associated with DiGeorge Syndrome, but has a great deal of phenotypic variation. It is associated with mild intellectual disability in about one-third of patients, and is the second most common source of congenital heart defects behind Down Syndrome [37]. Three-quarters of these 22q11.2 deletion patients have some type of heart defect; the more common include Tetrology of Fallot, Truncus Arteriosus, Interrupted Aortic Arches, VSDs, and other anomalies of the aortic arch. Frequently, these conditions require repair within the first year of life. Adults with a conotruncal defect—a defect of the ventricular outflow system—which was repaired in childhood have similar cardiac complications and outcomes whether or not they also have an intellectual disability. Right ventricular–pulmonary artery conduits can develop both pulmonary regurgitation and valvular stenosis. Typically, these present with dyspnea and varied amounts of fluid overload, pulmonary edema, and heart failure. Treatment is highly lesion dependant, and cardiology consultation is often required for echocardiography.

Repaired interrupted aortic arches may have recoarctation of the reconstructed aortic arch, though the rate decreases as time passes after repair. These present in a similar manner to a late presentation of an inborn coarctation—often with murmur and hypertension, more rarely with headaches, chest pain, fatigue, claudication, or intracranial hemorrhage. With the exception of intracranial hemorrhage, these generally do not require true emergent treatment. The emergency physician can perform a lifesaving intervention by simply diagnosing this condition and referring the patient for future repair [37, 45].

Additionally, left ventricular outflow obstruction at the level of the aortic valve, truncal valve (valve at the base of a tetrology outflow tract), or subaortic region may develop. These lesions impose increased afterload on the left ventricle and eventually result in hypertrophy, dilatation, and failure of the left ventricle. The patient will present with typical symptoms of left-sided heart failure, but should be carefully managed as some outflow lesions can be very volume-dependent. These lesions also carry a high risk of infectious endocarditis, which must be considered both for prophylaxis and as a potential diagnosis in a patient with fever [43]. Lastly, Tetralogy of Fallot is frequently associated with late post-operative atrial tachyarrhythmias, ventricular tachyarrhythmias, and heart block [37, 45].

Turner Syndrome, characterized by a female with a single X chromosome, is also classically associated with cardiac anomalies, largely types of left heart obstruction, including bicuspid aortic valves and coarctation of the aorta. Aside from the typical post-operative complications, adult Turner's patients have been recognized to have some unique cardiac risk factors. First, they can have a subtle bicuspid aortic valve or aortic coarctation that may be unrecognized in childhood. More worrisome, recent population-based studies have demonstrated that Turner Syndrome can be associated with perhaps a 100-fold increased incidence in the rate of thoracic aortic dissection in comparison to the general population [40]. The emergency physician must be acutely aware of this correlation, which is reminiscent of the relationship of Marfan's disease and dissection, and have a low threshold for ordering imaging studies to assess for this critical condition in this patient population. These patients should also have aortic imaging at least every 5 years to assess for the development of thoracic aortic pathology [37].

Lastly, Williams–Beuren Syndrome is a microdeletion related form of mild intellectual disability associated with dysmorphic facies and musculoskeletal deformities. These patients are very likely to have supravalvular aortic stenosis, often requiring surgical repair or serial balloon dilatation in childhood [41]. As adults, aside from continued issues with this stenosis, they are at special risk of stenosis of the coronary ostia, likely due to medial hyperplasia, which has been implicated in numerous episodes of sudden death in these patients. This specific lesion can be difficult to detect using standard cardiac imaging, and these patients are often unable to complete typical exercise stress tests. These patients should be admitted for further cardiac workup if their presenting symptoms are compatible with acute coronary syndrome (ACS); their initial treatment is no different than a standard patient with ACS [37].

Pulmonary

Unlike the cardiovascular system, few forms of intellectual disability have direct correlations to anatomic variants in the pulmonary system. However, respiratory concerns, often related to aspiration, are the second most common cause of mortality in patients with intellectual disability [46, 47]. These common respiratory infections are multifactorial: some patients with severe intellectual disability have problems with pulmonary toilet, some have related facial abnormalities that can impair proper swallowing, and many patients are unable to voice their symptoms until they become severe and obvious to outsiders. Health care providers must recall that many patients with intellectually disability live in institutionalized settings, which can change the recommended antibiotic coverage for pneumonia. Also, secondary to their anatomic dysmorphism, many patients with intellectual disability have chest radiographs that are difficult to interpret. In our clinical opinion, the clinician must consider the risk and benefit of treating without clear radiographic evidence of infection versus the use of advancing imaging techniques, such as CT.

Gastrointestinal

Gastroesophageal reflux disease is a common cause of sore throat, choking, coughing, and behavioral changes in patients with intellectual disability. They often lack the verbal ability to explain the sensation, and appropriate diagnostic radiologic studies can be difficult to obtain in these patients [33].

Constipation is also common in patients with intellectual disability, up to 70% in some studies [48]. Constipation can present as simple behavioral changes, a presentation it shares with reflux disease [46]. Predictors of constipation include limited mobility, anticonvulsant therapy, severe intellectual disability, cerebral palsy, and refusal to eat. This can occur despite the frequent use of standing laxatives in this population [48].

Parasites, including *Strongyloides stercoralis* and *Enterobius vermicularis* (pinworm), are also more prevalent in the intellectually disabled population and should be considered in the diagnosis of unexplained diarrhea, discomfort, or eosinophilic leukocytosis [49].

Patients with severe intellectual disability or concomitant dementia frequently require gastrostomy or jejunostomy tubes for their nutritional needs. These can trigger frequent ED visits. Often, if the presenting complaint involves the displacement of the tube, the emergency physician can place another tube into the tract and verify placement with radiography. Occasionally, the emergency physician is left with a choice between placing a temporary place-holding tube, such as a foley catheter, or contacting a specialist for assistance. This choice must be made based on institutional preferences and the patient's need and ability to follow-up for definitive management [28].

In patients with Down Syndrome, there is an increasingly diverse body of literature suggesting they are at higher risk for symptomatic gall bladder disease, including sludge, cholelithiasis, and acute cholecystitis. Some of these studies have noted that while obesity and Down Syndrome often occur together, the chromosomal abnormality alone does seem to confer added risk of cholelithiasis. This risk includes children, in whom gallbladder disease is classically rare [50–52]. Apart from a higher pre-test probability, the ED evaluation and treatment of Down Syndrome patients with gallbladder disease is similar to the general patient population.

Endocrine

The most prevalent endocrine disease associated with intellectual disability is hypothyroidism, with a prevalence of 29%, increasing to 46% in patients with Down Syndrome [30]. While rarely resulting in an acute emergency, this problem can precipitate visits to acute care providers and should be considered in many differential diagnoses.

Obesity is a well-publicized epidemic in recent decades. Patients with certain intellectual disabilities have an even higher rate of obesity than the baseline population, including high rates during their youth. Patients with Down Syndrome or autism have rates as high as double or triple the general population during adolescence [53]. Obesity serves as both a causative agent and surrogate marker for many conditions. Research demonstrates that patients with intellectual disability and concomitant obesity have higher rates of asthma, high blood pressure, high blood cholesterol, diabetes, depression, and pressure sores [54]. Obesity is also an independent risk factor for worsening outcomes from serious blunt trauma, including increased length of stay and increased mortality [55].

Patients with Down Syndrome have high rates of both hypothyroidism and obesity. These two conditions have been noted in tandem in clusters of Down Syndrome patients suffering from slipped capital femoral epiphysis, and patients noted to have this orthopedic disease should be screened for hypothyroidism [56].

Genitourinary and gynecologic

Sexual activity is a little-explored topic within the realm of the intellectually disabled. However, multiple studies document a normal rate of consensual sexual activity in the mildly intellectually disabled and a higher rate of rape and incest [57]. Some studies suggest that the rate of abuse in this population is 4–10 times as high as the general population [58]. The abuser is usually a person known to the victim, most frequently service providers or family members [59]. Emotional insecurities, ignorance of sexuality, and powerless position in society have been the noted causes of frequent exploitation of the intellectually disabled [60]. As such, emergency physicians must remain aware of the real possibility of sexually transmitted diseases, HIV, and pregnancy in this population. They also must remain conscious of the subtle clues and presentations that could be related to abuse. Many of these victims are able to communicate the nature of the abuse, making it important to draw on them for the history beyond that given by family or service providers [58]. Laws vary by state and often involve complex determinations on the ability to consent when determining the need to report possible abuse [60]. The emergency physician has a key role in recognizing abuse and sexually related disorders in this vulnerable population.

Incontinence of bowel or bladder is common in a number of severe forms of intellectual disability. It is a key measure of functional status, and poor functional status correlates with the rate of presentation to ED with acute health problems [28]. The severity of function status impairment is also an independent predictor of multiple health problems, including obesity, gastroesophageal reflux, and urinary tract infections [61].

Musculoskeletal

Multiple studies have demonstrated that the intellectually disabled have a higher rate and earlier onset of osteoporosis, necessitating earlier screening and increased attention to minor trauma [62]. This is especially true in patients on long-term anticonvulsant therapy, those with limited mobility or those with Down or Prader–Willi Syndromes [63]. Fractures due to osteoporosis are the most frequent musculoskeletal reason for ED presentation in patients with intellectual disability. One chart review demonstrated that a third of women with intellectual disability had a diagnosed fracture as an adult, suggesting they may benefit from earlier commencement of bone mineral supplements [64]. Intellectual disability has been strongly associated with vitamin D deficiency, though this has not been proven to be a causative factor in their increased risk of fractures [65]. It is important to consider the patient's baseline functional status when deciding on the eventual treatment of any fracture, as some patients with limited functional status will prefer conservative management versus operative fixation.

Joint contractures are another musculoskeletal disorders frequently associated with the intellectually disabled. The effects of contractures are variable, but often limit ambulation, impair posture, cause discomfort, and predispose to the development of osteoarthritis, as well as decubitus ulcers [11]. The aforementioned obesity epidemic also leads to a number of orthopedic complications, including increased rates of degenerative joint disease and slipped capital femoral epiphysis [56].

Hematology and oncology

Despite the fact that the standardized incidence of malignancy in patients with Down Syndrome is identical to the general population, they have a 10–20-fold higher risk of leukemia and a markedly lower risk of solid organ tumors [66]. Patients with Down Syndrome are at higher risk of acquiring three hematologic disorders: transient myeloproliferative disorder (TMD), acute megakaryoblastic leukemia (AML), and acute lymphoblastic leukemia (ALL). TMD is a unique disease to patients with Down Syndrome and is a clonal expansion of megakaryocytes, which appears very similar to AML. However, in TMD, the condition spontaneously regresses after some number of months. It can be seen in up to 10% of infants with Down Syndrome, and symptoms vary from solitary laboratory abnormalities to death from acute leukemia with organ failure. In AML, Down syndrome patients have a better prognosis than the general population, but are more prone to treatment side effects. Lastly, in ALL, Down Syndrome patients once again have a higher chemotherapy-associated side effect profile [66].

Other population studies have shown an equal rate of most cancers between the general population and the intellectually disabled and do not suggest a variation in screening techniques. However, the one exception is cervical cancer, which has a markedly lower rate in the intellectually disabled population, presumably related to a lower rate of sexual activity in the more severely intellectually disabled [1].

Pharmacology

Lastly, like the elderly, intellectually disabled patients often have an extensive medication list. Polypharmacy complications can be found in both the presenting complaint or develop due to new medications used in the ED. It is especially important to note drug–drug interactions related to antiepileptic and cardiovascular medications [11]. One emerging concern is the increased rate of prolonged QT intervals in patients with Turner Syndrome. Clinicians should use caution prescribing any drugs that have QT prolongation effects in these patients [37]. Lastly, polypharmacy itself is an independent predictor of the need for hospitalization in ED patients with intellectual disability [28].

Emergency department management

Personal interactions and obtaining patient history

Many health care providers are uncomfortable interacting with individuals who have an intellectual disability, which can carry over to the assessment and management of these patients in the ED. One manifestation of this is the difficulty in taking a history from a patient who may have limited, if any, verbal skills. Often a clinician will discuss the case only with the attendant service provider and not the patient [67]. This can worsen the clinician–patient relationship [68].

A number of suggestions can improve physician–patient communication. The patient should be evaluated in a quiet area, preferably one time by a single health care provider team. Before entering the room, the emergency physician should review any accompanying data, such as baseline level of functioning, medical history, vital signs, and presenting complaints. It is also important to formally note the patient's code status, primary physician, and legal guardian and health care proxy.

The provider should specifically introduce themselves to the patient and any family or service personnel who accompany them. The patient should give as much history as possible, even employing non-verbal communication such as signs or picture boards as needed. The provider should assume the patient can understand, and the patient should feel included when spoken to, even if there is no outward sign of cognition [68]. Physicians should use clear and age-appropriate language. Any of the caregivers present should be asked to supplement the history since caregivers as well as primary physicians can often give valuable clues to the diagnosis, especially in patients presenting with subtle and non-specific complaints such as altered mental status. If the provider has any concern for abuse, the patient should also be interviewed separately from any caregivers. Special attention should be given to non-specific changes in personality, activity, food and water intake, mobility, bowel habits, or acute changes in cognition [3, 11].

Strategies in physical examination and laboratory evaluations

The physical examination in the intellectually disabled takes on increased importance, due to the often incomplete history given to the physician. However, there are also new difficulties encountered during the examination such as agitation. Frequently, having a caregiver or family member assist with the examination will calm the patient and allow the physician a better examination.

The emergency physician must perform a detailed examination as guided by the history or chief complaint. Frequent inspection of the oral cavity is required to look for dental abscesses or periodontic disease. The aforementioned frequent otitis media can only be evaluated with careful exam. Also, considering the frequency of co-morbid heart conditions, cardiac auscultation should be mandatory. Pulmonary and abdominal examination may give clues to occult infections. A rectal exam should be considered to evaluate both constipation and occult blood loss. Extremities should be assessed for signs of trauma, both accidental and secondary to abuse. Occult fractures can be the cause of many non-specific presentations. The patient should also be disrobed, to fully inspect the skin for potential ulcerations or bruising. Care should be taken with any pelvic exam, as such examination is frequently indicated, but the patient may have had few, or none, in the past [11].

Once a thorough history and examination are complete, the physician will often need additional information. Laboratory data and other studies should be ordered as with any patient. It may be wise to consider the need for evaluation of levels of any antiepileptic drugs and EKGs for patients with congenital heart disease. The indication for lumbar puncture and CT of the brain can be obfuscated in a patient with a baseline abnormal exam; knowledge of the patient's prior studies and status can help determine which tests should be done and interpret the results of these tests. Other times, baseline anatomy can make a test less sensitive or specific than usual, such as in the case of chest X-ray examination in patients who have severe kyphoscoliosis or even EKG after a complex heart repair.

One consideration that is frequently encountered is that many tests and procedures are invasive and painful. In a patient with compromised understanding, this can create a tense and even violent environment. In addition to the above mentioned communication techniques, the emergency physician should consider anxiolytics or even conscious sedation when appropriate.

Several studies have shown that propofol, midazolam, thioridazine, chloral hydrate, and, most recently, ketamine can be used for conscious sedation in patients with intellectual disability with minimal side effects [69–71]. Despite these advances in conscious sedation, some procedures that are routinely performed without any sedation in other patients may require general anesthesia in patients with intellectual disability. These include painful procedures, such as abscess drainage and orthopedic reductions.

Familial and social issues: informed consent

The intellectually disabled not only present with complex medical conditions, but also with complex social situations. As this population ages, there will be an increasing number of adults with intellectual disability who do not have living parents serving in the traditional role of guardians. ED nurses have noted difficulties with informed consent when the patient has difficulty with communication, especially when there are no guardians to rely upon [72].

In the case of an adult with an intellectual disability, one should assume they have the ability to provide consent for their own treatment choices, while ensuring that this is correct. Most ethicists agree that consent is valid when it is given freely, is informed and specific, and given by someone competent to consent. This competence is often questioned in patients with intellectual disability. Depending on the complexity of the situation, the patient may be able to consent for some procedures and not for others.

To ensure the patient has the capacity to consent, the emergency physician must check that the patient has the ability to comprehend, weigh information, and have a rationale for any decision that the he makes. In the case of a patient without ability to consent for treatment, local and regional laws vary with regards to guardianship. In the case of emergency, or uncertainty, the physician should proceed as they would with any patient who is unable to consent: prudently provide the lifesaving interventions that any reasonable person would desire, while employing whatever means they have (social work, case management, local agencies) to determine the patient's true legal status.

If the ability to consent is unclear, the emergency physician can try a number of strategies to assess the patient's capacity for medical decision-making. The patient can be asked to paraphrase the choices. They can be asked to compare the differences between two choices. The practitioner should always use whatever communication adjuncts are needed by a certain patient. Physicians should also be aware that a patient may have the capacity to make decisions on certain health care topics, but not on others that are more complex. It is also important to ensure that the patient makes their own decision, even if their family or other caregiver is needed to communicate with the patient. If the patient is deemed to lack capacity, the physician should cautiously proceed forward with the patient's "best interests" in mind [73].

The next five years

For many years, treatment of intellectual disability has focused on behavioral therapy and discrete medical interventions targeting individual symptoms. Sometimes anatomic variants are amenable to surgical repair. Prevention has been limited to public health campaigns targeting alcohol consumption and seat-belt use as well as prenatal screening for known metabolic disorders such as phenylketonuria. However, with the rapid emergence of molecular biology and genetics, the future promises novel diagnostic testing and treatment options.

One condition that demonstrates these emerging technologies is Fragile X Syndrome. This condition is characterized by a range of learning problems, intellectual disability, autism, and anxiety. It is caused by absent or decreased levels of Fragile X Mental Retardation Protein (FMRP). On a genetic level, this is triggered by either a genetic microdeletion, or more commonly, an expansion of a trinucleotide sequence that causes a failure to express the protein. This trinucleotide sequence expansion can range widely in size and can also be methylated in different amounts, both of which lend variability to the exact symptoms and level of disability caused by this condition [74].

Researchers have spent decades identifying this genetic mutation and also trying to explain its downstream effects. A lack of FMRP leads to a number of changes in the biochemistry of the brain, including lack of regulation of the *mGluR5* pathway [74]. Recently, a small study was undertaken looking at the effect of an *mGluR5* anatagonist (fenobam) on adults with Fragile X. Surprisingly, with a single dose they recorded improved scores on a behavior and attention assay. Despite the fact that this study only involved 12 patients and was non-randomized, it immediately sparked public interest and widespread news coverage [75]. Even if this therapy is eventually disproven, it demonstrates the promise of molecular biology to offer novel therapies to individuals with intellectual disability. With little difficulty, one can imagine how gene therapy, fetal testing, and novel pharmaceuticals could lead to markedly improved outcomes in the near future for intellectually disabled patients with an identifiable genetic or metabolic abnormality.

Conclusion

With improvements in medical care, greater social acceptance, and integration of the intellectually disabled, this patient population will become more prevalent in the ED. Emergency physicians will need to gain a greater understanding of the range of pathology that can cause the intellectually disabled to require acute care. Along with this medical knowledge, sensitivity to the special considerations in assessing the intellectually disabled will allow improved care and outcomes for this challenging and emerging patient population.

References

1. Schalock RL, Borthwick-Duffy SA, Buntinx WH, Coulter DL, Craig EM. *Intellectual Disability: Definition, Classification, and Systems of Supports*. 11th ed. American Association on Intellectual and Developmental Disabilities; 2009.
2. Closing the Gap. *A National Blueprint to Improve the Health of Persons with Mental Retardation–Report of the Surgeon General's Conference on Health Disparities and Mental Retardation* [Internet]. 2001 Feb; Available at: http://www.nichd.nih.gov/publications/pubs/closingthegap/, accessed June 5, 2010.
3. Levy SE, Hyman SL. Pediatric assessment of the child with developmental delay. *Pediatr Clin North Am* 1993; 40(3): 465–477.
4. Leonard H, Wen X. The epidemiology of mental retardation: challenges and opportunities in the new millennium. *Mental Retardation and Developmental Disabilities Research Reviews* 2002; 8(3): 117–134.

5. World Health Organization, editor. *Ageing and Intellectual Disabilities – Improving Longevity and Promoting Healthy Ageing: Summative Report* [Internet]. 2000; Available at: http://www.who.int/mental_health/media/en/20.pdf, accessed September 1, 2010.

6. Woodruff TJ, Axelrad DA, Kyle AD, Nweke O, Miller GG, Hurley BJ. Trends in environmentally related childhood illnesses. *Pediatrics* 2004; 113(4): 1133–1140.

7. Batshaw ML. Mental retardation. *Pediatr Clin North Am* 1993; 40(3): 507–521.

8. Scheerenberger R. *History of Mental Retardation*. Baltimore: Brookes Publishing Company; 1983.

9. Netherton SD, Holmes D, Walker CE. *Child and Adolescent Psychological Disorders: A Comprehensive Textbook*. 1st ed. Oxford, NY: Oxford University Press; 1999.

10. Yang Q, Rasmussen SA, Friedman JM. Mortality associated with Down's syndrome in the USA from 1983 to 1997: a population-based study. *Lancet* 2002; 359(9311): 1019–1025.

11. Grossman SA, Richards CF, Anglin D, Hutson HR. Caring for the patient with mental retardation in the emergency department. *Ann Emerg Med* 2000; 35(1): 69–76.

12. Brosco JP, Mattingly M, Sanders LM. Impact of specific medical interventions on reducing the prevalence of mental retardation. *Arch Pediatr Adolesc Med* 2006; 160(3): 302–309.

13. Harris JC. Intellectual disability: understanding its development, causes, classification, evaluation, and treatment. Oxford, NY: Oxford University Press; 2006.

14. Gravholt CH, Juul S, Naeraa RW, Hansen J. Prenatal and postnatal prevalence of Turner's syndrome: a registry study. *BMJ* 1996; 312(7022): 16–21.

15. Winter S, Autry A, Boyle C, Yeargin-Allsopp M. Trends in the prevalence of cerebral palsy in a population-based study. *Pediatrics* 2002; 110(6): 1220–1225.

16. Schwartz RA, Fernández G, Kotulska K, Jóźwiak S. Tuberous sclerosis complex: advances in diagnosis, genetics, and management. *J Am Acad Dermatol* 2007; 57(2): 189–202.

17. Public Health Genomics at CDC. Genomics|Resources|Books|HuGE|Part 4, Chapter 23 [Internet]. Available at: http://www.cdc.gov/genomics/resources/books/HuGE/chap23.htm, accessed September 14, 2010.

18. Driscoll DA, Salvin J, Sellinger B, et al. Prevalence of 22q11 microdeletions in DiGeorge and velocardiofacial syndromes: implications for genetic counselling and prenatal diagnosis. *J Med Genet* 1993; 30(10): 813–817.

19. Belay ED, Bresee JS, Holman RC, Khan AS, Shahriari A, Schonberger LB. Reye's syndrome in the United States from 1981 through 1997. *N Engl J Med* 1999; 340(18): 1377–1382.

20. Sanders T, Liu Y, Buchner V, Tchounwou PB. Neurotoxic effects and biomarkers of lead exposure: a review. *Rev Environ Health* 2009; 24(1): 15–45.

21. Visootsak J, Graham JM. Klinefelter syndrome and other sex chromosomal aneuploidies. *Orphanet J Rare Dis* 2006; 1:42.

22. Basel-Vanagaite L. Clinical approaches to genetic mental retardation. *Isr Med Assoc J* 2008; 10(11): 821–826.

23. Mulcahy M, Reynolds A. Demographic factors and the incidence of Down's syndrome in Ireland. *Journal of Intellectual Disability Research* 1985; 29(2): 113–123.

24. Curry CJ, Stevenson RE, Aughton D, et al. Evaluation of mental retardation: Recommendations of a consensus conference. *American Journal of Medical Genetics* 1997; 72(4): 468–477.

25. Eicher PS, Batshaw ML. Cerebral palsy. *Pediatr Clin North Am* 1993; 40(3): 537–551.

26. Senecky Y, Inbar D, Diamond G, Basel-Vanagaite L, Rigler S, Chodick G. Fetal alcohol spectrum disorder in Israel. *Isr Med Assoc J* 2009; 11(10): 619–622.

27. Rosin A. The long-term consequences of exposure to lead. *Isr Med Assoc J* 2009; 11(11): 689–694.

28. Venkat A, Pastin RB, Hegde GG, Shea JM, Cook JT, Culig C. An analysis of ED utilization by adults with intellectual disability. *The American Journal of Emergency Medicine* [Internet]. [In press, corrected proof] Available at: http://www.sciencedirect.com/science/article/B6W9K-4YXKFP8-1/2/9b649bd073a9eb9bf17d32162f466fe9, accessed June 7, 2010.

29. Strauss D, Eyman RK, Grossman HJ. Predictors of mortality in children with severe mental retardation: the effect of placement. *Am J Public Health* 1996; 86(10): 1422–1429.

30. Beange H, McElduff A, Baker W. Medical disorders of adults with mental retardation: a population study. *Am J Ment Retard* 1995; 99(6): 595–604.

31. Kapell D, Nightingale B, Rodriguez A, Lee JH, Zigman WB, Schupf N. Prevalence of chronic medical conditions in adults with mental retardation: comparison with the general population. *Ment Retard* 1998; 36(4): 269–279.

32. Morgan CL, Baxter H, Kerr MP. Prevalence of epilepsy and associated health service utilization and mortality among patients with intellectual disability. *Am J Ment Retard* 2003; 108(5): 293–300.

33. Prater CD, Zylstra RG. Medical care of adults with mental retardation. *Am Fam Physician* 2006; 73(12): 2175–2183.

34. Kerker BD, Owens PL, Zigler E, Horwitz SM. Mental health disorders among individuals with mental retardation: challenges to accurate prevalence estimates. *Public Health Rep* 2004; 119(4): 409–417.

35. Costello H, Bouras N. Assessment of mental health problems in people with intellectual disabilities. *Isr J Psychiatry Relat Sci* 2006; 43(4): 241–251.

36. Merrick J, Merrick E, Lunsky Y, Kandel I. A review of suicidality in persons with intellectual disability. *Isr J Psychiatry Relat Sci* 2006; 43(4): 258–264.

37. Lin AE, Basson CT, Goldmuntz E, et al. Adults with genetic syndromes and cardiovascular abnormalities: clinical history and management. *Genet Med* 2008; 10(7): 469–494.

38. Pierpont ME, Basson CT, Benson DW, et al. Genetic basis for congenital heart defects: current knowledge: a scientific statement from the American Heart Association Congenital Cardiac Defects Committee, Council on Cardiovascular Disease in the Young: endorsed by the American Academy of Pediatrics. *Circulation* 2007; 115(23): 3015–3038.

39. Lin AE, Basson CT, Goldmuntz E, et al. Adults with genetic syndromes and cardiovascular abnormalities: clinical history and management. *Genet. Med* 2008; 10(7): 469–494.

40. Matura LA, Ho VB, Rosing DR, Bondy CA. Aortic dilatation and dissection in Turner syndrome. *Circulation* 2007; 116(15): 1663–1670.

41. Eronen M, Peippo M, Hiippala A, et al. Cardiovascular manifestations in 75 patients with Williams syndrome. *J Med Genet* 2002; 39(8): 554–558.
42. Hayes A, Batshaw ML. Down syndrome. *Pediatr Clin North Am* 1993; 40(3): 523–535.
43. Aboulhosn J, Child JS. Left ventricular outflow obstruction: subaortic stenosis, bicuspid aortic valve, supravalvar aortic stenosis, and coarctation of the aorta. *Circulation* 2006; 114(22): 2412–2422.
44. Marino B, Digilio MC, Di Donato R. Health supervision for children with Down syndrome. *Pediatrics* 2001; 108(6): 1384; author reply 1385.
45. Gatzoulis MA, Balaji S, Webber SA, et al. Risk factors for arrhythmia and sudden cardiac death late after repair of tetralogy of Fallot: a multicentre study. *Lancet* 2000; 356(9234): 975–981.
46. Sullivan WF, Heng J, Cameron D, et al. Consensus guidelines for primary health care of adults with developmental disabilities. *Can Fam Physician* 2006; 52(11): 1410–1418.
47. Patja K, Mölsä P, Iivanainen M. Cause-specific mortality of people with intellectual disability in a population-based, 35-year follow-up study. *J Intellect Disabil Res* 2001; 45(Pt 1): 30–40.
48. Böhmer CJ, Taminiau JA, Klinkenberg-Knol EC, Meuwissen SG. The prevalence of constipation in institutionalized people with intellectual disability. *J Intellect Disabil Res* 2001; 45(Pt 3): 212–218.
49. Schupf N, Ortiz M, Kapell D, Kiely M, Rudelli RD. Prevalence of intestinal parasite infections among individuals with mental retardation in New York State. *Ment Retard* 1995; 33(2): 84–89.
50. Chen M, Chen S. Cholelithiasis in Down syndrome. *Acta Paediatr Taiwan* 2004; 45(5): 269–271.
51. Boëchat MCB, Silva KSD, Llerena JC, Boëchat PRM. Cholelithiasis and biliary sludge in Downs syndrome patients. *Sao Paulo Med J* 2007; 125(6): 329–332.
52. Tyler CV, Zyzanski SJ, Runser L. Increased risk of symptomatic gallbladder disease in adults with Down syndrome. *Am J Med Genet A* 2004; 130A(4): 351–353.
53. Stewart L, Van de Ven L, Katsarou V, et al. High prevalence of obesity in ambulatory children and adolescents with intellectual disability. *Journal of Intellectual Disability Research* 2009; 53(10): 882–886.
54. Rimmer JH, Yamaki K, Lowry BMD, Wang E, Vogel LC. Obesity and obesity-related secondary conditions in adolescents with intellectual/developmental disabilities. *Journal of Intellectual Disability Research* 2010; 54(9): 787–794.
55. Christmas AB, Reynolds J, Wilson AK, et al. Morbid obesity impacts mortality in blunt trauma. *Am Surg* 2007; 73(11): 1122–1125.
56. Bosch P, Johnston CE, Karol L. Slipped capital femoral epiphysis in patients with Down syndrome. *J Pediatr Orthop* 2004; 24(3): 271–277.
57. Chamberlain A, Rauh J, Passer A, McGrath M, Burket R. Issues in fertility control for mentally retarded female adolescents: I. sexual activity, sexual abuse, and contraception. *Pediatrics* 1984; 73(4): 445–450.
58. Morano JP. Sexual abuse of the mentally retarded patient: medical and legal analysis for the primary care physician. *Prim Care Companion J Clin Psychiatry* 2001; 3(3): 126–135.

59. Grossman SF, Lundy M, Bertrand C, et al. Service patterns of adult survivors of childhood versus adult sexual assault/abuse. *J Child Sex Abus* 2009; 18(6): 655–672.

60. Furey EM. Sexual abuse of adults with mental retardation: who and where. *Ment Retard* 1994; 32(3): 173–180.

61. Henderson CM, Rosasco M, Robinson LM, et al. Functional impairment severity is associated with health status among older persons with intellectual disability and cerebral palsy. *J Intellect Disabil Res* 2009; 53(11): 887–897.

62. Wilkinson JE, Culpepper L, Cerreto M. Screening tests for adults with intellectual disabilities. *J Am Board Fam Med* 2007; 20(4): 399–407.

63. Tyler CV, Snyder CW, Zyzanski S. Screening for osteoporosis in community-dwelling adults with mental retardation. *Ment Retard* 2000; 38(4): 316–321.

64. Schrager S, Kloss C, Ju AW. Prevalence of fractures in women with intellectual disabilities: a chart review. *J Intellect Disabil Res* 2007; 51(Pt 4): 253–259.

65. Vanlint S, Nugent M. Vitamin D and fractures in people with intellectual disability. *J Intellect Disabil Res* 2006; 50(Pt 10): 761–767.

66. Rabin KR, Whitlock JA. Malignancy in children with trisomy 21. *Oncologist* 2009; 14(2): 164–173.

67. Millar L, Chorlton MC, Lennox N. People with intellectual disability. Barriers to the provision of good primary care. *Aust Fam Physician* 2004; 33(8): 657–658.

68. The Royal Australian College of General Practitioners. RACGP | Overcoming communication barriers – Working with patients with intellectual disabilities [Internet]. Available at: http://www.racgp.org.au/afp/200901/30043, accessed June 8, 2010.

69. Oei-Lim LB, Vermeulen-Cranch DM, Bouvy-Berends EC. Conscious sedation with propofol in dentistry. *Br Dent J* 1991; 170(9): 340–342.

70. Fukuta O, Braham RL, Yanase H, Atsumi N, Kurosu K. The sedative effect of intranasal midazolam administration in the dental treatment of patients with mental disabilities. Part 1. The effect of a 0.2 mg/kg dose. *J Clin Pediatr Dent* 1993; 17(4): 231–237.

71. Green SM, Rothrock SG, Hestdalen R, Ho M, Lynch EL. Ketamine sedation in mentally disabled adults. *Acad Emerg Med* 1999; 6(1): 86–87.

72. Sowney M, Barr OG. Caring for adults with intellectual disabilities: perceived challenges for nurses in accident and emergency units. *J Adv Nurs* 2006; 55(1): 36–45.

73. Department of Health. Seeking consent: working with people with learning disabilities [Internet]. Available at: http://www.dh.gov.uk/en/Publicationsand statistics/Publications/PublicationsPolicyAndGuidance/DH_4007861, accessed September 14, 2010.

74. Hagerman RJ, Berry-Kravis E, Kaufmann WE, et al. Advances in the treatment of Fragile X syndrome. *Pediatrics* 2009; 123(1): 378–390.

75. Harris G. Promise seen in drug for retardation syndrome [Internet]. The New York Times. 2010 Apr 29. Available at: http://www.nytimes.com/2010/04/30/health/research/30fragile.html?_r=1&ref=health, accessed August 3, 2010.

CHAPTER 16

Adults with conditions causing chronic pain

Victoria L. Thornton[1,2] and Lauren T. Southerland[2]
[1]Duke University Medical Center, Durham, NC, USA
[2]Duke University School of Medicine, Durham, NC, USA

Introduction

Between 50% and 70% of the over 119 million emergency department (ED) visits each year in the United States involved pain as one of their chief symptoms [1, 2]. Of the top 12 categories of pain treated in the ED, 60% are of medical cause rather than due to trauma or injury (Table 16.1). Yet while pain and chronic pain are so prevalent in the ED patient population, the treatment of these conditions is often difficult in the acute care setting.

Emergency physicians often receive inadequate training in the essentials of pain management, such as the interpretation of the subjective nature of pain assessment and multimodal treatments for pain. Even if they have been fortunate to have received training in acute pain management, a relatively new addition to medical school and residency curricula, they may be particularly unprepared to assess and treat chronic pain and manage acute exacerbations of chronic pain syndromes [3]. There is also the ever present dread of being duped by a so-called "drug seeker" or of causing addiction, drug abuse, or misuse. Many emergency physicians have confusion about dependence, tolerance, addiction, and pseudoaddiction, as well as substantiated concern about the adverse effects that can occur with pain medications.

In general, emergency physicians are fairly intolerant of patients presenting with any kind of chronic problems, especially chronic pain. Many emergency physicians have the perception that the ED is an environment strictly for acute and critical care treatment [4, 5]. Yet a recent survey of US adults found that 15% reported an ED visit for chronic or recurrent

Challenging and Emerging Conditions in Emergency Medicine, First Edition. Edited by Arvind Venkat.
© 2011 by John Wiley & Sons, Ltd. Published 2011 by Blackwell Publishing Ltd.

Table 16.1 Summary of the discharge diagnoses of patients presenting to an academic ED with a pain complaint

	N (%)
Wound, abrasion, or contusion	91 (11)
Sprain or strain	90 (11)
Back or neck pain	85 (10)
Abdominal pain	71 (9)
Fracture or dislocation	48 (6)
Headache	47 (6)
Chest pain (non-cardiac)	40 (5)
Upper respiratory infection	30 (4)
Abscess or cellulitis	25 (3)
Toothache	19 (2)
Urinary tract infection	16 (2)
Renal colic	14 (2)
Other diagnoses	243 (30)
Total with ICD-9 diagnosis	819 (100)

Source: Redrawn from Todd KH, Ducharme J, Choiniere, M, et al. Pain in the emergency department: results of the Pain and Emergency Medicine Initiative [PEMI] Multicenter Study. *J Pain* 2007; 8(6): 460–466, Copyright © 2007, with permission from Elsevier.

pain. When this figure is applied to the overall US adult population, it suggests that during the 2 years preceding this study, more than 34 million adults were seen in EDs for chronic or recurrent pain [6]. Of these patients, more than 60% had chronic pain syndromes currently treated by a primary care physician, and over 40% had recurrent pain [7]. This represents a significant proportion of all ED patients seen. Adding in the increasing population of older adults and the continuing increases in the number of annual ED visits of all types, visits for chronic pain will continue to increase in number. Therefore, it seems clear that emergency physicians will have to become more facile with the management of acute and chronic pain. This chapter discusses the principles of management of patients with chronic pain in the ED setting with a particular emphasis on patients with back pain, migraine syndromes, and abdominal pain of various etiologies as well as pain management in the elderly.

Pain assessment in the emergency department

Prior to discussing the management of specific conditions that cause chronic pain, it is necessary to understand the broader basis for and terminology of pain management. Gender, ethnicity, and age issues affect pain assessment and management in the ED. Studies have found shorter times to pain relief for better educated, older, Caucasian men. The best single factor determining time to pain relief continues to be *physician* assessment of pain, rather than patient self-report [8]. This is pertinent to chronic pain sufferers, who often do not exhibit the typical signs of moderate to severe pain seen in patients who have acute pain, such as behavioral (facial grimacing, splinting, crying) or sympathomimetic signs (accelerated blood pressure or heart rate, mydriasis, or pallor). There are numerous means of assessing acute pain, including visual analog scales (VAS), numerical rating scales (NRS), graphical or picture scales (GRS), the Face, Legs, Activity, Cry and Consolability (FLACC) observational scale for use in very young children or non-verbal adults, and the Pain Assessment IN Advanced Dementia (PAINAD) scale for use in the setting of older patients with cognitive impairment. These may not accurately reflect a chronic pain state in which patients continually reside at a moderate level of pain. Additionally, patients with chronic pain and dementia or delirium may have difficulty in explaining pain *or* differentiating chronic pain from acute pain in the ED. Pain scales based on observation of the patient at rest and with activity may provide a better assessment of pain in patients with chronic pain syndromes. For example, observational pain scales such as the PAINAD and Abbey Pain Scale were found to be helpful in elderly patients with chronic osteoarthritic pain [9]. Even when pain is appropriately assessed at triage, reassessments after pain treatment are inconsistent [10].

In addition to appropriately assessing pain, physicians must understand and assess the physiologic state of the patient with chronic pain. *Dependence* is the progressive development of a physiologic tolerance to the same dosing and an increasing need for higher dosing to achieve the same effect. This condition generally develops whenever opioids are administered for over 2 weeks. When drug dosage is rapidly reduced or discontinued in a patient who is dependent, or when an antagonist is administered, a *withdrawal state* develops. Withdrawal symptoms include irritability, anxiety, tachycardia, lacrimation, nausea, vomiting, or diarrhea. *Addiction* is a primary neurobiological disease state in which the patient exhibits a psychological dependence associated with a compulsion and craving for the drug(s), despite the adverse impact of the drug use. *Pseudoaddiction* is another state commonly encountered in the ED. Pseudoaddiction may resemble the behaviors associated with addiction, but differs from addiction in that all of the behaviors disappear when the patient is provided adequate medication to treat the pain-causing syndrome. Due to confusion around these terms, patients may have fears of addiction even with minimal or short-term use of opioids. Clearly, there is a significant problem of drug use, misuse, and abuse within American society; however, emergency physicians are also faced in the ED with patients with chronic pain problems interfacing with a relative shortage of available pain management specialists. Many of the patients frequently termed "drug seekers" more likely represent patients suffering from pseudoaddiction with lack of access to physicians able to treat their conditions [11].

Chronic pain syndromes are the summation of multiple factors producing a disordered pattern of pain perception. *Nociceptive pain* results from contact with a noxious stimulus that alerts the nervous system via pain pathways extending from the periphery to the spinal cord and onto the brainstem, thalamus, and cerebral cortex. *Inflammatory pain* is part of the healing process that causes us to protect the injured part until that healing has been accomplished. It is mainly mediated by cytokines and the immune system. The maladaptive pain response that occurs with *neuropathic pain*, as seen in diabetes, HIV, cancer, stroke, spinal cord injury, and following surgery or other trauma is a result of lack of inhibition of these pain processes resulting in increased sensitivity and chronic or recurrent pain. *Allodynia*, a painful response to a non-painful stimulus, and *hyperalgesia*, an exaggerated painful response to normally painful stimuli, are common features of neuropathic pain. *Functional pain* is the most difficult to characterize, but is also related to abnormal nociceptive responses. It results from induced genetic changes that alter the chemical character or phenotype of the neuron, resulting in hypersensitivity, amplified responses, and propagation of the signal to uninjured areas. This phenomenon of peripheral and central sensitization demonstrates the ability, or plasticity, of the nervous system to modify itself based on varying feedback, in this case tissue injury. Unfortunately, both neuropathic and functional pain can occur spontaneously without a noxious stimulus or tissue injury as well [12].

Assessment of the patient with chronic pain should aim to determine the etiology when possible and the predominant pain pathways involved, as well as some consideration of disability [13]. Disability is the effect of the pain on activities of daily living. For example, an assessment of disability after an ankle sprain includes the patient's ability to bear weight. Disability for a patient with chronic pain may include the patient's ability to participate in social functions or bathe. The Brief Pain Inventory (BPI) is a short tool that provides information on pain in the preceding 24 hours, the degree of pain relief from current pain regimen and interruption of usual activities [14, 15]. Evaluation of mood and psychological co-morbidities, such as depression, attention deficit hyperactivity disorder (ADHD), or bipolar disorder may also impact decisions in the initiation or modification of treatments. Physical examination should be thorough in assessing areas of tenderness, hyperalgesia, allodynia, numbness, or weakness. A pain assessment that accounts for biological, psychological, social, and cultural elements, as well as subjective perceptions and personal stressors (often financial), will help to build a successful and comprehensive multimodal approach to pain treatment.

Pain treatment in the emergency department: multimodal therapy

The goal of treatment of the chronic pain patient in the ED is to successfully relieve pain, defined as a reduction of at least 30% or two points in the pain intensity numerical rating scale (PI-NRS), using medications directed to the mechanism of pain while anticipating and lowering or avoiding adverse effects and safety risks [16]. Choosing the correct medication combinations, routes of administration, and adjuncts involves consideration of the significant side effects and safety profiles of each medication. Physicians must also consider safety in and outside of the ED. The majority of patients will be discharged, and their driving status, the ability to fill prescriptions and necessary adjuncts, such as antiemetics or a bowel regimen, must be considered.

The route of administration is an important factor. If the patient is able to swallow, and there are no concerns about bowel motility, oral preparations are preferred. Enteric treatments are convenient, allow for flexibility in dosing, and, when prescribed on a time-dependent, around the clock, rather than pain-dependent schedule, allow for steady blood levels. Immediate release (IR) and controlled release (CR) formulations are available. For patients with chronic, persistent pain, a longer acting analgesic combined with a short-acting medication for breakthrough pain often provides the best results. Intramuscular injections are a common method of administration; however, this route has a lack of consistent absorption, long times to onset, rapid offset, and potential necrosis of nerves and muscle. Subcutaneous administration, when intravenous access cannot be achieved, is a much more desirable alternative [11]. The onset is only somewhat slower than the intravenous route and the offset somewhat quicker. Opioids such as morphine, fentanyl, hydrocodone, methadone, oxycodone, and codeine have all been successfully used subcutaneously, particularly in palliative medicine settings [17]. Subcutaneous morphine administered in high doses should be avoided due to local histamine release. Intravenous bolus dosing or infusions in combination with patient controlled anesthesia (PCA) can provide good relief of severe pain. Repeated bolus dosing is necessary if insignificant relief is achieved at the time of peak effect. In severe exacerbations of cancer pain and chronic non-malignant pain, boluses every 10–20 minutes may be needed to achieve a significant reduction of pain. Infusions provide consistent blood levels of opioids. Transdermal opioid preparations are a convenient method of providing analgesia, and their lipophilic characteristics allow for good absorption. Transdermal preparations cause less constipation than other equianalgesic CR oral preparations. They have an extended lag time, 12–16 hours, before any substantial therapeutic effect is noted. Topical nonsteroidal anti-inflammatory drug (NSAID) preparations are available with

Table 16.2 Parental opioid dosing for opioid naive patients

IV opioid	Weight-based dosing	Time to onset of action (min)	Duration of action	Side effects
Fentanyl	1 mcg/kg	1–5	30–45 min	Rigidity at high doses
Hydromorphone	0.02 mg/kg	5–6	2–3 h	Least vagal effect; significant euphoria
Morphine	0.15 mg/kg	15–30	3–4 h	Vagal symptoms; histamine release; dose adjustment in patients with renal insufficiency

the same conveniences of transdermal opioids [18]. Many transdermal and topical analgesic preparations are costly however and may be a financial burden to patients.

Fentanyl, hydromorphone, and morphine are the mainstays of opioid analgesia in the ED. These drugs differ in their analgesic and side effect profiles, and best results are achieved with weight-based dosing (Table 16.2) that helps avoid over- or undertreatment of pain. Dosage increases are required in patients who are opioid tolerant, and decreases are required in patients who are elderly, dehydrated, or have renal insufficiency. A starting regimen in opioid-dependent patients of an equi-analgesic dose based on 20% of their overall daily opioids is often sufficient [19]. PCAs should be considered for patients with severe pain, such as sickle cell vaso-occlusive crisis, or admitted patients with moderate to severe pain expected to last more than 12 hours. Patients must be able to self-administer and understand the relationship between the pain and pushing the button. Hourly sedation assessment, such as the Richmond Agitation and Sedation Scale (RASS), is required.

Many chronic pain patients on daily opioids will present to the ED with complaints related to side effects. Constipation is the one side effect to which tolerance does not develop; therefore, most patients on chronic opioids must be prescribed a daily bowel regimen that includes a stool softener, such as docusate, and a stimulant laxative, such as senna or bisacodyl. Osmotic agents such as lactulose or sorbitol may be needed for acute exacerbations of constipation [11]. Sedation and respiratory depression are two of the major adverse effects of opioid usage. Excessive sedation occurs when opioids are combined with other sedating drugs, such as antiemetics and benzodiazepines. Respiratory depression occurs more commonly in opioid naive patients, patients who are sleeping, patients with existing pulmonary disease or obstructive sleep apnea, and those who are obese [11, 20]. PCAs, intrathecal, or epidural pumps also increase the risk [21]. Pulse oximetry should be continuous, and capnography is important for assessing ventilatory effort. Opioid tolerant patients who have been on scheduled therapy for a week or more rarely develop respiratory depression as tolerance to this side effect develops rather quickly over time. If excessive sedation and/or respiratory depression occur, a dilute solution of naloxone (1 mg in 10 cc saline) should be administered in small bolus doses until adequate respiratory effort and/or awakening are achieved. Caution must be exercised to avoid intense withdrawal or seizures, pulmonary edema and severe pain. The relative short half-life of naloxone requires that patients be observed for return of respiratory depression or need for a naloxone infusion dosed at an hourly rate of two-third of the initial dose required to produce awakening and increased ventilatory effort. Other opioid side effects include nausea and vomiting. This is best treated with non-sedating antiemetics, such as ondansetron, metoclopramide, or prochlorperazine. Meclizine or transdermal scopolamine might be considered in motion-exacerbated nausea due to opioid vestibular effects. Pruritus is another common complaint with opioid usage, which often resolves on its own within a few days or may improve with a low-dose naloxone infusion [11].

Multimodal analgesia also reduces the occurrence of these adverse effects. Dose sparing agents, such as an NSAID, or coanalgesics, such as acetaminophen, topical NSAIDs, and lidocaine, may help. Stimulant drugs, such as caffeine or modafinil, anticonvulsant drugs, such as carbamazepine, gabapentin, or pregabalin, and antidepressants, including the tricyclic antidepressants, serotonin selective reuptake inhibitors, and serotonin norepinephrine reuptake inhibitors can also decrease the dosage of opioids. Adjuncts such as heat or cold, physical therapy, ambulatory assist devices, and therapies involving relaxation or cognitive behavioral approaches may also allow the dose of the opioid analgesic to be lowered. Changing the route of delivery or the type of opioid may also help reduce side effects [22].

Management of conditions causing chronic pain in the emergency department

Chronic back pain

Acute and persistent low back pain is one of the most frequently-cited reasons for ED visits, and painful episodes can lead to significant disability, ongoing disruption of daily functioning, and psychological distress. Approximately 80% of adults experience low back pain problems at some point in their lives. In 2006, EDs reported 3.3 million patient visits for back symptoms, about half of which were for low back pain symptoms, ranking back-related symptoms among the top 20 reasons for ED visits [2]. Studies have shown that back pain is frequently recurrent and that organic pathologies are rarely identified. Approximately 30% of patients seen in primary care for back pain continue to have persistent problems 12 months later. Combined medical and disability compensation costs for back pain in the United States are estimated at over $50 billion annually [23].

Clinical practice guidelines for persistent low back pain were developed over a decade ago by the Agency for Health Care Policy and Research and state that physicians should, among other recommendations, educate patients about their symptoms and the role of behavioral self-management in managing these symptoms [24]. These guidelines note that the vast majority of low back pain patients who experience persistent pain and pain-related disability are unlikely to require extensive diagnostic workups or other physician-initiated interventions. For example, even with acute back pain and certainly with persistent low back pain, lumbar radiographs are only advised when certain "red flags" are present (e.g., history of recent trauma or symptoms suggestive of fracture, unexplained fever or weight loss, history of cancer, use of steroids, and age greater than 55) that would suggest a more serious back problem. Despite evidence that persistent low back pain responds better to behavioral strategies, such as exercise, activity pacing, and time-contingent, that is around the clock, scheduled medication dosing, the majority of emergency physicians continue to prescribe "light activity" and bed rest when patients present with acute exacerbations of pain [25, 26]. Persistent pain is a complex biopsychosocial problem. Effective management requires attention to patients' beliefs, attitudes, coping abilities, and social environment, among other factors [27].

Understandably with ED overcrowding, it may be difficult to implement clinical practice guidelines that seemingly require more time with each patient. Providers may not be trained to routinely assess these factors when patients present to the ED, nor are they trained to deliver recommendations for behavioral self-management. Patients treated for persistent low back pain in the ED are typically provided only general medical recommendations for self-management, and little is known about the extent to which discharged patients appropriately implement those recommendations. Emergency physicians should emphasize the importance of returning to normal activities, increasing physical activity levels and taking pain medications on a time-contingent, rather than pain-contingent, basis. These patients may benefit most from an approach that fosters appropriate use of behavioral self-management skills. Analgesics that address the mechanisms of pain present—inflammatory, nociceptive, and even neuropathic—and that also account for the muscle spasm that frequently accompanies the pain, should be used. Topical 1% diclofenac which has a < 1% systemic absorption rate can be quite useful when used regularly at least 3–4 times per day. Orphenadrine can assist for muscle relaxation, and appropriate opioid and other adjuncts are needed for more severe or radicular pain. In the case of the latter, interventional injections of epidural steroids and radiofrequency ablation may be needed. Most importantly, the drug regimen should be administered on an around-the-clock scheduled basis, and patients should be encouraged to maintain and gradually increase activities and to alternate periods of rest and activity throughout the day [28].

Chronic headaches and migraines

Recurrent episodes of headaches and migraines result from a variety of inflammatory, neuropathic, and functional mechanisms and can be associated with objective neurologic findings. EDs remain a mainstay location of treatment for these recurrent episodes. Much research has been developed over the past decade to evaluate these pathways and determine appropriate analgesic treatments [29, 30]. Treatment should include rapid relief of symptoms with as few adverse effects as possible, prevention of recurrence and identification of headaches with life-threatening etiologies. Associated symptoms such as nausea, photophobia, and otophobia may be soothed by modification of environmental stimuli. Dehydration may make all these symptoms worse; so parenteral hydration is often a first step in treatment. Non-narcotic treatments of migraines, and other recurrent headaches, despite differences in mechanism, have shown good therapeutic results with the use of triptans, metoclopramide, prochlorperazine and other phenothiazines, and dopamine antagonist antiemetics. Benadryl is often added to prevent the akathesia and dystonic reactions that can occur with these medications [31, 32]. The addition of NSAIDs, such as parenteral ketorolac, can serve as abortive therapy alone or in combination with other medications [32]. The use of triptans, given their potential side effect profile and the time-consuming task of evaluating potential cardiovascular and cerebrovascular risks, should likely be reserved for those who have an established diagnosis of migraine and who report a good outcome from prior triptan use.

Research identifying phases of migraine with and without cutaneous allodynia has led to the observation that there are different mechanisms at work that respond to triptans when allodynia has not yet developed and to NSAIDs when allodynia is already present [33]. It is notable that in one study, NSAIDs relieved 100% of migraines unless the patient had already taken a narcotic analgesic. Caffeine intake should be assessed, and caffeine infusion, especially in combination with NSAID and a dopamine antagonist antiemetic, can be useful in those patients who may in fact have a caffeine withdrawal-induced headache or are in another phase of migraine suffering [34]. Resistant headaches may also respond to parenteral dihydroergotamine (DHE), valproic acid, and intravenous steroids [29, 35, 36]. Finally, the use of parenteral opioids is always a tool in the management of moderate to severe pain of all types, although in the management of chronic headaches this should be considered only after non-narcotic treatment of headache has failed, given the potential for the narcotic to lessen efficacy of non-narcotic treatment and/or cause rebound headache [37, 38].

Chronic abdominal pain

Chronic abdominal pain may be the most difficult category of chronic pain to assess and treat. These patients frequently undergo extensive and often invasive diagnostic testing to exclude acute diagnoses, such as diverticulitis, appendicitis, or abdominal tumors. Abdominal pains and gastrointestinal complaints are common areas of somatization. A study of patients at a gastroenterology clinic found that those ultimately diagnosed with a functional gastrointestinal disorder (FGID) had higher levels of somatization traits than those diagnosed with a structural illness. Multiple somatization complaints and a history of psychiatric illness together had a high predictive value for FGID [39]. Therefore, physicians must broaden their differential to include psychosocial influences on pain in this patient population and be diligent in treating all causes.

Chronic pancreatitis

A recent study following patients for up to 20 years found that 16% of patients with acute pancreatitis progress to chronic pancreatitis, with the risk increased in patients who smoke or consume alcohol [40]. The incidence of chronic pancreatitis is approximately 8/100,000 in the United States and is increasing worldwide [41]. The pain in pancreatitis is classically epigastric and often radiates to the back. It may worsen with eating or be associated with nausea, vomiting, or diarrhea with light-colored stools. Episodes can be triggered by alcohol or high-fat foods. These patients are at risk of hemorrhagic pancreatitis, sepsis, and pancreatic adenocarcinoma. The pathophysiology of pancreatitis pain is thought to be a combination of autodigestion from pancreatic enzyme release, pancreatic ductal hypertension, inflammation and sensitization, or damage of the pancreatic visceral nerves [42]. Bioactive enzymes and inflammatory cytokines are released causing a self-perpetuating inflammatory cascade. Conditions that increase the release of inflammatory molecules, such as smoking or inflammatory bowel diseases, can also exacerbate chronic pancreatitis [40, 43].

Management requires identifying precipitating causes, ruling out complications and treating symptoms. Surgical complications, such as pseudocyst or obstruction, must be excluded, especially if the pain is worsening or different than the patient's typical exacerbation pain. CT of the abdomen is helpful in assessing disease progression and evaluating for pseudocyst or obstruction [44]. Pancreatic enzymes may provide an estimate of disease severity, but may not correlate to symptomatology as many patients lose endocrine and exocrine function. Basic electrolytes are helpful in assessing dehydration from vomiting and diarrhea. Blood glucose should be monitored, as these patients are at risk of hyper- and hypoglycemia due to lower levels of glucagons and insulin and dysregulation in the pancreas [45].

Intravenous fluid resuscitation, antiemetics, and opioid pain control are usually required for acute exacerbations. Despite the inflammatory component of pancreatitis, NSAIDs should be used cautiously and not prescribed to patients with alcohol-induced exacerbations. This could worsen coexisting alcoholic gastritis and cause gastrointestinal bleeding. Additionally, high-dose naprosyn increased pancreatic fibrosis in a mouse model of chronic pancreatitis [46]. However, selective cycloxygenase-2 (COX2) inhibition decreased the inflammation and progression of chronic pancreatitis in another mouse study, suggesting that COX2 inhibitors may be an appropriate treatment for chronic pancreatitis [47]. Further studies in humans are needed. Abstinence from alcohol, tobacco, and high-fat foods should be counseled at every presentation. In patients with known autoimmune pancreatitis, steroids are first-line treatment and should be given in conjunction with discussion with the patient's gastroenterologist. Although some patients may require inpatient admission for symptom control, most patients with uncomplicated chronic pancreatitis can be stabilized symptomatically in the ED and discharged. For long-term suppression of illness, several medications can be prescribed at discharge. Pancreatic enzyme supplementation, such as Creon©, may help decrease stool symptoms. They should be prescribed with an H2 inhibitor to reduce gastric acid degradation of the capsules [44, 48]. Antioxidants may decrease pain episodes and narcotic use in patients with alcohol-induced pancreatitis. Studies have examined pancreatitis-specific antioxidant preparations of vitamin C, alpha-tocopherol (vitamin E), vitamin A, selenium, and the essential amino acid methionine [49, 50]. The preparation used is not currently available in the United States as one pill but included almost ten times the recommended dietary allowance (RDA) of vitamin C, nine times the RDA of vitamin E, almost twice the RDA of vitamin A, and 8.5 times the RDA of selenium, which are available individually at health food stores. Further treatments under development include specific anti-inflammatories such as anti-interleukin 6, which would theoretically decrease the inflammatory cascade [42]. Some patients may benefit from daily subcutaneous octreotide injections. This inhibits pancreatic enzyme secretion and may help control pain and improve quality of life [51]. Octreotide and additional treatments such as ERCP, celiac plexus block, long-term nasojejunal feedings or pancreatectomy with islet cell transplantation are strategies available to patients through their gastroenterologist. Emergency physicians may consider admission of these patients if pain and vomiting remain uncontrolled despite ED treatment with parenteral hydration, analgesics, and antiemetics, or if the obstructive or hemorrhagic complications described above are suspected. If discharged, patients should be prescribed pancreatic enzyme supplements in conjunction with an H2 gastric acid blocker as well as supplemental antioxidant vitamins, and be referred to a gastroenterologist with specific expertise in these chronic and progressive pancreatic entities.

Irritable bowel syndrome

Irritable bowel syndrome (IBS) is the most common of the FGIDs. IBS is a chronic and episodic disease characterized by periods of exacerbation and remission. While the diagnosis of IBS can be difficult to make in the ED, the Rome II and III consensus criteria have helped clarify this syndrome [52]. Symptoms consist of abdominal pain that is relieved with defecation and associated with changes in stool frequency or consistency. Patients may present with right or left lower quadrant pain. Upper abdominal pain is rare. Bloating, abdominal distension, mucus in the stools, bowel urgency, and straining may occur. Up to 20% of adults in the United States are affected [53]. Almost 75% of patients diagnosed are women. Increased visceral hypersensitivity is thought to be the underlying cause of the pain. Patients with IBS, even in asymptomatic periods, have higher pain scores from colonoscopy compared with patients with other GI disorders [54]. Altered GI tract motility and intestinal secretion production may cause the bowel changes.

A thorough history of previous events and bowel habits must be obtained, especially in patients without a formal diagnosis of IBS by a gastroenterologist. Further physical exam, screening labs, or radiographic testing, such as abdominal CT, pelvic exam, or pelvic ultrasound, may be necessary to rule out appendicitis, diverticulitis, or pelvic inflammatory disease. Treatment is symptomatic, with stool softeners or laxatives as needed. Rice-based meals, less allergenic and inflammatory than wheat, are recommended during flairs [55]. Alpha$_2$-adrenergic agonists, such as clonidine, and calcium channel blockers, such as verapamil or nicardipine, can relieve rectosigmoid spasms and decrease rectal tone. Octreotide decreases visceral pain and intestinal response to distension. Several serotonergic agents targeting the gastrointestinal 5-HT$_4$ and 5-HT$_5$ receptors have been developed. Tegaserod, a 5-HT$_4$ agonist, is prescribed for IBS with constipation (IBS-C). However, Tegaserod is currently being investigated due to concerns about increased cardiovascular events. Alosetron, a 5-HT$_3$ agonist, is used in IBS with diarrhea (IBS-D) for uncontrollable diarrhea. Newer serotonergic pharmaceuticals are under development. A recent Cochrane review found insufficient high-quality trials to recommend herbal treatments for IBS [56]. Enteric coated peppermint capsules may provide some anti-spasmodic and analgesic effects from the methyl salicylate, but may also exacerbate any coexisting GERD. Low-dose erythromycin may help with GI complaints [57]. IV hydration, antispasmodics such as dicyclomine (Bentyl©), especially for diarrhea prone IBS, and analgesics are the mainstays of ED treatment. If discharged, recommendations regarding diet are equally important. The most essential part of IBS treatment in the ED is reassurance to the patient that symptoms are treatable and that there is no danger to their overall health from this disorder. Prompt and frequent primary care follow-up is important [58].

Chronic pelvic pain

Chronic pelvic pain (CPP) is a term applied to a variety of syndromes that can occur in women or men. It may have specific cause or be another type of visceral pain syndrome. In female CPP, the most common causes found during laparoscopy are adhesions (40%), endometriosis (14%–18%), pelvic congestion syndrome (12%–18%), and sequelae of pelvic inflammatory disease (20%) [59]. Previous caesarean section, endometriosis, or pelvic inflammatory disease (PID) increases the risk [60].

Assessment of the woman with CPP includes obtaining a history of the pain and the relationship with the menstrual cycle, sexual intercourse, and bowel symptoms. Ovarian torsion, pregnancy, acute PID, and sexual abuse must be considered. Treatment of female CPP is targeted to the cause of the pain. Cyclical pain with menstruation is likely endometriosis or dysmenorrheal. Oral contraceptives or hormone modulators are the first-line therapy, with NSAIDs as needed for pain. Results of GnRH agonist treatment have been mixed [61]. Leiomyomata may cause constant pressure or acute pain with necrosis. These are seen on abdominal ultrasound or CT and treated surgically. Adhesions may cause pain with movement or associated with bowel movements. Treatment is with NSAIDs or surgery. Screening for abuse and treating any concurrent gastrointestinal symptoms may help. Additionally, physical therapy can aid with the musculoskeletal component of pelvic pain that some women experience [62]. Tricyclic antidepressants and pregabalin can also decrease pain, but require close follow-up after prescription in the ED. Nerve blocks, such as ganglion impar block or sympathomimectomy may provide lasting pain relief, but are invasive and usually performed by a gynecologist or pain management specialist. ED care involves excluding diagnoses requiring immediate intervention, such as obstruction, ectopic pregnancy, ovarian torsion, or tubo-ovarian abscess, controlling nausea and pain, and ensuring appropriate and timely specialist follow-up.

Male pelvic pain is a syndrome of chronic non-bacterial prostatitis complicated by bladder spasms or pelvic floor dysfunction [63]. Patients may present with waxing and waning urinary symptoms, pain, and ejaculatory dysfunction. Management in the ED involves evaluating for acute prostatitis and urinary tract infection. Male CPP is treated with fluoroquinolone antibiotics, antispasmodics, and NSAIDs [64]. Referral to a urologist is also appropriate if the patient has long-standing symptoms or is resistant to antibiotic treatment.

CPP with referred urinary symptoms may be interstitial cystitis/bladder pain syndrome (IC/BPS). IC/BPS is a syndrome of chronic pelvic pain, urinary urgency, frequency, and nocturia in the absence of infection or other cause [65]. Thirty percent of women suffering with IC/BPS are less than 50 years old; however, it is most common in women older than 65 years [66]. It has similar features to overactive bladder, with the addition of pain. There are three pain pathways involved. First, a defect in the glycosaminoglycan layer of the urothelium allows urinary irritants to affect the bladder wall cells. Secondly, hyperalgesia occurs from bladder nerve sensitization, and thirdly, mast cell activation causes inflammation [67]. Management involves evaluating for urinary tract infection, prostatitis, and urinary retention. Bladder ultrasound, pre- and post-voiding, quantifies retention. First-line treatment is with dietary changes and fluid monitoring. Elimination of triggering foods, such as spicy foods or chocolate, may help. Medical treatment with pentosan polysulfate sodium (PPS), which chemically resembles glycosaminoglycans, may decrease symptoms but requires weeks to months of therapy. Significant relief from symptoms occurs in about one-third of patients [68]. Anticholinergics, such as oxybutinin, may also help. Patients with chronic or uncontrolled symptoms should be referred to an urologist for discussion of hydrodistension, intravesicular injections, and other long-term therapies, such as pelvic floor therapy and neuromodulators.

Chronic post-operative abdominal pain

Up to 18% of woman who undergo caesarean sections report chronic post-operative pain [69]. Numbness at the incision site acutely post-operatively and emergent caesarean are risk factors for persistent pain [70]. Pain may be from adhesions or nerve entrapment within the incision. Inguinal hernia repair is another surgery with a high rate of post-operative pain. Risk factors for the development of chronic inguinal pain include age (younger adults are at higher risk), pre-existing pain or pain syndromes and history of multiple surgeries. Laparoscopic procedure versus open repair was not associated with chronic pain [71]. High ratings of pain immediately post-operatively increase the risk of chronic pain, suggesting that better treatment of pain acutely may prevent chronic post-operative pain [72]. In patients with concern for incisional nerve entrapment, treatment with topical lidocaine patches, capsaicin, or systemic gabapentin or pregabalin is first line. Abdominal wall physical therapy can also help reduce pain.

Other causes of chronic abdominal pain

Other causes of chronic abdominal pain not covered above include angioedema, porphyria, cyclic vomiting syndrome, abdominal migraines, superior mesenteric artery syndrome, sexual assault, and domestic violence. These syndromes may be waxing and waning without evidence of disease on screening labs or imaging. With these difficult patients who present with recurrent pain and no identifiable cause, it is important to remember that the resources of the ED are limited and that there are many causes of pain that cause significant morbidity, but are not apparent on commonly obtained exams. If symptoms are not able to be well controlled in the ED setting, or you suspect a serious underlying cause, or have concerns about follow-up, hospital admission may be the pathway to distinguish these often elusive diagnoses. As the ED is often better equipped to diagnosis and manage acute life-threatening problems or acutely manage symptoms more so than chronic issues, appropriate outpatient follow-up for further workup including colonoscopy, ERCP, small bowel follow through, laparoscopy, and metabolic workup may be required.

Chronic pain in the geriatric patient

The many difficulties of chronic pain management in the ED setting are further complicated in the older adult patient. Older adults are at risk of chronic pain conditions such as cancer pain, osteoarthritis, rheumatologic disorders, peripheral neuropathies, and compression fractures. The prevalence of chronic pain in long-term care facilities ranges from 49%–83% [73]. In the community, 63% of older adults report daily pain [74]. Cancer pain is the most common cause of chronic pain. The probability of developing an invasive cancer after 60 years of age is 10%–15%, and up to 26%–37% in patients over 70 [20]. Of those currently battling cancer, 64% report daily pain and 33% of patients who have achieved a cure still report pain [75]. Additionally, up to 43% of men and 54% of women older than 65 report arthritis pain in at least one joint [76]. This creates a population of patients who require long-term pain control that may present to the ED.

Older patients are also at higher risk for secondary problems from chronic pain, such as falls, immobilization, delirium, polypharmacy, inappropriate over-the-counter drug use, and constipation. A study of community dwelling older adults found that musculoskeletal pain in two or more sites or any severe daily pain significantly increased their risk of falls [77]. Even 2 days of immobilization or bed rest while in pain after a fall can result in muscle atrophy, dehydration, or pressure ulcers. Other common causes of pain exacerbations include disease progression, medication changes, social stressors, and depression.

The physiologic changes of aging alter pain sensation and complicate treatment. Increased gastrointestinal transit time predisposes older adults to constipation and gastritis. Liver mass and liver blood flow decrease with aging, resulting in decreased albumin synthesis and phase I drug metabolism. Cyclobenzaprine, buprenorphine, hydrocodone, oxycodone, and methadone are all metabolized by the cytochrome P450 system and, therefore, will have longer half-lives. Impaired renal function is also very common in older patients. The serum creatinine level may not give an accurate measurement of their renal function due to alterations in muscle mass. Renal insufficiency decreases the clearance of morphine and oxycodone metabolites, hydromorphone, most benzodiazepines, gabapentin, pregabalin and baclofen. Dementia and delirium may obscure symptoms and confuse the medical history. Untreated pain increases the risk of delirium. In a study of hip fracture patients who developed delirium, the patients with delirium received significantly less pain medicine prior to the onset of delirium than matched non-delirious controls [78]. Additionally, delirium in the ED is an independent risk factor for patient decline and death within 6 months [79]. Therefore, pain control in this at risk population is not only appropriate symptomatic treatment, but also an essential intervention to reduce short- and long-term morbidity.

There are several classes of pain medications that should be prescribed cautiously or not at all in older adults. NSAIDs are inexpensive, but have many concerning side effects, including cardiovascular risks, renal function compromise, and GI bleeding. Patients already on a daily aspirin for cardioprotection are at especially high risk of bleeding [80]. Propoxyphene and tramadol are also not recommended. Propoxyphene is a weak mu-opioid receptor agonist that also affects acetylcholine and serotonin reuptake. Propoxyphene and derivatives (Darvocet©, Darvon©) are only as effective as acetaminophen in studies of chronic pain, but have more side effects. In addition to the anticholinergic and opiate effects, propoxyphene is a class 1c antiarrhythmic more potent than its classmate lidocaine. It decreases the heart rate via sodium channel blocking, widens the QRS interval, and may result in arrhythmias [81]. Tramadol is another mu-opioid receptor agonist that has additional antagonistic effects on norepinephrine and serotonin reuptake. It also lowers the seizure threshold. For acute pain, tramadol is only as effective as acetaminophen [82]. Corticosteroids must be prescribed cautiously as their usual side effect profile of fluid retention, hyperglycemic effects, steroid psychosis, bone demineralization, immunosuppression, and cardiovascular effects are amplified in the older patient. Corticosteroids may be helpful in inflammatory conditions such as rheumatoid arthritis, malignant compression fractures, or the crystal arthropathies. They are not recommended for osteoarthritis, and the use of steroids for chronic back pain remains controversial [83].

The current American Geriatrics Society guidelines recommend first-line use of acetaminophen for treating chronic pain [83]. In the ED, many non-medication adjuvants, such as physical therapy, cognitive behavioral therapy, acupuncture, and heat pads, are unavailable or difficult to arrange. Adjuvant medications, such as selective serotonin reuptake inhibitors, are not appropriate to initiate during an acute flair of chronic pain as they require drug monitoring and weeks to take effect. Other faster acting opioid alternatives are topical lidocaine patches, topical NSAIDs, or transdermal buprenorphine.

The ED is not the appropriate place to initiate CR opioids unless there is prompt and reliable outpatient follow-up. Short-acting opioids are therefore recommended for patients who require further pain control after acetaminophen and adjuvant therapies [83]. The best opioid depends on the patient's co-morbidities and pain needs as described above. Over- and underuse must be discussed. Patients should adjust their dosing schedule so that medication is taken before painful travel or exercise and before sleep. It is not unreasonable to check renal and liver functions before prescribing these medications. Elderly patients, especially the opioid naive, should be monitored in the ED for delirium or other side effects after the initial dose of opioids and discharged on a bowel regimen that includes daily docusate (stool softener) and laxatives, such as the sennosides, lactulose, or sorbitol as needed.

Overall, treating chronic pain in the older adult population is a difficult task that is compounded in the acute care setting. However, it can be highly rewarding when done appropriately as one has the satisfaction of relieving pain, restoring functional status, and reducing the long-term morbidity and mortality of these patients.

The next five years

There are many new mechanisms being developed to help in the attack on drug misuse and abuse. The use of electronic medical records within an institution or health system will assist in the important information sharing critical to making good decisions. Additionally, departmental policies that restrict prescribing more than 24–72 hours of opioid analgesics to patients not followed within that health system where information can be shared is also useful. Next is the advent of many state prescription drug management programs (PDMPs), which allow physicians and pharmacists in real time to be aware of prescribing, dispensing, and usage of controlled substances [84]. As of 2009, nearly 40 states had legislation to allow for PDMPs, and 32 programs were operational. The federally sponsored PDMP Information Exchange (PMIX) allows for sharing of this information across state lines. Access to this information allows the emergency physician to make a better judgment about prescribing substances that could be abused or diverted.

Finally, pharmaceutical companies are using new technologies to find novel ways to package opioid analgesics so that they are tamper-proof and do not allow them to be used for unintended routes of intranasal or intravenous administration. These newer formulations incorporate antagonists that help lower the potential for tolerance and addiction (Embeda©) and contain substances that cause release of a gel when exposed to solvents

(Extended Release Oxycontin©), and some are being combined with substances, such as niacin, with unpleasant side effects when consumed in excess (Acurox©).

The problems of access to health care, and to primary care, and pain specialist physicians in particular, must be addressed on a local as well as global level. Emergency medicine leadership must work in conjunction with their physician colleagues to ensure appropriate follow-up, case management, and coordination with long-term care settings, as the care of pain and opioid-dependent patients requires a multidisciplinary approach [85]. However, this care often begins in the ED, where concerned and educated physicians can truly make a difference in the lives of patients living with chronic pain and suffering.

Conclusion

Management of patients with conditions causing chronic pain in the ED, for better or for worse, is becoming more relevant to the practice of emergency medicine. A thorough understanding of the anatomical and pathophysiologic basis of chronic pain can aid the emergency physician in the management of these patients. Ideally, interaction and consultation with specialists in pain management, occupational and physical therapy, behavioral psychology, and psychiatry would optimize the care of this population; however, this often requires approaches initiated by ED, institutional, and community leaders. For emergency physicians, careful attention to the history, physical examination, and underlying diagnoses of the patient with chronic pain can allow optimal outcomes for this challenging and emerging ED patient population.

References

1. Tanabe P, Buschmann M. A prospective study of ED pain management practices and the patient's perspective. *J Emerg Nurs* 1999; 25(3): 171–177.
2. 2007 National Hospital Ambulatory Medical Care Survey. In: *National Center for Health Statistics*, ed.: Hyattsville, MD: U.S. Department of Health and Human Services; 2010.
3. Wilsey BL, Fishman SM, Ogden C, Tsodikov A, Bertakis KD. Chronic pain management in the emergency department: a survey of attitudes and beliefs. *Pain Med* 2008; 9(8): 1073–1080.
4. Wilsey BL, Fishman SM, Tsodikov A, Ogden C, Symreng I, Ernst A. Psychological co-morbidities predicting prescription opioid abuse among patients in chronic pain presenting to the emergency department. *Pain Med* 2008; 9(8): 1107–1117.
5. Miner J, Biros MH, Trainor A, Hubbard D, Beltram M. Patient and physician perceptions as risk factors for oligoanalgesia: a prospective observational study

of the relief of pain in the emergency department. *Acad Emerg Med* 2006; 13(2): 140–146.

6. Todd KH. Pain management in the emergency department. In: Fishman SM, Ballantyne JC, Rathmell JP (eds.) *Bonica's Management of Pain.* Lippincott Williams & Wilkins; 2010.

7. Todd KH, Cowan P, Kelly N. Chronic or recurrent pain in the emergency department: a national telephone survey of patient experience. *Ann Emerg Med* 2007; 50(3): S37.

8. Patton KR, Bartfield JM, McErlean M. The effect of practitioner characteristics on patient pain and embarrassment during ED internal examinations. *Am J Emerg Med* 2003 May; 21(3): 205–207.

9. Liu JY, Briggs M, Closs SJ. The psychometric qualities of four observational pain tools (OPTs) for the assessment of pain in elderly people with osteoarthritic pain. *J Pain Symptom Manage* 2010 Oct; 40(4): 582–598.

10. Cordell WH, Keene KK, Giles BK, Jones JB, Jones JH, Brizendine EJ. The high prevalence of pain in emergency medical care. *Am J Emerg Med* 2002 May; 20(3): 165–169.

11. Miaskowski C. *Principles of Analgesic Use in Acute and Cancer Pain.* 6th ed. IASP Press; 2008.

12. Woolf CJ. American college of physicians; American psychological society. Pain: moving from symptom control to mechanism-specific pharmacologic management. *Ann Intern Med* 2004; 140(6): 441–451.

13. Broglio K. Multidimensional assessment of chronic pain. In: Fine PG (ed.) *Chronic Pain and Risk Management Compendium.* Albert Einstein College of Medicine and Montefiore Medical Center and Asante Communications; 2010.

14. Tan G, Jensen MP, Thornby JI, Shanti BF. Validation of the brief pain inventory for chronic non-malignant pain. *J Pain* 2004; 5(2): 133–137.

15. Keller J, Bann CM, Dodd SL, Schein J, Mendoza TR, Cleeland CS. Validity of the brief pain inventory for use in documenting the outcomes of patients with non-cancer pain. *Clin J Pain* 2004; 20(5): 309–318.

16. Farrar JT, Young JP, LaMoreaux L, Werth JL, Poole RM. Clinical importance of changes in chronic pain intensity measured on an 11-point numerical pain rating scale. *Pain* 2001; 94: 149–158.

17. Parsons HA, Shukkoor A, Quan H, et al. Intermittent subcutaneous opioids for management of cancer pain. *J Pall Med* 2008; 11(10): 1319–1324.

18. Massey T, Derry S, Moore RA, McQuay HJ. Topical NSAIDs for acute pain in adults. *Cochrane Database of Systematic Reviews* 2010; 16(6): CD007402.

19. Mercadante S, Villari P, Ferrera P, Mangione S, Casuccio A. The use of opioids for breakthrough pain in acute palliative care unit by using doses proportional to opioid basal regimen. *Clin J Pain* 2010; 26(4): 306–309.

20. Winters BA. Older adults with traumatic rib fractures: an evidence-based approach to their care. *J Trauma Nurs* 2009; 16(2): 93–97.

21. Galer BS, Coyle N, Pasternak GW, Portenoy RK. Individual variability in the response to different opioids: report of five cases. *Pain* 1992; 49: 87–91.

22. Mercadante S. Opioid switching: a systematic and critical review. *Cancer Treat Rev* 2006; 32(4): 304–315.

23. Wipf JE, Deyo RA. Low back pain. *Med Clin N Am* 1995; 79: 231.

24. Bigos SJ, Davis GE. Scientific application of sports medicine principles for acute low back problems. The Agency for Health Care Policy and Research Low Back Guideline Panel (AHCPR, Guideline #14). *J Orthop Sports Phys Ther* 1996; 24(4): 192–207.

25. Hagen KB, Hilde G, Jamtvedt G, Winnem M. Bed rest for acute low back pain and sciatica. *Cochrane Database of Systematic Reviews* 2000; 6: CD001254.

26. Hagen KB, Hilde G, Jamtvedt G, Winnem MF. The Cochrane review of advice to stay active as a single treatment for low back pain and sciatica. *Spine* 2002; 27(16): 1736–1741.

27. Keefe FJ, Block AR, Williams RB Jr, Surwit RS. Behavioral treatment of chronic low back pain: clinical outcome and individual differences in pain relief. *Pain* 1981; 11(2): 221–231.

28. Waddell G. *The Back Pain Revolution*. 2nd ed. Churchill Livingstone, Elsevier Limited; 2004.

29. Friedman BW, Grosberg BM. Diagnosis and management of the primary headache disorders in the emergency department setting. *Emerg Med Clin North Am* 2009; 27(1): 71–87, viii.

30. Friedman BW. Review: phenothiazines relieve acute migraine headaches in the ED and are better than other active agents for some outcomes. *Ann Intern Med* 2010; 152(8): JC4–JC11.

31. Friedman BW, Esses D, Solorzano C, et al. A randomized controlled trial of prochlorperazine versus metoclopramide for treatment of acute migraine. *Ann Emerg Med* 2008; 52(4): 399–406.

32. Jakubowski M, Levy D, Goor-Aryeh I, Collins B, Bajwa Z, Burstein R. Terminating migraine with allodynia and ongoing central sensitization using parenteral administration of COX1/COX2 inhibitors. *Headache* 2005; 45(7): 850–861.

33. Burstein R, Yarnitsky D, Goor-Aryeh I, Ransil BJ, Bajwa ZH. An association between migraine and cutaneous allodynia. *Ann Neurol* 2000; 47(5): 614–624.

34. Ghelardini C, Galeotti N, Vivoli E, Grazioli I, Uslenghi C. The central analgesia induced by antimigraine drugs is independent from Gi proteins: superiority of a fixed combination of indomethacin, prochlorperazine and caffeine, compared to sumatriptan, in an in vivo model. *J Headache Pain* 2009; 10(6): 435–440.

35. Stillman MJ, Zajac D, Rybicki LA. Treatment of primary headache disorders with intravenous valproate: initial outpatient experience. *Headache* 2004; 44(1): 65–69.

36. Friedman BW, Greenwald P, Bania TC, et al. Randomized trial of IV dexamethasone for acute migraine in the emergency department. *Neurology* 2007 Nov 27; 69(22): 2038–2044.

37. Ward TN, Levin M, Phillips JM. Evaluation and management of headache in the emergency department. *Med Clin N America* 2001 Jul; 85(4): 971–985.

38. Ward TN. Medication overuse headache. *Prim Care* 2004; 31(2): 369–380.

39. Sayuk GS, Elwing JE, Lustman PJ, Clouse RE. High somatic symptom burdens and functional gastrointestinal disorders. *Clin Gastroenterol Hepatol* 2007; 5(5): 556–562.

40. Lankisch PG, Breuer N, Bruns A, Weber-Dany B, Lowenfels AB, Maisonneuve P. Natural history of acute pancreatitis: a long-term population-based study. *Am J Gastroenterol* 2009; 104(11): 2797–2805.

41. Jupp J, Fine D, Johnson CD. The epidemiology and socioeconomic impact of chronic pancreatitis. *Best Practice & Research Clinical Gastroenterology* 2010; 24: 219–231.

42. Vardanyan M, Melemedjian OK, Price TJ, et al. Reversal of pancreatitis-induced pain by an orally available, small molecule interleukin-6 receptor antagonist. *Pain* 2010; 151(2): 257–265. [Epub July 4, 2010]

43. Pitchumoni CS, Rubin A, Das K. Pancreatitis in inflammatory bowel diseases. *J Clin Gastroeneterol* 2010; 44(4): 246–253.

44. Chauhan S, Forsmark CE. Pain management in chronic pancreatitis: a treatment algorithm. *Best Practice & Research Clinical Gastroenterology* 2010; 24: 323–335.

45. DK Anderson. Mechanisms and emerging treatments of the metabolic complications of chronic pancreatitis. *Pancreas* 2007; 35(1): 1–15.

46. Zhang W, Gao J, Zhao T, et al. High-dose naproxen aggravates pancreatic fibrosis in a rat model of chronic pancreatitis. *Pancreas* 2010; 39(3): 293–300.

47. Reding T, Bimmler D, Perren A, et al. A selective COX-2 inhibitor suppresses chronic pancreatitis in an animal model (WBN/Kob rats): significant reduction of macrophage infiltration and fibrosis. *Gut* 2006; 55(8): 1165–1173.

48. Waljee AK, Dimagno MJ, Wu BU, Schoenfeld PS, Conwell DL. Systematic review: pancreatic enzyme treatment of malabsorption associated with chronic pancreatitis. *Alimentary Pharmacol Ther* 2009; 29: 235–246.

49. Shah NS, Makin AJ, Sheen AJ, Siriwardena AK. Quality of life assessment in patients with chronic pancreatitis receiving antioxidant therapy. *World J Gastroeneterol* 2010; 16(32): 4066–4071.

50. Bhardwaj P, Garg PK, Maulik SK, Saraya A, Tandon RK, Anderson, SK. A randomized controlled trial of antioxidant supplementation for pain relief in patients with chronic pancreatitis. *Gastroenterology* 2009; 136(1): 149–159.

51. Lieb JG 2nd, Shuster JJ, Theriaque D, Curington C, Cintrón M, Toskes PP. A pilot study of Octreotide LAR vs. octreotide tid for pain and quality of life in chronic pancreatitis. *JOP* 2009; 10(5): 518–522.

52. Drossman DA. *Rome III: The Functional Gastrointestinal Disorder.* 3rd ed. McLean, VA: Degnon Associates, Inc; 2006.

53. Drossman DA, Li Z, Andruzzi E, et al. US householder survey of functional gastrointestinal disorders: prevalence, sociodemography, and health impact. *Dig Dis Sci* 1993; 38: 1569–1580.

54. Kim ES, Cheon JH, Park JJ, et al. Colonoscopy as an adjunctive method for the diagnosis of irritable bowel syndrome: focus on pain perception. *J Gastroenterol Hepatol* 2010; 25(7): 1232–1238.

55. Gonlachanvit S. Are rice and spicy diet good for functional gastrointestinal disorders? *J Neurogastroenterol Motil* 2010; 16(2): 131–138.

56. Liu JP, Yang M, Liu YX, Wei ML, Grimsgaard, S. Herbal medicines for treatment of irritable bowel syndrome. *Cochrane Database of Systematic Reviews* 2006; (1): CD004116.

57. Pimentel M, Morales W, Lezcano S, Sun-Chuan D, Low K, Yang J. Low-dose nocturnal tegaserod or erythromycin delays symptom recurrence after treatment of irritable bowel syndrome based on presumed bacterial overgrowth. *Gastroenterol Hepatol* 2009; 5(6): 435–442.

58. Grover M, Drossman DA. Functional abdominal pain. *Curr Gastroenterol Rep* 2010; 12(5): 391–398.

59. Sharma D, Dahiya K, Duhan N, Bansal R. Diagnostic laparoscopy in chronic pelvic pain. *Arch Gynecol Obstet* 2010 Jan 14. [Epub ahead of print]

60. Almeida EC, Nogueira AA, Candido dos Reis FJ, Rosa e Silva JC. Cesarean section as a cause of chronic pelvic pain. *Int J Gynaecol Obstet* 2002; 79(2): 101–104.

61. Green IC, Cohen SL, Finkenzeller D, Christo PJ. Interventional therapies for controlling pelvic pain: what is the evidence? *Curr Pain Headache Rep* 2010; 14(1): 22–32.

62. Montenegro ML, Vasconcelos EC, Candido Dos Reis FJ, Nogueira AA, Poli-Neto OB. Physical therapy in the management of women with chronic pelvic pain. *Int J Clin Pract* 2008; 62(2): 263–269.

63. Westesson KE, Shoskes DA. Chronic prostatitis/chronic pelvic pain syndrome and pelvic floor spasm: can we diagnose and treat? *Curr Urol Rep* 2010; 11(4): 261–264.

64. Murphy AB, Nadler RB. Pharmacotherapy strategies in chronic prostatitis/chronic pelvic pain syndrome management. *Expert Opin Pharmacother* 2010; 11(8): 1255–1261.

65. Hanno P, Dmochowski R. Status of international consensus on interstitial cystitis/bladder pain syndrome/painful bladder syndrome: 2008 snapshot. *Neurourol Urodyn* 2009; 28: 274–286.

66. Anger JT, Zabihi N, Clemens JQ, Payne CK, Saigal CS, Rodriguez LV. Treatment choice, duration, and cost in patients with interstitial cystitis and painful bladder syndrome. *Int Urogynecol J Pelvic Floor Dysfunct* 2010.

67. Patel BN, Evans RJ. Overactive bladder and pain: Management strategies. *Curr Urol Rep* 2010; 11(6): 379–384.

68. Shoskes DA, Nickel JC, Kattan MW. Phenotypically directed multimodal therapy for chronic prostatitis/chronic pelvic pain syndrome: a prospective study using UPOINT. *Urology* 2010; 75(6): 1249–1253.

69. Kainu JP, Sarvela J, Tiippana E, Halmesmäki E, Korttila KT. Persistent pain after caesarean section and vaginal birth: a cohort study. *Int J Obstet Anesth* 2010; 19(1): 14–19.

70. Loos MJ, Scheltinga MR, Mulders LG, Roumen RM. The Pfannenstiel incision as a source of chronic pain. *Obstet Gynecol* 2008; 111(4): 839–846.

71. Dickinson KJ, Thomas M, Fawole AS, Lyndon PJ, White CM. Predicting chronic post-operative pain following laparoscopic inguinal hernia repair. *Hernia* 2008; 12(6): 597–601.

72. Al Samaraee A, Rhind G, Saleh U, Bhattacharya V. Factors contributing to poor post-operative abdominal pain management in adult patients: a review. *Surgeon* 2010; 8(3): 151–158.

73. Fox PL, Raina P, Jadad AR. Prevalence and treatment of pain in older adults in nursing homes and other long-term care institutions: a systematic review. *CMAJ* 1999; 160(3): 329–333.

74. Eggermont L, Bean JF, Guralnik JM, Leveille SG. Comparing pain severity versus pain location in the MOBILIZE Boston study: chronic pain and lower extremity function. *J Gerontol* 2009; 64A(7): 763–770.

75. Van Den Beuken-van Everdingen MH, de Rijke JM, Kessels AG, Schouten HC, van Kleef M, Patijn J. Prevalence of pain in patients with cancer: a systematic review of the past 40 years. *Ann Oncol* 2007; 18(9): 1437–1449.

76. Older Americans 2008. Key Indicators of Well-Being. Federal Interagency Forum on Aging-Related Statistics; 2008; Washington, DC: U.S. Government Printing Office; 2008.

77. Leveille SG, Jones RN, Kiely DK, et al. Chronic musculoskeletal pain and the occurrence of falls. *JAMA*; 302(20): 2214–2221.

78. Robinson S, Vollmer C. Undermedication for pain and precipitation of delirium. *Medsurg Nurs* 2010; 19(2): 79–83.

79. Han JH, Shintani A, Eden S, et al. Delirium in the emergency department: an independent predictor of death within 6 months. *Ann Emerg Med* 2010. [Epub ahead of print]

80. Barber JB, Gibson SJ. Treatment of chronic non-malignant pain in the elderly: safety considerations. *Drug Saf* 2009; 32(6): 457–474.

81. Barkin RL, Barkin SJ, Barkin DS. Propoxyphene (dextropropoxyphene): a critical review of a weak opioid analgesic that should remain in antiquity. *Am J Ther* 2006; 13(6): 534–542.

82. Akcali GE, Iskender A, Demiraran Y, et al. Randomized comparison of efficacy of paracetamol, lornoxicam, and tramadol representing three different groups of analgesics for pain control in extracorporeal shockwave lithotripsy. *J Endourol* 2010; 24(4): 615–620.

83. Pharmacologic Management of Persistent Pain in Older Persons. *AGS Panel on the Pharmacological Management of Persistent Pain in Older Persons.* JAGS; 2009: 1331–1346.

84. Fishbain D, Johnson S, Webster L, Greene L, Faysal J. Review of regulatory programs and new opioid technologies in chronic pain management: balancing the risk of medication abuse with medical need. *J Manag Care Pharm* 2010; 16(4): 276–287.

85. Ruetsch C. Practice strategies to improve compliance and patient self-management. *J Manag Care Pharm* 2010; 16(1 Suppl. B): S26–S27.

Index

Note: Page numbers followed by italicized *f*'s and *t*'s indicate figures and tables, respectively.

Challenging and Emerging Conditions in Emergency Medicine, First Edition. Edited by Arvind Venkat.
© 2011 by John Wiley & Sons, Ltd. Published 2011 by Blackwell Publishing Ltd.

Keep up with critical fields

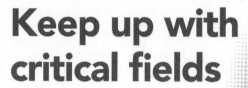

Would you like to receive up-to-date information on our books, journals and databases in the areas that interest you, direct to your mailbox?

Join the **Wiley e-mail service** - a convenient way to receive updates and exclusive discount offers on products from us.

Simply visit **www.wiley.com/email** and register online

We won't bombard you with emails and we'll only email you with information that's relevant to you. We will ALWAYS respect your e-mail privacy and NEVER sell, rent, or exchange your e-mail address to any outside company. Full details on our privacy policy can be found online.

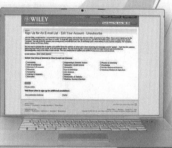

WILEY-BLACKWELL

www.wiley.com/email